Clinical Epidemiology
The Essentials

FOURTH EDITION

Clinical Epidemiology
The Essentials

Robert H. Fletcher, M.D., M.Sc.

Professor
Department of Ambulatory Care and Prevention
Harvard Medical School
Boston, Massachusetts

Adjunct Professor
Departments of Epidemiology and Social Medicine
The University of North Carolina at Chapel Hill
Chapel Hill, North Carolina

Suzanne W. Fletcher, M.D., M.Sc.

Professor
Department of Ambulatory Care and Prevention
Harvard Medical School
Boston, Massachusetts

Adjunct Professor
Departments of Epidemiology and Social Medicine
The University of North Carolina at Chapel Hill
Chapel Hill, North Carolina

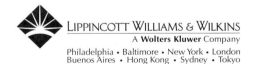

LIPPINCOTT WILLIAMS & WILKINS
A **Wolters Kluwer** Company
Philadelphia • Baltimore • New York • London
Buenos Aires • Hong Kong • Sydney • Tokyo

Acquisitions Editor: Betty Sun
Developmental Editor: Emilie Linkins
Marketing Manager: Joe Schott
Associate Production Manager: Kevin P. Johnson
Designer: Holly McLaughlin
Services/Compositor: Seven Worldwide Publishing Solutions
Printer: Quebecor/Versailles

Copyright © 2005 Lippincott Williams & Wilkins

351 West Camden Street
Baltimore, MD 21201

530 Walnut Street
Philadelphia, Pennsylvania 19106-3621 USA

The publisher is not responsible (as a matter of product liability, negligence, or otherwise) for any
injury resulting from any material contained herein. This publication contains information relating
to general principles of medical care that should not be construed as specific instructions for individual
patients. Manufacturers' product information and package inserts should be reviewed for current
information, including contraindications, dosages, and precautions.

Printed in the United States of America

First Edition, 1982
Second Edition, 1988
Third Edition, 1996

Library of Congress Cataloging-in-Publication Data

Fletcher, Robert H.
    Clinical epidemiology: the essentials/Robert H. Fletcher, Suzanne W. Fletcher.—4th ed.
        p. ; cm.
    Includes bibliographical references and index.
    ISBN 0-7817-5215-9 (alk. paper)
    1. Clinical epidemiology. I. Fletcher, Suzanne W. II. Title.
        [DNLM: 1. Epidemiologic Methods. WA 950 F614c 2005]
RA652.2.C55F57 2005
614.4—dc22
    2004029660

*The publishers have made every effort to trace the copyright holders for borrowed material.
If they have inadvertently overlooked any, they will be pleased to make the necessary arrangements
at the first opportunity.*

To purchase additional copies of this book, call our customer service department at **(800) 638-3030**
or fax orders to **(301) 824-7390.** International customers should call **(301) 714-2324.**

Visit Lippincott Williams & Wilkins on the Internet: http://www.LWW.com. Lippincott Williams
& Wilkins customer service representatives are available from 8:30 am to 6:00 pm, EST.

04 05 06 07 08
1 2 3 4 5 6 7 8 9 10

ACKNOWLEDGMENTS

Our thanks first go to Ed Wagner, co-author for the first three editions and a wonderful colleague in any season. Ed did not join us this time; his professional life was too full to participate in another round of revisions. He helped develop much of the original content of this book while we all taught together at the University of North Carolina. We missed the opportunity to write with Ed once again, but at least we still work together on research programs.

We are fortunate to have learned clinical epidemiology from its founders. Kerr White, our mentor during postgraduate studies at Johns Hopkins, taught us that what really matters are "the benefits of medical interventions in relation to their hazards and costs." Alvan Feinstein taught a generation of young clinician-scholars about the "architecture of clinical research" and the dignity of clinical scholarship. Archie Cochrane opened our eyes to "effectiveness and efficiency." David Sackett asserted that clinical epidemiology is a "basic science for clinical medicine" and helped the world to understand. There were more, of course. These founders, each in their own way, created an exciting intellectual environment as we entered medicine. Because of them, we believed that clinical epidemiology would be in the mainstream of medicine some day—and now it is.

Like all teachers, we have learned the most from our students, who have been clinicians of all ages and all specialties wanting to learn for themselves how to judge the validity of clinical observations and research. Recently, they have included students at Harvard Medical School and the University of North Carolina School of Public Health, faculty in the International Clinical Epidemiology Network (INCLEN), and participants in the Evidence-Based Health Care Workshop held each summer in Colorado. In the past, fellows in the Robert Wood Johnson Clinical Scholars Program and Harvard's General Medicine Fellowship have been important parts of our lives. Our friends in the Society of General Internal Medicine have found new ways to make clinical epidemiology grow. Fellow editors of *UpToDate* have made common cause in efforts to bring the best available evidence to busy clinicians. We continue to draw inspiration from our friends in the World Association of Medical Editors (WAME), who are asking authors to make the strengths and limitations of research methods explicit in articles and are sending this message out to the world.

Our colleagues at Lippincott Williams & Wilkins have represented the best of publishing by any standards. Betty Sun patiently helped us through plans for this edition in a rapidly changing publishing environment. Emilie Linkins' suggestions for improvements were remarkably insightful, especially for a newcomer to clinical epidemiology. Kathy Jaeger patiently drew and re-drew figures, helping us to clarify our thoughts in the process. Like many involved in publishing these days, all are part of a vast international enterprise, yet they gave this particular project individual care and attention.

We are especially grateful to readers all over the world for their encouraging comments and practical suggestions. They have sustained us through the rigors of preparing this, the fourth edition of a textbook first published 23 years ago.

PREFACE

When the first edition of this book was published in the 1980s, clinical epidemiology was on the fringes of medicine. Patient-centered research, the kind that should guide patient care decisions, was poorly developed. Epidemiology was so separate from clinical medicine that we were told it would be a bad idea to include "epidemiology" in the title of a book for clinicians.

Now, clinical epidemiology is in the mainstream. Clinicians are more sophisticated consumers of research information. They have a far better understanding of how to find the best information and to judge its validity and generalizability for themselves. Their efforts are now supported by an extraordinary array of clinically useful electronic databases, clinical practice guidelines, systematic reviews, articles selected for their scientific strength and clinical applicability, and courses in research methods and knowledge management. Many clinical practice guidelines are based on rigorous rules of evidence and provide a rationale for their recommendations, including grades for scientific strength. Editors of textbooks, such as *UpToDate* and *ACP Medicine,* now expect authors to incorporate into their chapters critical evaluations of evidence and modern, quantitative descriptions of the benefits and risks of treatments.

The clinical research community has built clinical epidemiology into all phases of its work. Grants are judged by study sections guided largely by the principles described in this book. Serious clinical investigators in many different specialties are pursuing formal postgraduate training in research methods, often in departments of epidemiology. Research teams increasingly comprise the full range of expertise in design, measurement, and analysis that bears on their work. Clinical epidemiology is the language of journal peer review and "hanging committees" in which decisions are made about research results that should or should not be published and how the completeness and balance of articles can be improved. The National Library of Medicine now includes (in Medline searches) terms for methodologic strength, such as

randomized controlled trial and sensitivity/specificity. In short, clinical medicine and epidemiology are making common cause. "Healing the schism" is what Kerr White called it.

For these reasons, readers expect more from an entry-level textbook of clinical epidemiology than they did when earlier editions were published. We have made changes in this new edition to take these expectations into account. Many topics are covered in greater depth, such as the credibility of observational studies of treatment effects, gold standards for studies of screening test accuracy, Bayesian reasoning, and large simple trials. Systematic reviews (and meta-analyses when warranted) have become an especially powerful way of summarizing the results of individual studies, which often seem to disagree with one another. We cover systematic reviews more completely in this edition. We have added a new chapter on knowledge management (Chapter 13) to help clinicians cope more effectively and efficiently with the vast body of research results. In this chapter, we take into account clinicians' practical needs for rapid access to information and for delegating to others some of the responsibility of finding information and selecting and summarizing the best studies. We continue to use clinical examples to illustrate concepts. Some of the facts in these examples have been modified by subsequent research, as expected, and we have updated those examples. Most underlying concepts have not changed, although some are described in greater depth.

Many clinicians (and even students) have difficulty finding adequate time with an uncluttered mind for reading. We have tried to make their job easier by highlighting key words and listing them at the beginning of each chapter. At the end of each chapter, we provide questions to assist readers who wish to review in this way. We hope the clinical examples throughout the book continue to anchor abstract concepts in real-life application. The publisher has done its part by creating a more modern, reader-friendly layout, adding color, and choosing a larger trim size and a two-column format.

This book is for clinicians of all sorts, whether they are physicians, nurses, physicians' assistants, dietitians, psychologists, veterinarians, and others who care for patients and want to understand for themselves the strength of the information base of clinical decisions. Some students of epidemiology and public health may find this book a refreshing complement to the many wonderful textbooks on epidemiology itself.

Some scholars who used to identify themselves with "clinical epidemiology" now also identify themselves with "evidence-based medicine." This new label recognizes the importance, in addition to judging the validity and generalizability of research results, of finding the best available information, and of applying this information in practice. We have always considered these additional competencies important, and we give them even more attention in this edition of the book.

While we assert that clinical epidemiology is now in the mainstream, we do not wish to imply that clinicians have taken its lessons completely to heart. Adoption is spotty, and much more is to be done. But the principles of clinical epidemiology have become a standard of excellence in clinical research and bedside reasoning. As health professionals internalize the message and methods of clinical epidemiology, many have come to regard these concepts as a basis for good clinical research conduct and interpretation. Clinical educators have built this discipline into existing educational activities such as residency and fellowship training, the formal and informal curricula of medical schools, and continuing medical education for postgraduate physicians. The principles are so extensively integrated into medicine that clinical epidemiology itself is starting to lose some of its separate identity. Is there any better sign of success?

Robert H. Fletcher
Suzanne W. Fletcher

CONTENTS IN BRIEF

CONTENTS

CHAPTER **7**
Prognosis   105

CHAPTER **8**
Treatment   125

CHAPTER **12**
Systematic Reviews   205

CHAPTER **13**
Knowledge Management   221

APPENDIX **A**
Answers to Review Questions   233

APPENDIX **B**
Additional Readings   241

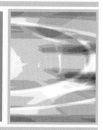

CHAPTER 1

Introduction

KEY WORDS

Biologic sciences	Clinical epidemiology	Bias
Clinical sciences	Evidence-based medicine	Selection bias
Population sciences	Variables	Measurement bias
Epidemiology	Independent variable	Confounding bias
Health services research	Dependent variable	Random variation
Quantitative decision making	Extraneous variables	Internal validity
Cost-effectiveness analyses	Populations	External validity
Decision analyses	Sample	Generalizability
Social sciences	Inference	Shared decision making

We should study "the benefits of medical interventions in relation to their hazards and costs."

— Kerr L. White

EXAMPLE

A 51-year-old man asks to see you because of chest pain. He was well until 2 weeks ago, when he noticed tightness in the center of his chest while walking uphill. The tightness stopped after 2 to 3 minutes of rest. A similar discomfort has occurred several times since then, sometimes during exercise and sometimes at rest. He smokes one pack of cigarettes per day and has been told that his blood pressure is "a little high." He is otherwise well and takes no medications, but he is worried about his health, particularly about heart disease. A complete physical examination and resting electrocardiogram are normal except for a blood pressure of 150/96.

This patient is likely to have many questions. Am I sick? How sure are you? If I am sick, what is causing my illness? How will it affect me? What can be done about it? How much will it cost?

As the clinician caring for this patient, you have the same kinds of questions although yours reflect greater understanding of the possibilities. Is the probability of serious, treatable disease high enough to proceed immediately beyond simple explanation and reassurance to diagnostic tests? How well do various tests distinguish among the possible causes of chest pain: angina pectoris, esophageal spasm, muscle strain, anxiety, and the like. For example, how helpful will an exercise stress test be in either confirming or ruling out coronary artery disease? If coronary disease is found, how long can the patient expect to have the pain? How likely is it that other complications—congestive heart failure, myocardial infarction, or atherosclerotic disease of other organs—will occur? Will the condition shorten his life? Will reduction of his risk factors for coronary disease (from cigarette smoking and hypertension) reduce his risk? If medications control the pain, would a coronary revascularization procedure add benefit—for example, by preventing future attacks or cardiovascular death?

Clinicians need the best possible answers to these questions. They use various sources of information: their own experiences, the advice of their colleagues, and reasoning from their knowledge of the biology of disease. In many situations, the most credible source is clinical research, which involves the use of past observations on other similar patients to predict what will happen to the patient at hand. The manner in which such observations are made and interpreted determines whether the conclusions reached are valid, and thus how helpful the conclusions will be to patients.

THE SCIENTIFIC BASIS FOR CLINICAL MEDICINE

Clinical epidemiology is one of the basic sciences that clinicians rely on in the care of patients. Other sciences are also integral to patient care, and these are summarized in Figure 1.1.

Biologic sciences, studies of the sequence of biologic events that lead from health to disease, are a powerful way of knowing how clinical phenomena may play out at the human level. Anatomy explains nerve entrapment syndromes and their cause and relief. Physiology and biochemistry guide the management of diabetic ketoacidosis. Molecular genetics predicts the occurrence of diseases ranging from common cardiovascular diseases and cancer to rare inborn errors of metabolism, such as phenylketonuria and cystic fibrosis.

Understanding the biology of disease, however, is often not, in itself, a sound basis for prediction in intact humans. Too many other factors contribute to health and disease. For one thing, mechanisms of

disease may be incompletely understood. For example, the notion that blood sugar in diabetic patients is more affected by ingestion of simple sugars (sucrose or table sugar) than by complex sugars such as starch (as in potatoes or pasta) has been dispelled by rigorous studies comparing the sugars' respective effects. Also, it is becoming clear that the effects of single genetic abnormalities are often modified by their genetic environment, as well as by a complex physical and social environment involving the individual's diet, exposure to infectious and chemical agents, and prevailing ways of reacting to illness in the family or community. The gene for phenylketonuria, for example, is expressed only in children who ingest phenylalanine in their diets (which happens to be everyone unless this amino acid is purposefully excluded). Therefore, knowledge of the biology of disease produces hypotheses, often very good ones, about what might happen in patients. But these hypotheses need to be tested by strong studies of intact human beings before they are accepted as clinical facts.

The **clinical sciences** provide information that can be used to care for individual patients. Foremost among them is clinical epidemiology (described below). Some biologic sciences, such as anatomy and

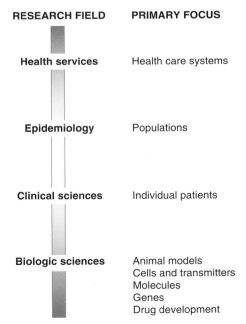

RESEARCH FIELD	PRIMARY FOCUS
Health services	Health care systems
Epidemiology	Populations
Clinical sciences	Individual patients
Biologic sciences	Animal models Cells and transmitters Molecules Genes Drug development

FIGURE 1.1 ■ The health sciences and their complementary relationships

physiology, as mentioned earlier, are "clinical" to the extent that they provide sound information to guide clinical decisions. Distinctions among the sciences are by no means sharp. In fact, bridging disciplines, as is done in clinical epidemiology, can be enormously fruitful.

The **population sciences** study large groups of people. **Epidemiology** is the "study of disease occurrence in human populations" (1); by counting health-related events in people in relation to the naturally occurring groups (populations) of which they are a member. The results of many such studies are directly applicable to the care of individual patients. For example, such studies are used as the basis for advice about avoiding behaviors such as smoking and inactivity that place patients at increased risk. Other epidemiologic studies, such as those showing harmful effects of passive smoking and other environmental and occupational hazards, are the basis for public health recommendations. Clinical epidemiology is a subset of the population sciences because not all epidemiologic studies are directly useful in the care of individual patients.

Health services research is the study of how nonbiologic factors (such as clinical workforce and facilities, how care is organized and paid for, and clinicians' beliefs and patients' cooperation) affect patients' health. Such studies have shown, for example, that medical care differs substantially from one small geographic area to another (without corresponding differences in patients' health); that surgery in hospitals that often perform a specific procedure tends to have better outcomes than hospitals in which the procedure is done infrequently; and that relatively few patients with heart disease take aspirin during the hours following the onset of chest pain, even though this simple practice has been shown to reduce the number of subsequent vascular events by about 30%. These kinds of studies guide clinicians in their efforts to apply existing knowledge about the best clinical practices.

Other sciences also guide patient care. **Quantitative decision making** includes **cost-effectiveness analyses,** which describe the financial costs required to achieve a good outcome such as prevention of death or disease and **decision analyses,** which set out the rational basis for clinical decisions and the consequences or choices. The **social sciences** describe how the social environment affects health-related behaviors and the use of health services.

CLINICAL EPIDEMIOLOGY

Clinical epidemiology is the science of making predictions about individual patients by counting clinical events in groups of similar patients and using strong scientific methods to ensure that the predictions are accurate. The purpose of clinical epidemiology is to develop and apply methods of clinical observation that will lead to valid conclusions by avoiding being misled by systematic error and the play of chance. It is one important approach to obtaining the kind of information clinicians need to make good decisions in the care of patients.

The term "clinical epidemiology" is derived from its two parent disciplines: clinical medicine and epidemiology. It is "clinical" because it seeks to answer clinical questions and to guide clinical decision making with the best available evidence. It is "epidemiology" because many of the methods used to answer these questions have been developed by epidemiologists and because the care of individual patients is seen in the context of the larger population of which the patient is a member.

Evidence-based medicine is a modern term for the application of clinical epidemiology to the care of patients. It includes formulating specific clinical questions, finding the best available research evidence bearing on those questions, judging whether the information is strong enough to base clinical decisions on, and actually using this information in the care of patients. (2) This book will deal with many aspects of evidence-based medicine.

Clinicians have long depended on research evidence to some extent. But understanding clinical evidence is more important in modern times than it was in the past for several reasons. An extraordinary amount of information is available. Diagnostic and therapeutic interventions have the potential for great effectiveness, as well as risk and cost, so the stakes in choosing among them are high. Clinical research at its best is much stronger and, thus, a sounder basis for clinical decisions. The credibility of clinical research varies from study to study, so clinicians must have an approach to sorting out strong from weak evidence. Also, there is growing evidence that many physicians, not just the "bad" ones, do not practice according to the best available evidence.

Clinical epidemiology is just one of many sciences basic to clinical medicine, but an especially important one because it bears so directly on the care of individual patients. At best, the various health-related sciences complement one another. Discoveries in one are confirmed in another; discoveries in the other lead to new hypotheses in the first.

EXAMPLE

The drug amantadine was being used for the treatment of Parkinson's disease when an observant neurologist noticed that patients treated with this drug seemed to have less severe symptoms of influenza A during an epidemic. The hypothesis that amantadine was effective in preventing influenza was confirmed by more rigorous research, clinical trials in patients without Parkinson's disease. However, patients taking amantadine had a high rate of central nervous system side effects (such as anxiety, impaired thinking, insomnia, and even hallucinations). Scientists developed a structurally related drug, rimantadine, in the laboratory, and trials of that drug showed similar effectiveness against influenza but fewer side effects. In this example, clinicians, epidemiologists, clinical epidemiologists, and laboratory scientists all contributed to a new way of preventing and treating influenza and confirming its effectiveness.

In real-life clinical settings, other kinds of "evidence" compete for clinicians' attention and can influence medical decisions. Table 1.1 describes some of them in a parody of evidence-based

TABLE 1.1 ■ Factors Other Than Evidence-based Medicine that May Influence Clinical Decisions

Eminence-based medicine	Senior colleagues who believe experience trumps evidence
Vehemence-based medicine	Substitution of volume and stridency for evidence
Eloquence (or elegance)-based medicine	Sartorial elegance and verbal eloquence
Providence-based medicine	The decision is best left in the hands of the Almighty
Diffidence-based medicine	The diffident doctor does nothing from a sense of despair
Nervousness-based medicine	Fear of litigation is a powerful stimulus to over-investigation and over-treatment
Confidence-based medicine	Bravado

Modified from Isaacs D, Fitzgerald D. Seven alternatives to evidence-based medicine. BMJ 1999; 319: 1618.

TABLE 1.2 ■ Clinical Issues and Questions*

Issue	Question
Abnormality (Ch. 2)	Is the patient sick or well?
Diagnosis (Ch. 3)	How accurate are tests used to diagnose disease?
Frequency (Ch. 4)	How often does a disease occur?
Risk (Chs. 5 and 6)	What factors are associated with an increased risk of disease?
Prognosis (Ch. 7)	What are the consequences of having a disease?
Treatment (Ch. 8)	How does treatment change the course of disease?
Prevention (Ch. 9)	Does an intervention on well people keep disease from arising? Does early detection and treatment improve the course of disease?
Cause (Ch. 11)	What conditions lead to disease? What are the origins of the disease?

*Three chapters—chance, systematic reviews, and knowledge management—pertain to all of these issues.

medicine. These less reliable alternatives to evidence-based medicine can be very compelling at the emotional level, and may provide a convenient way of coping with uncertainty, but are a weak substitute for research evidence.

BASIC PRINCIPLES

The purpose of clinical epidemiology is to foster methods of clinical observation and interpretation that lead to valid conclusions and better patient care. The most credible answers to clinical questions are based on a few basic principles.

Clinical Questions

Types of questions addressed by clinical epidemiology are listed in Table 1.2. These are the same questions confronting the doctor and patient in the example presented at the beginning of this chapter. One or more of these questions are at issue in most doctor-patient encounters (and each is also the topic of chapters in this book).

Variables

Researchers call the attributes of patients and clinical events **variables**—things that vary and can be measured. In a typical study, there are two main kinds of variables. One is a purported cause or predictor variable, sometimes called the **independent variable**. The other is the possible effect, sometimes called the **dependent variable**. Other variables may be part of the system under study and may affect the relationship between these two. These are called **extraneous variables** because they are extraneous to the main question (though perhaps very much a part of the phenomenon under study).

Health Outcomes

The clinical events of primary interest in clinical epidemiology are the health outcomes of particular concern to patients and those caring for them, such as symptoms, disability, and death. (Table 1.3). These are the events doctors try to understand, predict, interpret, and change when caring for patients. They can be studied directly only in intact humans and not in parts of humans (such as humeral transmitters, tissue cultures, cell membranes, and genetic sequences) or in animals.

During their training, clinicians are steeped in the biology of disease, the sequence of events that leads to clinically apparent effects. Although very important to clinical medicine, these biologic mechanisms cannot be substituted for clinical outcomes unless there is strong clinical evidence confirming that the two are related.

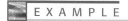

E X A M P L E

Figure 1.2 summarizes some biologic and clinical outcomes for the treatment of a patient with ventricular arrhythmias. Frequent and complex ventricular premature depolarizations (VPDs) are associated with an increased risk of sudden death (from a fatal ventricular arrhythmia), especially in people with other evidence of heart disease. Therefore, it seems logical that preventing these depolarizations with drugs would prevent sudden death. Reduction in the rate of depolarizations might be a convenient marker of therapeutic success because it can be observed right away whereas the real clinical outcome, sudden death, occurs infrequently and, in most cases, long after treatment was started. However, studies have shown that treatment with arrhythmia-suppressing drugs often does not prevent sudden death. In fact, some drugs that suppress the depolarizations actually increase the rate of sudden death. In this situation, ventricular depolarizations, an intermediate, biologic outcome, are an unreliable marker of the clinical outcome—sudden death.

Numbers and Probability

Clinical science, like all other sciences, depends on quantitative measurements. Impressions, instincts and beliefs are important in medicine too, but only when added to a solid foundation of numerical information. This foundation allows better confirmation, more precise communication among clinicians and between clinicians and patients, and estimation of error. Clinical outcomes, such as occurrence of disease, death, symptoms, or disability, can be counted and expressed as numbers.

In most clinical situations the diagnosis, prognosis, and results of treatment are uncertain for an individual patient. An individual will either experience a clinical outcome or will not; a prediction that is seldom exact. Therefore, prediction must be expressed as a probability. The probability for an individual patient is best estimated by referring to past experience with groups of similar patients—for example, that cigarette smoking doubles one's risk of dying at all ages, that blood tests for troponins detect about 96% of myocardial infarctions in patients with acute chest pain, and that 2%–6 % of patients undergoing surgery for abdominal aortic aneurysm will die within 30 days of the procedure.

TABLE 1.3 ■ **Outcomes of Disease (the Five Ds)**[a]	
Death	A bad outcome if untimely
Disease[b]	A set of symptoms, physical signs, and laboratory abnormalities
Discomfort	Symptoms such as pain, nausea, dyspnea, itching, and tinnitus
Disability	Impaired ability to go about usual activities at home, work, or recreation
Dissatisfaction	Emotional reaction to disease and its care, such as sadness or anger

[a] Perhaps a sixth D, destitution, belongs on this list because the financial cost of illness (for individual patients or society) is an important consequence of disease.
[b] Or illness, the patient's experience of disease.

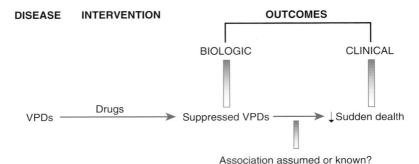

FIGURE 1.2. ■ Clinical and biologic outcomes. Does suppression of ventricular premature depolarizations by drugs prevent sudden death?

Populations and Samples

Populations are all people in a defined setting (such as North Carolina) or with certain defined characteristics (such as being age >65 years or having a thyroid nodule). Unselected people in the community are the usual population for epidemiologic studies of cause. On the other hand, clinical populations include all patients with a clinical characteristic such as all those with community-acquired pneumonia or aortic stenosis. Thus, one speaks of the general population, a hospitalized population, or a population of patients with a specific disease.

A **sample** is a subset of people in the defined population. Clinical research is ordinarily carried out on samples. One is interested in the characteristics of the defined population but must, for practical reasons, estimate them by describing the characteristics of people in a sample (Figure 1.3). One then makes an **inference**, a reasoned judgment based on

data, that the characteristics of the sample resemble those of the parent population.

The extent to which a sample represents its population, and thus is a fair substitute for it, depends on how the sample was selected. Methods in which every member of the population has an equal (or known) chance of being selected can produce samples that are extraordinarily similar to the parent population, at least in the long run and for large samples. An everyday example is opinion polls using household sampling based on census data. In our own clinical research, we often use a computer to select a representative sample from all patients in our large, multispecialty group practice, each of which has the same chance of being selected. On the other hand, samples taken haphazardly or for convenience (i.e., by selecting patients who are easy to work with or happen to be visiting the clinic when data are being collected) may misrepresent their parent population and so be misleading.

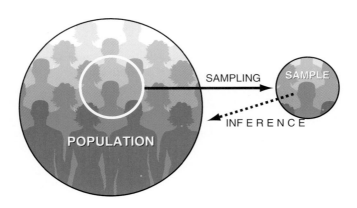

FIGURE 1.3 ■ Population and sample

Bias (Systematic Error)

Bias is "a process at any stage of inference tending to produce results that depart systematically from the true values." (3) It is "any trend in the collection, analysis, interpretation, publication, or review of data that can lead to conclusions that are systematically different from the truth." (4)

 E X A M P L E

Patients with inguinal hernia who get laparoscopic repair seem to have less postoperative pain and more rapid return to work than those who get the traditional, open surgery. The careful clinician asks: "Are the results of laparoscopic surgery really better or might they only appear better as a result of biases in the way the information was collected?" Perhaps laparoscopic repair is offered to patients who are in better health or who seem to have better tissue strength because of age or general health. Perhaps surgeons and patients are more inclined to think that the procedure should cause less pain, because it is new and the scar is smaller, and so the patients report less pain and the surgeons are less likely to ask about it or are less likely to record pain in the medical record. Perhaps patients who get laparoscopic surgery are usually instructed to return to work earlier than those who get open surgery. If any of these were so, the favorable results could be related to systematic differences in how patients are selected for the laparoscopic procedure, how they report their symptoms, or how they were told what they can do—rather than a true difference in success rates. As we shall see later (in Chapter 8), there are ways to protect against these potential biases. Studies that avoided these biases have found that patients who undergo laparoscopic surgery in fact do experience less pain and a more rapid return to work, everything else being equal. (5)

Observations of patients (whether for patient care or research) are particularly susceptible to bias. The process tends to be just plain untidy. As participants in a study, human beings have the disconcerting habit of doing as they please and not necessarily what would be required for producing scientifically rigorous answers. When researchers attempt to conduct an experiment with them, as one might in a laboratory, things tend to go wrong. Some people refuse to participate, while others drop out or choose another treatment. In addition, clinicians are inclined to believe that their therapies are successful. (Most patients would not want a physician who felt otherwise.) This attitude, so important in the practice of medicine, makes clinical observations particularly vulnerable to bias.

Although dozens of biases have been defined, (6) most fall into one of three broad categories (Table 1.4). **Selection bias** occurs when comparisons are made between groups of patients that differ in ways other than the main factors under study, ones that affect the outcome of the study. Groups of patients often differ in many ways—age, sex, severity of disease, the presence of other diseases, the care they receive, and so on. If one compares the experience of two groups that differ on a specific characteristic of interest (for example, a treatment or a suspected cause of disease) but are dissimilar in these other ways and the differences are themselves related to outcome, the comparison is biased and little can be concluded about the independent effects of the characteristic of interest. In the herniorrhaphy example, selection bias would have occurred if patients receiving the laparoscopic procedure were healthier than those who had open surgery.

Measurement bias occurs when the methods of measurement are dissimilar in different groups of patients.

 E X A M P L E

Studies associating use of birth control pills with thrombophlebitis are examples of the potential for measurement bias. Information about the use of birth control pills and the occurrence of thrombophlebitis is typically taken from medical records. Suppose a study compared the frequency of oral contraceptive use among women admitted to a hospital because of thrombophlebitis and a group of women admitted for other reasons. It is entirely possible that if women with thrombophlebitis were aware

TABLE 1.4 ■ Bias in Clinical Observation

Selection bias	Occurs when comparisons are made between groups of patients that differ in determinants of outcome other than the one under study
Measurement bias	Occurs when the methods of measurement are dissimilar among groups of patients
Confounding bias	Occurs when two factors are associated (travel together) and the effect of one is confused with or distorted by the effect of the other

of the reported association between estrogens and thromboembolic events they might report use of oral contraceptives more completely than women without thrombophlebitis, because they had already heard of the association. For the same reasons, clinicians might obtain and record information about oral contraceptive use more completely for women with thrombophlebitis than for those without it. If so, an association between oral contraceptives and thrombophlebitis might be observed because of the way in which the history of exposure was reported, whether or not there is a true association.

Confounding bias can occur when one is trying to find out whether a factor, such as a behavior or drug exposure, is a cause of disease in and of itself. If that factor is associated or "travels together" with another factor, which is itself related to the outcome, that effect can be confused with or distorted by the effect of the other.

E X A M P L E

Potential for confounding bias is illustrated by a study of the relationship between diet and disease. Long-term folic acid intake (in the form of multivitamin supplements) is associated with lower rates of colon cancer. (7) However, people who take multivitamins are more likely to be health-conscious in other ways (see Figure 1.4). They may tend to eat a low fat, high fiber, high calcium diet; to exercise; and to refrain from smoking. These are behaviors that protect against developing colon cancer. Also, multivitamins contain up to 13 different vitamins, among them folic acid, as well as minerals and other food supplements; one or more of these other components might also be related to colon cancer risk. So the possibility exists, beyond the control of the investigators,

that other elements of the diet, ones related to both folic acid use and colon cancer, are responsible for the observed association. The investigators made efforts to take these other factors into account and found that the association between folic acid intake and colon cancer was independent of these other factors. That is, confounding did not account for the observed effects in this case.

A variable is not confounded if it is directly along the path from cause to effect. Nor does a confounding variable have to be a cause itself. It may be related to the suspected cause and the effect in a particular set of data at hand, because of selection bias or chance, but not related in nature. Whether just in the data or in nature, the consequences are the same: the mistaken impression that the factor of interest is a true, independent cause when it is not.

Selection bias and confounding bias are not mutually exclusive. They are described separately, however, because they present problems at different points in a clinical study. Selection bias is at issue primarily when patients are chosen for investigation and it is important in the design of a study. Confounding bias must be dealt with during analysis of the data, once the observations have been made.

Often in the same study more than one bias operates, as in the following hypothetical example.

E X A M P L E

A study was done to determine whether regular exercise lowers the risk of coronary heart disease (CHD). An exercise program was offered to employees of a plant, and

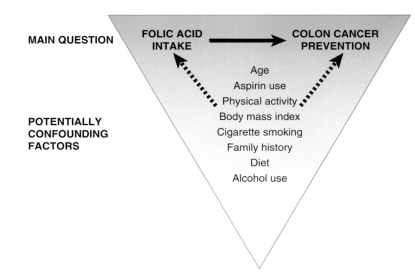

FIGURE 1.4 ■ Confounding. The relationship between folic acid intake and colon cancer risk is potentially confounded by other behaviors related to both folic acid use and colon cancer. (Source: Giovannucci E, Stampfer MJ, Colditz GA, Hunter DJ, Fuchs C, Rosner BA, Speizer FE, Willett WC. Multivitamin use, folate, and colon cancer in women in the Nurses' Health Study. Ann Intern Med 1998;129:517–524.)

the rates of subsequent coronary events were compared in employees who volunteered for the program and those who did not volunteer. Coronary events were determined by means of regular voluntary checkups, including a careful history, an electrocardiogram, and a review of routine health records. The group that exercised had lower rates of CHD. However, fewer of them smoked cigarettes.

In this example, selection bias could be present if volunteers for the exercise program were at lower risk for coronary disease even before the program began—for example, because they had lower serum lipids or less family history of coronary disease. Measurement bias might have occurred because the exercise group stood a better chance of having a coronary event detected, because more of them were examined routinely. Finally, the conclusion that exercise lowered the risk of coronary disease might be the result of a confounding bias if the association between exercise and coronary events in this particular study might result from the fact that smoking cigarettes is a risk factor for coronary disease and associated with less exercise.

The potential for bias does not mean that bias is actually present in a particular study or, if present, would have a big enough effect on the results to matter. For a researcher or reader to deal effectively with bias, it is first necessary to know where and how to look for it and what can be done about it. But one should not stop there. It is also necessary to determine whether bias is actually present and how large it is likely to be, and then decide whether it is important enough to change the conclusions of the study in a clinically meaningful way.

Chance

Observations about disease are ordinarily made on a sample of patients because it is not possible to study all patients with the disease in question. These samples, even if selected without bias, may misrepresent the situation in the population as a whole because of chance. However, results of an unbiased sample do tend to approximate the true value. If the observations were repeated on many such patient samples, results for the samples would cluster around the true value, with more of them close to, rather than far from, the true value. The divergence of an observation on a sample from the true population value, due to chance alone, is called **random variation**.

All of us are familiar with chance as an explanation for why a coin does not come up heads exactly 50% of the time when it is flipped, say, 100 times. The same effect, random variation, applies when comparing the effects of laparoscopic and open repair of inguinal hernia, discussed earlier. Suppose all biases were removed from a study of the effects of the two procedures. Suppose, further, that the two procedures are, in reality, equally effective, each followed by pain in 10% of patients. Even so, because of chance alone, a single study with small numbers of patients in each treatment group might easily find that patients do better with laparoscopy than with open surgery (or vice versa).

Chance can affect all the steps involved in clinical observations. In the assessment of the two ways of repairing inguinal hernia, random variation occurs in the sampling of patients for the study, the selection of treatment groups, and the measurements of pain and return to work.

Unlike bias, which tends to distort the situation in one direction or another, random variation is as likely to result in observations above the true value as below it. As a consequence, the mean of many unbiased observations on samples tends to approximate the true value in the population, even though the results of individual small samples may not.

Statistics can be used to estimate the extent to which chance (random variation) accounts for the results of a clinical study. Knowledge of statistics can also help reduce the role of chance by helping to create a better design and analyses. However, random variation can never be eliminated totally, so chance should always be considered when assessing the results of clinical observations. The role of chance in clinical observations will be developed in Chapter 10.

The Effects of Bias and Chance Are Cumulative

The two sources of error—bias and chance—are not mutually exclusive. In most situations, both are present. The relationship between the two is illustrated in Figure 1.5. The measurement of diastolic blood pressure on a single patient is taken as an example; each dot represents an observation of that patient. True blood pressure, which is 80 mm Hg for this patient, can be obtained by an intra-arterial cannula, but this method is not feasible for routine measurements. Blood pressure is ordinarily measured indirectly, using a sphygmomanometer (a blood pressure

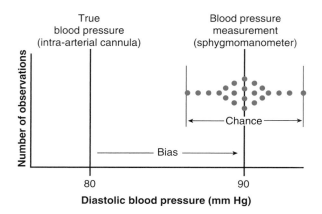

FIGURE 1.5. ■ Bias and chance. True blood pressure by intra-arterial cannula and clinical measurement by sphygmomanometer.

cuff). The simpler instrument is prone to error or deviations from the true value. In the figure, the error is represented by all of the sphygmomanometer readings falling to the right of the true value. The deviation of sphygmomanometer readings to the right (bias) may have several explanations—for example, a poorly calibrated sphygmomanometer, the wrong cuff size, or a deaf clinician. Bias could also result if different sounds were chosen to represent diastolic blood pressure. The usual end points—phase IV and phase V Korotkoff sounds—tend to be above and below the true diastolic pressure, respectively, and even that is unpredictable, especially in obese people. Individual blood pressure readings are also subject to error because of random variation in measurement, as illustrated by the spread of the sphygmomanometer readings around the mean value (90 mm Hg).

The main reason for distinguishing between bias and chance is that they are handled differently. In theory, bias can be prevented by conducting clinical investigations properly or can be corrected through proper data analysis. If not eliminated, bias often can be detected by the discerning reader. Most of this book is about how to recognize, avoid, or minimize bias. Chance, on the other hand, cannot be eliminated, but its influence can be reduced by proper design of research, and the remaining effect can be estimated by statistics. Chance is discussed primarily in Chapter 10. No amount of statistical treatment can correct for unknown biases in data. Some statisticians would go so far as to suggest that statistics should not be applied to data that are vulnerable to bias because of poor research design, for

fear of giving false respectability to fundamentally misleading work.

Internal and External Validity

When making inferences about a population from observations on a sample, clinicians need to make up their minds about two fundamental questions: First, are the conclusions of the research correct for the people in the sample? Second, if so, does the sample represent fairly the patients they are most interested in, such as the kind of patients they see or perhaps a specific patient at hand? (Figure 1.6)

Internal validity is the degree to which the results of a study are correct for the sample of patients being studied. It is "internal" because it applies to the conditions of the particular group of patients being observed and not necessarily to others. The internal validity of clinical research is determined by how well the design, data collection, and analyses are carried out and is threatened by all of the biases and random variation discussed earlier. For a clinical observation to be useful, internal validity is a necessary but not sufficient condition.

External validity is the degree to which the results of an observation hold true in other settings. Another term for this is **generalizability**. For an individual clinician, it is an answer to the question, "Assuming that the results of a study are true, do they apply to my patients as well?" Generalizability expresses the validity of assuming that patients in a study are similar to other patients.

Every study is generalizable to patients very much like the ones in the study. However, an unimpeach-

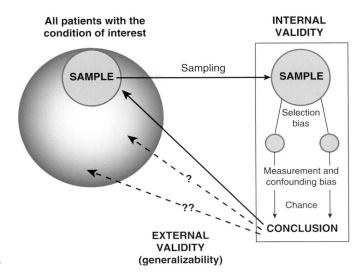

FIGURE 1.6 ▦ Internal and external validity

able study, with high internal validity, may be totally misleading if its results are generalized to the wrong patients.

EXAMPLE

What is the long-term death rate in anorexia nervosa, an eating disorder mainly afflicting young women? In a synthesis of 42 studies, estimated mortality was 15% in 30 years. (8) These studies, like most clinical research, were of patients identified in referral centers, where relatively severe cases are seen. A study of all patients developing anorexia in a defined population provided a different view of the disease. Researchers at the Mayo Clinic were able to identify all patients developing this disease in their city, Rochester, Minnesota, from 1935 to 1989 (Figure 1.7). (9) All-cause mortality at 30 years was 7%, half that of reported studies. The predicted mortality in these patients, taking into account their age and sex, was about the same, 6%. Therefore, while some patients do die of anorexia nervosa, published studies greatly overestimate the risk, presumably because they report experience with relatively severe cases.

The generalizability of clinical observations, even those with high internal validity, is a matter of personal judgment about which reasonable people might disagree.

EXAMPLE

In patients with colorectal cancer and regional spread, adjuvant chemotherapy (giving anticancer drugs after curative intent surgery) has been shown to reduce the

recurrence rate. However, it is uncertain whether adjuvant chemotherapy does more good than harm in the elderly, who comprise more than half of the patients with this cancer. Available studies supporting use of adjuvant chemotherapy either excluded elderly patients or have not reported effects in the different age groups separately, leaving a knowledge gap. Should the elderly be

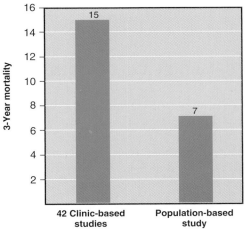

FIGURE 1.7 ▦ Sampling bias. 30-year mortality from all causes in patients with anorexia nervosa. Comparison of a synthesis of 42 published studies, mainly from referral centers, and a study of all patients with anorexia in the population. (Source: Sullivan PF. Mortality in anorexia nervosa. Am J Psychiatry 1995;152:1073–1074; and Korndorfer SR, Lucan AR, Suman VJ, Crowson CS et al. Long-term survival of patients with anorexia nervosa: A population-based study in Rochester, Minn. Mayo Clinic Proceedings 2003;78:278–284.)

offered this option even though there are no studies bearing directly on the benefits and harms in them? Some clinicians are willing to generalize from experience with younger patients and say "yes." Others, citing the absence of evidence for the elderly and reasons for believing that the older patients might be more likely to experience toxicity (because their organs have less reserve capacity) are reluctant to offer adjuvant chemotherapy to the elderly. In practice, the elderly are less likely to receive adjuvant chemotherapy. The case for generalizability from younger to older patients was strengthened by an analysis that pooled the results of existing studies of adjuvant chemotherapy and found no relationship between age and efficacy of treatment and no more toxicity in the elderly. (10)

Generalizability can rarely be dealt with satisfactorily in any one study. Even a defined, geographically based population is a biased sample of larger populations. For example, hospital patients are biased samples of county residents; counties, of states; states, of regions, and so on. The best a researcher can do about generalizability is to ensure internal validity, have the study population fit the research question, describe the study patients carefully, and avoid studying patients who are so unusual that experience with them generalizes to few others. It then remains for other studies, in other settings, to extend generalizability.

INFORMATION AND DECISIONS

The primary concerns of this book are the quality of clinical information and its correct interpretation. Making decisions is another matter. True, good decisions depend on good information; but they involve a great deal more as well, including value judgments and weighing competing risks and benefits.

In recent years, medical decision making has become a valued discipline in its own right. The field includes qualitative studies of how clinicians make decisions and how the process might be biased and can be improved. It also includes quantitative methods such as decision analysis, cost-benefit analysis, and cost-effectiveness analysis that present the decision-making process in an explicit way so that its components and the consequences of assigning various probabilities and values to them can be examined.

Patients and clinicians make clinical decisions. At best, they make decisions together, a process called **shared decision making**, recognizing that their expertise is complementary. Patients are experts in what they hope to achieve by care, given their unique experiences and preferences. They may have found a lot of information about their condition (for example, from the Internet) but are not grounded in how to sort out credible from fallacious claims. Doctors are experts in whether it is possible to achieve patients' goals and how to achieve them. For this they depend on the body of research evidence and the ability, based on the principles of clinical epidemiology, to distinguish stronger from weaker evidence. Of course, clinicians also bring to the encounter experience in how disease presents and the human consequences of care, such as what it is like to be intubated or to have an amputation, with which patients may have little experience. For clinicians to play their part on this team, they need to be experts in the interpretation of clinically relevant information.

Patients' preferences and sound evidence are the basis for choosing among care options. For example, a patient with valvular heart disease may prefer the possibility of long-term good health that surgery offers, even though surgery is associated with discomfort and risk of death in the short term. The clinician, armed with critical reading and communication skills, can help the patient understand how big those potential benefits and risks are and how surely they have been established.

Some aspects of decision analysis, such as evaluation of diagnostic tests, are included in this book. However, we have elected not to go deeply into medical decision making itself. Our justification is that decisions are only as good as the information used to make them, and we have found enough to say about the essentials of collecting and interpreting clinical information to, literally, fill a book. Readers who wish to delve more deeply into medical decision making can begin with some of the additional readings listed in the appendix at the end of this book.

ORGANIZATION OF THIS BOOK

In most textbooks on clinical medicine, information about each disease is presented as answers to traditional clinical questions: diagnosis, clinical course, treatment, and the like. On the other hand, most epidemiology books are organized around research strategies such as clinical trials, surveys, case-control studies, and the like. This way of organizing a book may serve those who perform clinical research, but it is often awkward for clinicians.

We have organized this book primarily according to the questions clinicians encounter when caring for patients (see Table 1.2). Figure 1.8 illustrates how these questions correspond to the book's chapters, taking infection with human immunodeficiency virus (HIV) as an example. The questions relate to the entire natural history of disease, from the time people without HIV infection are first exposed to risk, through when some acquire the disease and emerge as patients, until the results of disease are manifest.

In each chapter, we describe research strategies used to answer that chapter's clinical questions. Some strategies, such as cohort studies, are useful for answering several different kinds of clinical questions. For the purposes of presentation, we have discussed each strategy primarily in one chapter and have simply referred to the discussion when the method is relevant to other questions in other chapters.

REVIEW QUESTIONS

Questions 1–6 are based on the following clinical scenario. For each item, select the one best answer.

A 37-year-old-woman with low back pain for the past four weeks wants to know if you recommend surgery. You prefer to base your treatment recommendations on research evidence whenever possible. In the strongest study you can find, investigators reviewed the medical records of 40 consecutive men with low back pain under care at their clinic. Twenty-two had been referred for surgery and the other 18 patients had remained under medical care without surgery. The study compared rates of disabling pain after 2 months. All of the surgically treated patients and 10 of the medically treated patients were still being seen in the clinic throughout this time. Rates of pain relief were slightly higher in the surgically-treated patients.

For each of the following questions, circle the one response that represents the corresponding threat to validity.

1.1. Because there are relatively few patients in this study, it may give a misleading impression of the actual effectiveness of surgery.

  A. Selection bias
  B. Measurement bias
  C. Confounding
  D. Chance
  E. External validity (generalizability)

1.2. The results of this study may not apply to your patient, a woman, because all the patients in the study were men.

  A. Selection bias
  B. Measurement bias
  C. Confounding
  D. Chance
  E. External validity (generalizability)

1.3. The patients who were referred for surgery were younger and fitter than those who remained under medical care.

  A. Selection bias
  B. Measurement bias
  C. Confounding
  D. Chance
  E. External validity (generalizability)

1.4. Fewer patients who did not have surgery remained under care at the clinic two months after surgery.

  A. Selection bias
  B. Measurement bias
  C. Confounding
  D. Chance
  E. External validity (generalizability)

1.5. Compared with patients who had medical care alone, patients who had surgery might have been less likely to report whatever pain they had and the treating physicians less inclined to record pain in the medical record.

  A. Selection bias
  B. Measurement bias
  C. Confounding
  D. Chance
  E. External validity (generalizability)

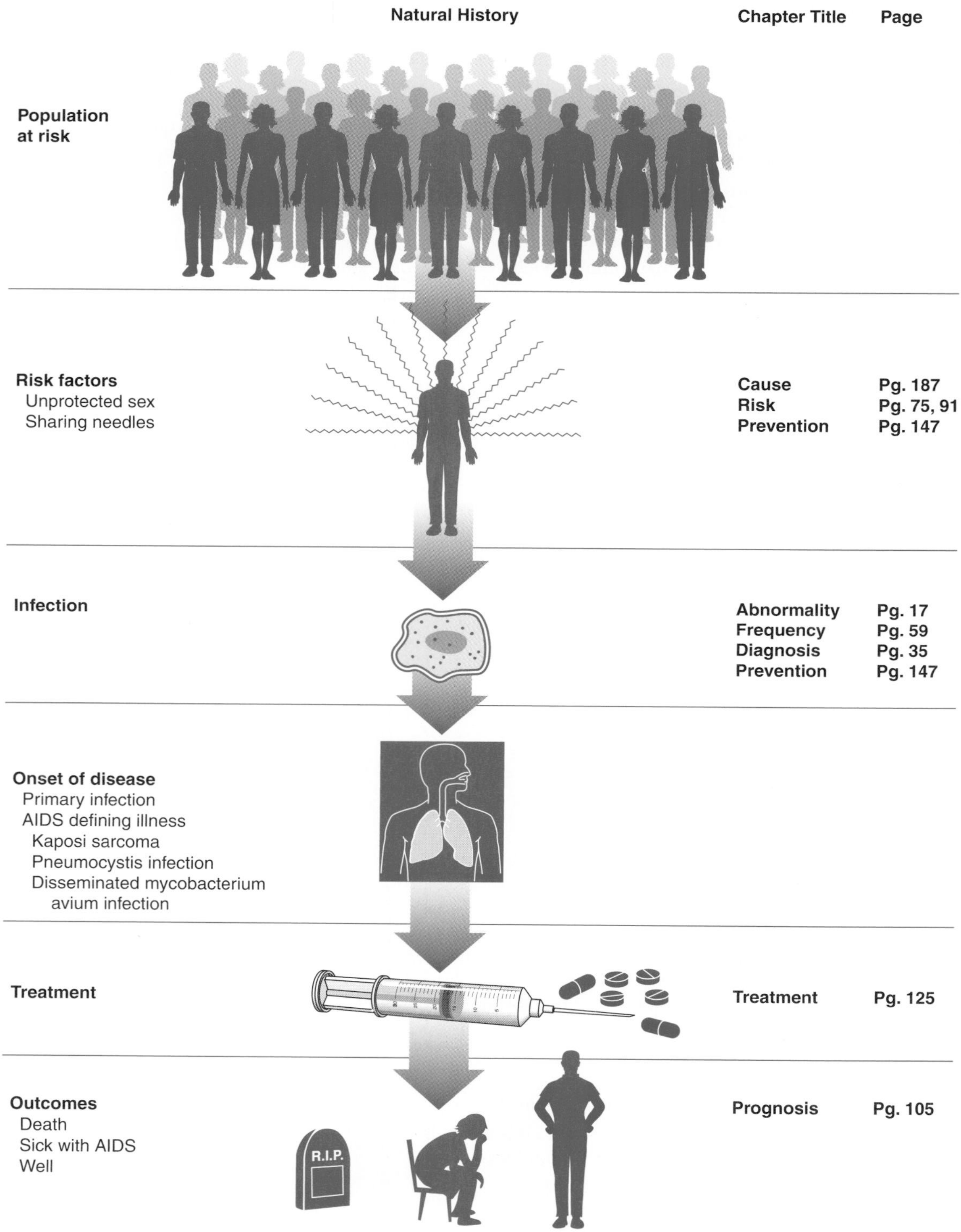

Natural History   **Chapter Title**   **Page**

Population at risk

Risk factors
  Unprotected sex
  Sharing needles

Cause   Pg. 187
Risk   Pg. 75, 91
Prevention   Pg. 147

Infection

Abnormality   Pg. 17
Frequency   Pg. 59
Diagnosis   Pg. 35
Prevention   Pg. 147

Onset of disease
  Primary infection
  AIDS defining illness
    Kaposi sarcoma
    Pneumocystis infection
    Disseminated mycobacterium
      avium infection

Treatment

Treatment   Pg. 125

Outcomes
  Death
  Sick with AIDS
  Well

Prognosis   Pg. 105

FIGURE 1.8 ■ Organization of this book in relation to the natural history of human immunodeficiency virus (HIV) infection. Chapters 10 (Chance), 12 (Systematic Reviews), and 13 (Knowledge Management) describe crosscutting issues related to all points in the natural history of disease.

1.6. Patients without other medical conditions were both more likely to recover and more likely to be referred for surgery.

- **A.** Selection bias
- **B.** Measurement bias
- **C.** Confounding
- **D.** Chance
- **E.** External validity (generalizability)

1.7. Histamine is a mediator of inflammation in patients with allergic rhinitis ("hay fever"). Based on this fact, which of the following is true?

- **A.** Drugs that block the effects of histamines will relieve symptoms.
- **B.** A fall in histamine levels in the nose is a reliable marker of clinical success.
- **C.** Antihistamines may be effective and their effects on symptoms (such as itching nose, sneezing and congestion) should be studied in patients with allergic rhinitis.
- **D.** Other mediators are not important.
- **E.** If laboratory studies of disease are convincing, clinical research is unnecessary.

Read the following statements about samples of populations and mark each one as True or False.

_____ **1.8.** Samples of populations may have characteristics that differ from the population because of random variation.

_____ **1.9.** Samples of populations are the only feasible way of studying the population.

_____ **1.10.** Samples of populations should be selected in a way that every member of the population has an equal chance of being chosen.

Read the clinical vignette below, then read each statement about the vignette and mark each one as True or False.

You are making a treatment decision with a 72-year-old man with colon cancer. You are aware of several good studies that have shown that a certain drug combination prolongs the life of patients with colon cancer. However, all the patients in these studies were much younger. Relying on those studies for your particular patient.

_____ **1.11.** Is a matter of personal judgment.

_____ **1.12.** Is called internal validity.

_____ **1.13.** Is affected by chance but not bias.

Answers are in Appendix A.

REFERENCES

1. Friedman GD. Primer of epidemiology. 5th Ed. New York: Appleton and Lange, 2003.
2. Sackett DL, Straus SE, Richardson WS, Rosenberg W, Haynes RB. Evidence-Based Medicine. How to Practice and Teach EBM. 2nd Ed. New York: Churchill Livingstone, 2000.
3. Murphy EA. The Logic of Medicine. Baltimore: Johns Hopkins University Press, 1976.
4. Last JM. A Dictionary of Epidemiology. 3rd Ed. New York: Oxford University Press, 1995.
5. EU Hernia Trialist Collaboration. Laparoscopic compared with open methods of groin hernia repair: Systematic review of randomized controlled trials. Brit J Surg 2000;87:860–867.
6. Sackett DL. Bias in analytic research. J Chronic Dis 1979;32:51–63.
7. Giovannucci E, Stampfer MJ, Colditz GA, Hunter DJ, Fuchs C, Rosner BA, et al. Multivitamin use, folate, and colon cancer in women in the Nurses' Health Study. Ann Intern Med 1998; 129:517–524.
8. Sullivan PF. Mortality in anorexia nervosa. Am J Psychiatry 1995;152:1073–1074.
9. Korndorfer SR, Lucas AR, Suman VJ, Crowson CS et al. Long-term survival of patients with anorexia nervosa: A population-based study in Rochester, Minn. Mayo Clinic Proceedings 2003;78:278–84.
10. Sargent DJ, Goldberg RM, Jacobson SD, Macdonald JS, Labianca R, Haller DG, et al. A pooled analysis of adjuvant chemotherapy for resected colon cancer in elderly patients. N Engl J Med 2001;345:1091–1097.

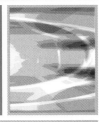

Abnormality

Nominal data
Dichotomous
Ordinal data
Interval data
Continuous data
Discrete data
Validity
Accuracy
Items

Constructs
Scales
Content validity
Construct validity
Criterion validity
Reliability
Reproducibility
Precision
Range

Responsiveness
Interpretability
Sampling fraction
Frequency distribution
Central tendency
Dispersion
Skewed
Normal distribution
Regression to the mean

. . . the medical meaning of "normal" has been lost in the shuffle of statistics.
— Alvan Feinstein

Clinicians spend a great deal of time distinguishing "normal" from "abnormal." Is the thyroid normal or slightly enlarged? Is the heart murmur "innocent" (of no health importance) or a sign of valvular disease? Is a slightly elevated serum alkaline phosphatase evidence of liver disease, unrecognized Paget disease, or nothing important?

When confronted with something grossly different from the usual, there is little difficulty telling the two apart. We are all familiar with pictures in textbooks of physical diagnoses showing massive hepatosplenomegaly, huge goiters, or hands severely deformed by rheumatoid arthritis. It takes no great skill to recognize this degree of abnormality. More often, however, clinicians must make subtler distinc-

tions between normal and abnormal. That is when skill, and a conceptual basis for deciding, become important.

Decisions about what is abnormal are most difficult among relatively unselected patients, usually found outside of hospitals. When patients have already been selected for special attention, as is the case in most referral centers, it is usually clear that something is wrong. The tasks are then to refine the diagnosis and to treat the problem. In primary care settings and emergency departments, however, patients with subtle manifestations of disease are mixed with those with the everyday complaints of basically healthy people. It is not possible to pursue all of these complaints aggressively. Which of many patients with abdominal

17

pain have self-limited gastroenteritis and which have early appendicitis? Which patients with sore throat and hoarseness have a viral pharyngitis and which have the rare but potentially lethal *Haemophilus* epiglottitis? These are examples of how difficult and important distinguishing various kinds of abnormalities can be.

The point of distinguishing normal from abnormal is to separate out those clinical observations that should be the basis for action from those that can be simply noted. Observations that are thought to be normal are usually described as "within normal limits," "unremarkable," or "noncontributory" and remain buried in the body of a medical record. The abnormal findings are set out in a problem list or under the heading "impressions" or "diagnoses" and are the basis for action.

Simply calling clinical findings normal or abnormal is undoubtedly crude and results in some misclassification. The justification for taking this approach is that it is often impractical or unnecessary to consider the raw data in all their detail. As Bertrand Russell put it, "To be perfectly intelligible one must be inaccurate, and to be perfectly accurate, one must be unintelligible." Physicians usually choose to err on the side of being intelligible—to themselves and others—even at the expense of some accuracy. Another reason for simplifying data is that each aspect of a clinician's work ends in a decision—to pursue evaluation or to wait, to begin a treatment or to reassure. Under these circumstances some sort of "present" or "absent" classification is necessary.

Table 2.1 is an example of how relatively simple expressions of abnormality are derived from more complex clinical data. On the left is a typical problem list, a statement of the patient's important med-

ical problems. On the right are some of the data on which the decisions to call them problems are based. Conclusions from the data, represented by the problem list, are by no means noncontroversial. For example, the mean of the four diastolic blood pressure measurements is 92 mm Hg. Some might argue that this level of blood pressure does not justify the label "hypertension," because it is not particularly high and there are some disadvantages to telling patients they are sick and recommending drugs. Others might consider the label fair, considering that this level of blood pressure is associated with an increased risk of cardiovascular disease and that the risk can be reduced by treatment. Although crude, the problem list serves as a basis for decisions— about diagnosis, prognosis, and treatment. And clinical decisions must be made, whether actively (by additional diagnostic tests and treatment) or passively (by no intervention).

This chapter describes some of the ways clinicians distinguish normal from abnormal. For them to do so, first it will be necessary to consider how biologic phenomena are measured, how they vary, and how they are summarized. Then, it will be possible to consider how these data are used as a basis for value judgments about what is worth calling abnormal.

TYPES OF DATA

Measurements of clinical phenomena yield three kinds of data: nominal, ordinal, and interval.

Nominal Data

Nominal data occur in categories without any inherent order. Examples of nominal data are characteristics that are determined by a small set of genes (such as, ABO blood type and sex) or are dramatic, discrete events (such as, death, dialysis, or surgery). These data can be placed in categories without much concern about misclassification. Nominal data that are divided into two categories (such as, present/absent, yes/no, alive/dead) are called **dichotomous**.

Ordinal Data

Ordinal data possess some inherent ordering or rank such as small to large or good to bad, but the size of the intervals between categories is not specified. Some clinical examples include 1+ to 4+ leg

---

TABLE 2.1 ■ Summary of Clinical Data: A Patient's Problem List and the Data on Which It Is Based	
Problem List	**Raw Data**
Hypertension	Several blood pressure measurements: 145/92, 149/93, 142/91
Diabetes mellitus	Fasting blood sugar 135 mg/dL
Renal failure	Serum creatinine 2.7 mg/dL
Obstructive pulmonary disease	Forced expiratory volume at 1 second (FEV1) 2.3 L

edema, heart murmurs grades I (heard only with special effort) to VI (audible with the stethoscope off the chest), and muscle strength grades 1 (no movement) to 5 (normal strength). The risk of birth defects from drugs during pregnancy is graded by the U.S. Food and Drug Administration on a 5-point scale ranging from "controlled studies show no risk" through "no evidence of risk in humans," "risk cannot be ruled out," and "positive evidence of risk" to "contraindicated in pregnancy."

Interval Data

For **interval data**, there is inherent order and the interval between successive values is equal, no matter where one is on the scale. There are two types of interval data. **Continuous data** can take on any value in a continuum, whether or not they are reported that way. Examples include most serum chemistries, weight, blood pressure, and partial pressure of oxygen in arterial blood. The measurement and description of continuous variables may in practice be confined to a limited number of points on the continuum, often integers, because the precision of the measurement, or its use, does not warrant greater detail. For example, a particular blood glucose reading may in fact be 193.2846573 . . . mg/100 mL but is simply reported as 193 mg/100 mL. **Discrete data** can take on only specific values and are expressed as counts. Examples of discrete data are the number of a woman's pregnancies and live births and the number of migraine attacks a patient has per month.

It is for ordinal and interval data that the question arises, "Where does normal leave off and abnormal begin?" When, for example, does a large normal prostate become too large to be considered normal? Clinicians are free to choose any cutoff point. Some of the reasons for the choices will be considered later in this chapter.

PERFORMANCE OF MEASUREMENTS

Whatever the type of measurement, its performance can be described in several ways:

Validity

Validity is the degree to which the data measure what they were intended to measure—that is, the results of a measurement correspond to the true state of the phenomenon being measured. Another word for validity is **accuracy**.

For clinical observations that can be measured by physical means, it is relatively easy to establish validity. The observed measurement is compared with some accepted standard. For example, serum sodium can be measured on an instrument recently calibrated against solutions made up with known concentrations of sodium. Laboratory measurements are commonly subjected to extensive and repeated validity checks. For example, it is common practice for blood glucose measurements to be monitored for accuracy by comparing readings against high and low standards at the beginning of each day, before each technician begins a day, and after any changes in the techniques, such as a new bottle of reagent or a new battery for the instrument. Similarly, accuracy of a lung scan for pulmonary embolus can be measured against pulmonary angiography, in which the pulmonary artery anatomy is directly visualized. The validity of a physical examination finding can be established by comparing it to the results of surgery or radiologic examinations.

Some other clinical measurements such as pain, nausea, dyspnea, depression, and fear cannot be verified physically. In patient care, information about these phenomena is usually obtained informally by "taking a history." More formal and standardized approaches, used in research, are structured interviews and questionnaires. Individual questions (**items**) are designed to measure specific phenomena (such as symptoms, feelings, attitudes, knowledge, beliefs) called **constructs** and these items are grouped together to form **scales**. Table 2.2 shows one such scale, a brief questionnaire used to detect heavy or problem drinking.

TABLE 2.2 ■ **The CAGE test for Detecting Heavy or Problem Drinking**
Have you ever felt the need to **c**ut down on drinking?
Have you ever felt **a**nnoyed by criticism of drinking?
Have you ever had **g**uilty feelings about your drinking?
Have you ever taken an **e**ye opener?
One "yes" response suggests the need for closer assessment
Two or more "yes" responses is strongly related to alcohol abuse, dependence, or both

Three general strategies are used to establish the validity of measurements that cannot be directly verified by the physical senses.

Content Validity

Content validity is the extent to which a particular method of measurement includes all of the dimensions of the construct one intends to measure and nothing more. For example, a scale for measuring pain would have content validity if it included questions about aching, throbbing, burning, and stinging but not about pressure, itching, nausea, and tingling.

Construct Validity

Construct validity is present to the extent that the measurement is related in a coherent way to other measures, also not physically verifiable, that are believed to be part of the same phenomenon. Thus, one might be more confident in the construct validity of a scale for depression to the extent that it is related to fatigue and headache—constructs thought to be different from but related to depression.

Criterion Validity

Criterion validity is present to the extent that the measurements predict a directly observable phenomenon. For example, one might see whether responses on a scale measuring pain bear a predictable relationship to pain of known severity: mild pain from minor abrasion, moderate pain from ordinary headache and peptic ulcer, and severe pain from renal colic. One might also show that responses to a scale measuring pain are related to other, observable manifestations of the severity of pain such as sweating, moaning, writhing, and asking for pain medications.

Validity of a scale is not, as is often asserted, either present or absent. Rather, with these strategies one can build a case for or against its validity under the conditions in which it is used, so as to convince others that the scale is more or less valid.

Because of their selection and training, physicians tend to prefer the kind of precise measurements that the physical and biologic sciences afford and may avoid or discount others, especially for research. Yet relief of symptoms and promoting satisfaction and a feeling of well-being are among the most important outcomes of patient care and are central concerns of patients and doctors alike. To guide clinical decisions, research must include them, lest the picture of medicine painted by the research be distorted.

As Feinstein (1) put it:

> The term "hard" is usually applied to data that are reliable and preferably dimensional (e.g., laboratory data, demographic data, and financial costs). But clinical performance, convenience, anticipation, and familial data are "soft." They depend on subjective statements, usually expressed in words rather than numbers, by the people who are the observers and the observed.
>
> To avoid such soft data, the results of treatment are commonly restricted to laboratory information that can be objective, dimensional, and reliable—but it is also dehumanized. If we are told that the serum cholesterol is 230 mg per 100 ml, that the chest X-ray shows cardiac enlargement, and that the electrocardiogram has Q waves, we would not know whether the treated object was a dog or a person. If we were told that capacity at work was restored, that the medicine tasted good and was easy to take, and that the family was happy about the results, we would recognize a human set of responses.

Reliability

Reliability is the extent to which repeated measurements of a stable phenomenon by different people and instruments at different times and places get similar results. **Reproducibility** and **precision** are other words for this property.

The reliability of laboratory measurements is established by repeated measures—for example, of the same serum or tissue specimen—sometimes by different people and with different instruments. The reliability of symptoms can be established by showing that they are similarly described to different observers under different conditions.

The relationships between reliability and validity are shown in simple form in Figure 2.1. Measurements can be valid (accurate) on the average but not be reliable, because they are widely scattered about the true value, as shown in C. On the other hand, measurements can be very reliable but inaccurate if they are systematically off the mark, as in B. Small numbers of measurements with poor reliability also have low validity because they are likely to be off the mark by chance alone. Therefore, reliability and

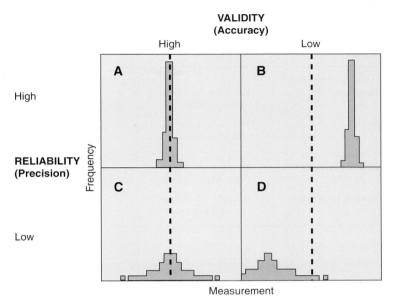

FIGURE 2.1 ■ Validity and reliability. A. High validity and high reliability. B. Low validity and high reliability. C. High validity and low reliability. D. Low validity and low reliability. The dotted lines represent the true values.

validity are not altogether independent concepts. Figure 2.1 is an approximation; in general, an unreliable measurement cannot be valid and a valid measurement must be reliable.

Range

An instrument may not register very low or high values of the phenomenon being measured; that is, it has limited **range**, which limits the information it conveys. For example, the Basic Activities of Daily Living scale that measures patients' ability in dressing, eating, walking, toileting, and maintaining hygiene does not measure ability to read, write, or play the piano (activities that might be very important to individual patients).

Responsiveness

An instrument demonstrates **responsiveness** to the extent that its results change as conditions change. For example, the New York Heart Association scale—classes I to IV (no symptoms, symptoms with slight exertion, with moderate exertion, and symptoms at rest)—is not sensitive to subtle changes in congestive heart failure, ones that might matter to patients. On the other hand, measurements of ejection fraction by echocardiography can detect changes so subtle that patients do not notice them.

Interpretability

Clinicians learn to interpret the significance of a PCO_2 of 50 or a blood sugar of 460 through experience, in which they repeatedly calibrate patients' current conditions and clinical courses against such test results. On the other hand, scales based on questionnaires may have little intuitive meaning to clinicians and patients who do not use them regularly. To overcome this **interpretability** disadvantage, researchers can "anchor" scale values to familiar states. For example, values of the Karnofsky Performance Status Scale, a measure of functional capacity commonly used in studies of cancer patients receiving chemotherapy, range from 100 (normal) to 0 (dead). Just how bad is it to have a value of 60? To help clinicians interpret scale values, the numbers are anchored to descriptions of everyday performance. At a scale value of 60, patients require occasional assistance but are able to care for most of their needs.

VARIATION

Clinical measurements of the same phenomenon can take on a range of values, depending on the circumstances in which they are made. To avoid erroneous

TABLE 2.3 ■ Sources of Variation	
Source of Variation	**Definition**
Measurement Variation	
Instrument	The means of making the measurement
Observer	The person making the measurement
Biologic Variation	
Within individuals	Changes a person with time and situation
Between individuals	Biologic differences from person to person

conclusions from data, clinicians should be aware of the reasons for variation in a given situation and know which are likely to play a large part, a small part, or no part at all in what has been observed. This is so not only for the interpretation of published research but also for the credibility of day-to-day clinical measurements.

Overall variation is the sum of variation related to the act of measurement, biologic differences

within individuals from time to time, and biologic differences among individuals (see Table 2.3).

Variation Resulting from Measurement

All observations are subject to variation because of the performance of the instruments and observers involved in making the measurements. The conditions of measurement can lead to a biased result (lack of validity) or simply random error (lack of reliability). It is possible to reduce this source of variation by making measurements with great care and by following standard protocols. However, when measurements involve human judgment, rather than machines, variation can be particularly large and difficult to control.

EXAMPLE

Fetal heart rate is often monitored by auscultation, which is subject to observer error. Electronic monitoring gives the true rate. Fetal heart rates that are unusually high or low are signs of fetal distress, suggesting a need for early delivery by Cesarean section.

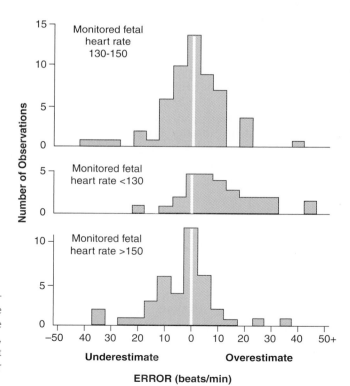

FIGURE 2.2 ■ Observer variability. Error in reporting fetal heart rate according to whether the true rate, determined by electronic monitor, is within the normal range, low, or high. (Redrawn from Day E, Maddern L, Wood C. Auscultation of foetal heart rate: An assessment of its error and significance. Br Med J 1968;4:422–424.)

Day et al. (2) compared fetal heart rates obtained by auscultation by hospital staff with rates obtained by electronic monitoring (Figure 2.2). When the true fetal heart rate was in the normal range, rates by auscultation were evenly distributed about the true value (i.e., there was only random error). But when the true fetal heart rate was unusually high or low, rates by auscultation were biased toward normal. Low rates tended to be reported as higher than the true rates, and high rates as lower than the true rates.

This study illustrates both random and systematic errors in clinical observations. In this case, the bias toward rates in the normal range might have arisen because the hospital staff hoped the fetus was well and were reluctant to undertake a major intervention based on their observation of an abnormally high or low heart rate.

Variations in measurements also arise because they are made on only a sample of the phenomenon being described, which may misrepresent the whole. Often, the **sampling fraction** (the fraction of the whole that is included in the sample) is very small. For example, a liver biopsy represents only about 1/100,000 of the liver. Because such a small part of the whole is examined, there is room for considerable variation from one sample to another.

If measurements are made by several different methods, such as different laboratories, technicians, or instruments, some of the measurements may be unreliable and may produce results that are systematically different from the correct value, which could contribute to the spread of values obtained.

Variation Resulting from Biologic Differences

Variation also arises because of biologic changes within individuals over time. Most biologic phenomena change from moment to moment. A measurement at a point in time is a sample of measurements during a period of time and may not represent the usual value of these measurements.

EXAMPLE

Clinicians estimate the frequency of ventricular premature depolarization (VPD) to help determine the need for and effectiveness of treatment. For practical reasons, they may do so by making relatively brief observations—perhaps feeling a pulse for 1 minute or reviewing an electrocardiogram recording several seconds. However, the frequency of VPDs in a given patient varies over time. To obtain a larger sample of VPD rate, a portable monitor is sometimes used. But monitoring even for extended periods of time can be misleading. Figure 2.3 shows observations on one patient with VPDs, similar to other patients studied. (3) VPDs per hour varied from less than 20 to 380 during a 3-day period, according to day and time of day. The authors concluded: "To distinguish a reduction in VPD frequency attributable to therapeutic intervention rather than biologic or spontaneous variation alone required a greater than 83% reduction in VPD frequency if only two 24-hour monitoring periods were compared." Much shorter periods of observation could be more misleading because of biologic variation.

Variation also arises because of differences among people. Biologic differences among people predomi-

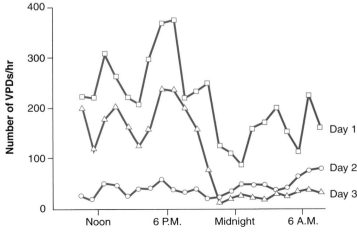

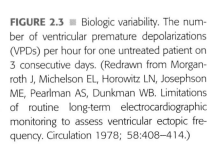

FIGURE 2.3 ■ Biologic variability. The number of ventricular premature depolarizations (VPDs) per hour for one untreated patient on 3 consecutive days. (Redrawn from Morganroth J, Michelson EL, Horowitz LN, Josephson ME, Pearlman AS, Dunkman WB. Limitations of routine long-term electrocardiographic monitoring to assess ventricular ectopic frequency. Circulation 1978; 58:408–414.)

nate in many situations. For example, several studies have shown that high blood pressure on single, casual measurements, although subject to all other forms of variation, is related to subsequent cardiovascular disease.

Total Variation

The several sources of variation are cumulative. Figure 2.4 illustrates this for the measurement of blood pressure. When looking at a population distribution, variation in measurement for individual patients is added to variation for those individuals from time to time, which is in turn added to variation among different patients. Measurement variation contributes relatively little, although it covers as much as a 12 mm Hg range among various observers. On the other hand, each patient's blood pressure varies a great deal from moment to moment throughout the day, so that any single blood pressure reading might

not represent the usual for that patient. Much of this variation is not random: blood pressure is generally higher when people are awake, excited, visiting physicians, or taking over-the-counter cold medications. Of course, we are most interested in knowing how an individual's blood pressure compares with that of his or her peers, especially if the blood pressure level is related to complications of hypertension and the effectiveness of treatment.

Effects of Variation

Another way of thinking about variation is in terms of its net effect on the validity and reliability of a measurement and what can be done about it.

Random variation—for example, by unstable instruments or many observers with various biases that tend to balance each other out—results on average in no net misrepresentation of the true state of a phenomenon, even though individual

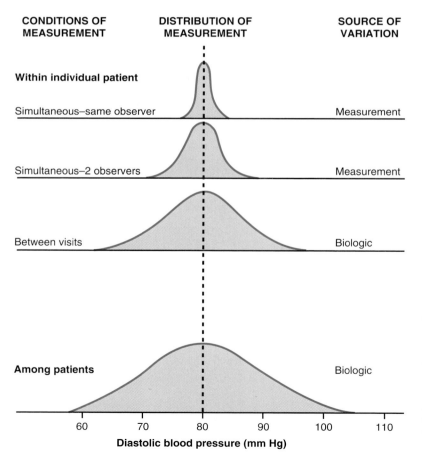

FIGURE 2.4 ■ Sources of variation in the measurement of diastolic (phase V) blood pressure. The dashed line indicates the true blood pressure. (Source: Fletcher RH and Fletcher SW (unpublished); and Boe J, Humerfelt S, Wedervang F, Oecon C. The blood pressure in a population [Special Issue]. Acta Med Scand 1957;321:5–313.)

measurements may be misleading. Inaccuracy resulting from random variation can be reduced by taking the average of a larger sample of what is being measured, for example, by counting more cells on a blood smear, examining a larger area of a urine sediment, or studying more patients. Also, the extent of random variation can be estimated by statistical methods (see Chapter 10).

On the other hand, biased results are systematically different from the true value, no matter how many times they are repeated. For example, measurement of fetal heart rate (the example shown in Figure 2.2) would remain off-target even if repeated many more times. Similarly, all of the high values for VPDs shown in Figure 2.3 were recorded on the first day, and most of the low values on the third. The days were biased estimates of each other, because of variation in VPD rate from day to day.

DISTRIBUTIONS

Data that are measured on interval scales are often presented as a figure, called a **frequency distribution**, showing the number (or proportion) of a defined group of people possessing the different values of the measurement. Figure 2.5 shows the distribution in

normal men of serum prostate-specific antigen (PSA), a test for prostate disease, especially cancer. Although PSA concentration ranges from 0 to 10, most measurement are in the 0 to 4 range. Presenting interval data as a frequency distribution conveys the information in relatively fine detail.

Describing Distributions

It is convenient to summarize distributions. Indeed, summarization is imperative when a large number of distributions are presented and compared.

Two basic properties of distributions are used to summarize them: **central tendency**, the middle of the distribution, and **dispersion**, how spread out the values are. Several ways of expressing central tendency and dispersion, along with their advantages and disadvantages, are illustrated in Figure 2.5 and summarized in Table 2.4.

Actual Distributions

Distributions of clinical phenomena have many different shapes. The frequency distributions of four common blood tests (for potassium, alkaline phosphatase, glucose, and hemoglobin) are shown in Figure 2.6. In general, most of the values appear near

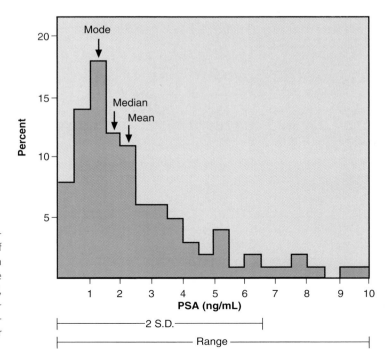

FIGURE 2.5 ■ Measures of central tendency and dispersion. The distribution of prostate-specific antigen (PSA) levels in presumably normal men. (Source: Kane RA, Littrup PJ, Babaian R, Drago JR, Lee F, Chesley A, Murphy GP, Mettlin C. Prostate-specific antigen levels in 1695 men without evidence of prostate cancer. Cancer 1992;69:1201–1207.)

TABLE 2.4 ■ **Expressions of Central Tendency and Dispersion**

Expression	Definition	Advantages	Disadvantages
Central Tendency			
Mean	$\dfrac{\text{Sum of values for observations}}{\text{Number of observations}}$	Well suited for mathematical manipulation	Affected by extreme values
Median	The point where the number of observations above equals the number below	Not easily influenced by extreme values	Not well suited for mathematical manipulation
Mode	Most frequently occurring value	Simplicity of meaning	Sometimes there are no, or many, most frequent values
Dispersion			
Range	From lowest to highest value in a distribution	Includes all values	Greatly affected by extreme values
Standard deviation[a]	The absolute value of the average difference of individual values from the mean[a]	Well suited for mathematical manipulation	For non-Gaussian distributions, (see below) does not describe a known proportion of the observations
Percentile, decile, quartile, etc.	The proportion of all observations falling between specified values	Describes "unusualness" of a value Does not make assumptions about the shape of a distribution	Not well suited for statistical manipulation

[a] $\sqrt{\dfrac{\Sigma(X - \bar{X})^2}{N - 1}}$ where X = each observation; $\bar{X}$ = mean of all observations; and N = number of observations

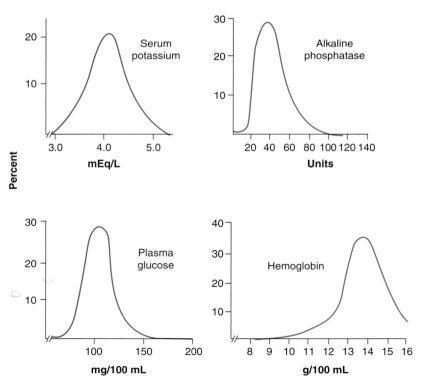

FIGURE 2.6 ■ Actual clinical distributions. (Source: Martin HF, Gudzinowicz BJ, Fanger H. *Normal values in clinical chemistry.* New York: Marcel Dekker, 1975.)

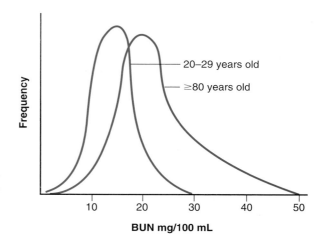

FIGURE 2.7. ▪ The distribution of clinical variables changes with age: BUN for people aged 20–29 versus those 80 or older. (Source: Martin HF, Gudzinowicz BJ, Fanger H. *Normal values in clinical chemistry.* New York: Marcel Dekker, 1975.)

the middle of the distribution, and except for the central part of the curves, there are no "humps" or irregularities. The high and low ends of the distributions stretch out into tails, with the tail at one end often being more elongated than the tail at the other (i.e., the curves are **skewed** toward the longer end). Whereas some of the distributions are skewed toward higher values, others are skewed toward lower values. In other words, all of these distributions are unimodal (have only one hump), are roughly bell shaped, though not necessarily symmetrical. Otherwise, they do not resemble one another.

The distribution of values for many laboratory tests changes with characteristics of the patients such as age, sex, race, and nutrition. Figure 2.7 shows

how the distribution of one such test, blood urea nitrogen (BUN, a test of kidney function), changes with age. A BUN of 25 mg/100 mL would be unusually high for a young person, but not particularly remarkable for an older person.

The Normal Distribution

Another kind of distribution is called the **normal distribution** (or "Gaussian," after the mathematician who first described it). The normal distribution, based in statistical theory, describes the frequency distribution of repeated measurements of the same physical object by the same instrument. Dispersion of values represents random variation alone. A normal curve is shown in Figure 2.8. The curve is

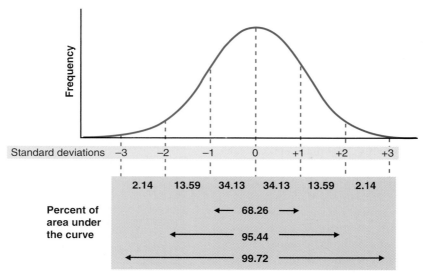

FIGURE 2.8 ▪ The Normal (Gaussian) distribution.

symmetrical and bell shaped. It has the mathematical property that about two-thirds of the observations fall within 1 standard deviation of the mean, and about 95% within 2 standard deviations.

Although clinical distributions often resemble a normal distribution the resemblance is superficial. As one statistician (4) put it, "The experimental fact is that for most physiologic variables the distribution is smooth, unimodal, and skewed, and that mean ±2 standard deviations does not cut off the desired 95%. We have no mathematical, statistical, or other theorems that enable us to predict the shape of the distributions of physiologic measurements."

The shapes of clinical distributions differ from one another because many differences among people, other than random variation, contribute to distributions of clinical measurements. Therefore, if distributions of clinical measurements resemble normal curves, it is largely by accident. Even so, it is often assumed, as a matter of convenience (because means and standard deviations are relatively easy to calculate and manipulate mathematically) that clinical measurements are "normally" distributed.

CRITERIA FOR ABNORMALITY

It would be convenient if the frequency distributions of clinical measurements for normal and abnormal people were so different that these distributions could be used to distinguish two distinct populations. This is actually the case for some abnormal genes. Sequences (genetic abnormalities coding) for the autosomal dominant condition Familial Adenomatous Polyposis are either present or absent. People with the abnormal gene develop hundreds of polyps in their colon whereas people without the gene rarely have more than a few. But this is the exception that proves the rule. Far more often, the various genetic abnormalities coding for the same disease produce a range of expressions. Even the expression of a specific genetic abnormality (such as substitution of a single base pair) differs substantially from one person to another, presumably related to differences in the rest of the genetic endowment as well as exposure to external causes of the disease.

Therefore, most distributions of clinical variables are not easily divided into "normal" and "abnormal." They are not inherently dichotomous and do not display sharp breaks or two peaks that characterize normal and abnormal results. This is because disease is usually acquired by degrees, so there is a smooth transition from low to high values with increasing degrees of dysfunction. Laboratory tests reflecting organ failure, such as serum creatinine for kidney failure or ejection fraction for heart failure, behave in this way.

Another reason why normals and abnormals are not seen as separate distributions is that even when people with and without a disease have substantially different frequency distributions, the distributions almost always overlap. When the two distributions are mixed together, as they are in naturally-occurring populations, the abnormals are usually not seen as separate because the abnormals comprise such a small proportion of the whole. The curve for people with disease is "swallowed up" by the larger curve for healthy, normal people.

EXAMPLE

Phenylketonuria (PKU) is an inherited disease characterized by progressive mental retardation in childhood. A variety of mutant alleles coding for phenylalanine hydroxylase results in dysfunction of the enzyme and, with a normal diet, accumulation of phenylalanine that results in symptoms. The genes are in principle either abnormal or not (Figure 2.9A). The diagnosis, which becomes apparent in the first year of life, is confirmed by persistently high phenylalanine levels (several times the usual range) and low tyrosine levels in the blood.

It is common practice to screen newborns for PKU with a blood test for phenylalanine a few days after birth, in time to treat before there is irreversible damage. However, even though the abnormal genes are present or absent (Figure 2.9A) the test misclassifies some infants because at that age there is an overlap in the distributions of serum phenylalanine concentrations in infants with and without PKU and because infants with PKU make up only a small proportion of those screened, less than 1/10,000 (Figure 2.9B). Some newborns with PKU are in the normal range either because they have not yet ingested enough phenylalanine-containing protein or because they have a combination of alleles associated with mild disease. Some children who are not destined to develop PKU have relatively high levels—for example, because their mothers have abnormal phenylalanine metabolism. The test is set to be positive at the lower end of the overlap between normal and abnormal levels, to detect most infants with the disease, even though only about 1 out of 5 infants with an abnormal screening test turns out to have PKU.

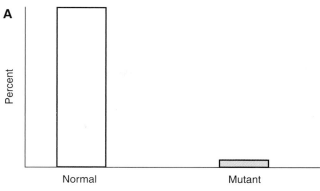

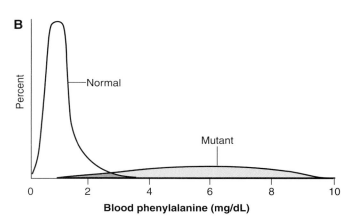

FIGURE 2.9 ■ Screening for phenylketonuria (PKU) in infants: dichotomous and overlapping distributions of normal and abnormal. A. Alleles coding for phenylalanine hydroxylase are either normal or mutant. B. The distributions of blood phenylalanine levels in newborns with and without PKU overlap and are of greatly different magnitude. (The prevalence of PKU, which is less than 1/10,000, is exaggerated so that its distribution can be seen in the figure.)

If there is no sharp dividing line between normal and abnormal, and the clinician can choose where the line is placed, what ground rules should be used to decide? Three criteria have proven useful: being unusual, being sick, and being treatable. For a given measurement, the results of these approaches bear no necessary relation to one another, so that what is considered abnormal by one criterion might be normal by another.

Abnormal = Unusual

Normal often refers to the frequently occurring or usual condition. Whatever occurs often is considered normal, and what occurs infrequently is abnormal. This is a statistical definition, based on the frequency of a characteristic in a defined population. Commonly, the reference population is made up of people without disease, but this need not be the case. For example, we may say that it is normal to have pain after surgery or itching with eczema.

It is tempting to be more specific by defining what is unusual in mathematical terms. One commonly used way of establishing a cutoff point between normal and abnormal is to agree, somewhat arbitrarily, that all values beyond 2 standard deviations from the mean are abnormal. On the assumption that the distribution in question approximates a normal distribution, 2.5% of observations would then appear in each tail of the distribution and be considered abnormally high or abnormally low.

Of course, as already pointed out, most biologic measurements are not normally distributed. So it is better to describe unusual values, whatever the proportion chosen, as a fraction (or percentile) of the actual distribution. In this way, it is possible to make a direct statement about how infrequent a value is without making assumptions about the shape of the distribution from which it came.

A statistical definition of normality is commonly used but it can be ambiguous or misleading for several reasons:

1. If all values beyond an arbitrary statistical limit, say the 95th percentile, were considered abnormal, then the frequency of all diseases would be the same (if one assumed the distribution was normal, 2.5% if we consider just the extreme high and low ends of the distribution). Yet it is common knowledge that diseases vary in frequency; diabetes and osteoarthritis are far more common than ovalocytosis and hairy cell leukemia.

2. There is no general relationship between the degree of statistical unusualness and clinical disease. The relationship is specific to the disease in question and the setting. Thus, obesity is quite common in the United States but uncommon in many developing countries. For some measurements, deviations from usual are associated with disease to an important degree only at quite extreme values, well beyond the 95th or even the 99th percentile. Failure of organs such as the liver and kidneys becomes symptomatic only when most of usual function is lost.

3. Sometimes extreme values are actually beneficial. For example, people with unusually low blood pressure are, on average, at lower risk of cardiovascular disease than people with more usual blood pressures. People with unusually high bone density are at lower than average risk of fractures.

4. Many measurements are related to risk of disease over a broad range of values, with no threshold dividing normal from increased risk. Blood pressure is an example.

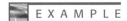

E X A M P L E

Figure 2.10 shows that higher than usual systolic blood pressure is related to higher rates of ischemic heart disease mortality throughout a broad range of blood pressures, from 115 to 185 mm Hg. For every 20 mm Hg, higher systolic blood pressure there is about a two-fold higher ischemic heart disease death rate, with no evidence of a threshold down to 115 mm Hg systolic pressure, the lowest level for which there are adequate data. (5) About 80% of the general population of adults has a blood pressure below 140 mm Hg, the point at which drug treatment is recommended.

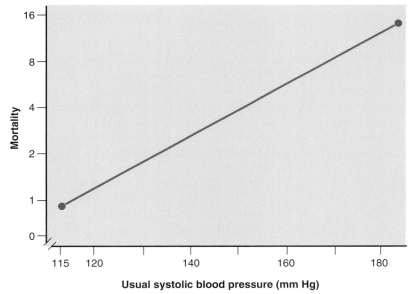

FIGURE 2.10 ■ Ischemic heart disease mortality for people age 40–49 years is related to systolic blood pressure throughout the range of values occurring in most people. There is no threshold between normal and abnormal, either for middle-aged and older people. "Mortality" is presented as a multiple of the baseline rate (Source: Prospective Studies Collaboration. Age-specific relevance of usual blood pressure to vascular mortality: A meta-analysis of individual data for one million adults in 61 prospective studies. Lancet 2002;360:1903–13.)

A

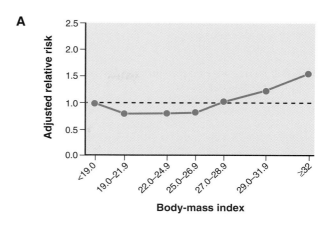

B

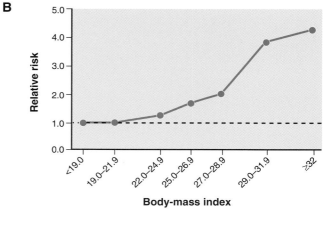

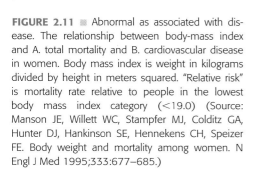

FIGURE 2.11 ▨ Abnormal as associated with disease. The relationship between body-mass index and A. total mortality and B. cardiovascular disease in women. Body mass index is weight in kilograms divided by height in meters squared. "Relative risk" is mortality rate relative to people in the lowest body mass index category (<19.0) (Source: Manson JE, Willett WC, Stampfer MJ, Colditz GA, Hunter DJ, Hankinson SE, Hennekens CH, Speizer FE. Body weight and mortality among women. N Engl J Med 1995;333:677–685.)

Abnormal = Associated with Disease

A sounder approach to distinguishing normal from abnormal is to call abnormal those observations that are clinically meaningful departures from good health—that is, associated with the risk of having or developing disease, disability, or death.

▨ E X A M P L E

At what point does higher than average weight for height become a health problem? Figure 2.11A shows the relationship between body mass index (BMI, weight in kilograms divided by height in meters squared) and the risk of death from all causes in women who never smoked. (6) The risk is about the same over a broad range of BMIs, and only at a BMI of 29 does the risk begin to rise. However, risk for cardiovascular disease begins to rise at lower BMIs (Figure 2.11B), illustrating that the cutoff point between normal and abnormal also depends on the disease in question.

Abnormal = Treatable

For some conditions, particularly those that are not troublesome in their own right (asymptomatic), it is better to consider a measurement abnormal only if treatment at that level leads to a better outcome. This is because not every condition that is associated with an increased risk can be successfully treated: the removal of the condition may not remove risk, either because the condition itself is not a cause of disease but is only related to a cause or because irreversible damage has already occurred. Also, to label people abnormal can cause worry and a sense of vulnerability that are not justified if treatment cannot improve the outlook.

What is considered treatable changes with time. At their best, therapeutic decisions are grounded on evidence from well-conducted clinical trials (Chapter 8). As new knowledge is acquired from the results of clinical trials, the level at which treatment is considered useful may change.

Folic acid, a vitamin that occurs mainly in green leafy vegetables, was discovered early in the last century. Diets low in folic acid were found to cause a vitamin deficiency syndrome mainly characterized by anemia. For many years, adequate intake of folic acid was defined in the "recommended dietary allowance" as the amount necessary to prevent anemia. Recently, however, reasons for a new and higher level of "normal" intake have emerged. Folic acid intake by women early in pregnancy, at levels lower than in many women but well above those needed to prevent anemia, have been linked to neural tube defects in their offspring. Folic acid supplementation in high-risk women prevented about three quarters of these malformations. Thus, a new level for "normal" folic acid intake has emerged because of new information about the levels needed to prevent disease. The optimal level is at least two times (and some suggest eight times) higher than the older criterion for normal intake. As a practical matter, these levels of intake are feasible in most people only by vitamin supplements, not by diet alone.

REGRESSION TO THE MEAN

When clinicians encounter an unexpectedly abnormal test result, they tend to repeat the test. Often, the second test result is closer to normal. Why does this happen? Should it be reassuring?

Patients selected because they represent an extreme value in a distribution can be expected, on the aver-

age, to have less extreme values on subsequent measurements. This phenomenon, called **regression to the mean,** occurs for purely statistical reasons, not because the patients have necessarily improved.

Regression to the mean arises in the following way (see Figure 2.12): People are selected for inclusion in a study or for further diagnosis or treatment because their initial measurement for a trait falls beyond an arbitrarily selected cutoff point in the tail of a distribution of values for all the patients examined. Some of these people will remain above the cutoff point on subsequent measurements, because their true values are usually higher than average. But others who were found to have values above the cutoff point during the initial screening usually have lower values. They were selected only because they happened, through random variation, to have a high value at the time they were first measured. When the measurement is made again, these people have lower values than they had during the first screening. This phenomenon tends to drag down the mean value of the subgroup originally found to have values above the cutoff point.

Thus, patients who are singled out from others because of a laboratory test result that is unusually high or low can be expected, on average, to be closer to the center of the distribution if the test is repeated. Moreover, subsequent values are likely to be more accurate estimates of the true value, which could be obtained if measurements were repeated for

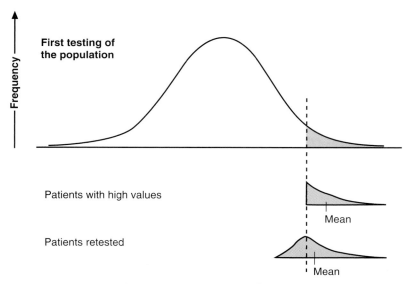

FIGURE 2.12 ■ Regression to the mean

a particular patient many times. So the time-honored practice of repeating laboratory tests that are found to be abnormal and of considering the second one the correct result is not merely wishful thinking. It has a sound theoretical basis. It also has an empirical basis. For example, it has been shown that half of serum T_4 tests found to be outside normal limits on screening were within normal limits when repeated. (7) However, the more extreme the initial reading is, the less likely it is to be normal when repeated.

REVIEW QUESTIONS

For each of the numbered clinical scenarios below (2.1–2.5), select from the lettered options the most appropriate term for the type of data. Each option can be used once, more than once, or not at all.

2.1. Deep tendon reflex grade 0 (no response), 1+ (somewhat diminished), 2+ (normal), 3+ (brisker than average), and 4+ (very brisk).

   A. Interval—Continuous
   B. Dichotomous
   C. Nominal
   D. Ordinal
   E. Interval—Discrete

2.2. Cancer recurrent/not recurrent 5 years after initial treatment.

2.3. Serum sodium 139 mg/dL.

2.4. Three seizures per month.

2.5. Causes of upper gastrointestinal bleeding: duodenal ulcer, gastritis, esophageal or other varices

2.6. When it is not possible to verify measurement of a phenomenon, such as itching, by the physical senses, which of the following can be said of its validity?

   A. It is questionable, and one should rely on "hard" measures such as laboratory tests
   B. It can be established by showing that the same value is obtained when the measurement is repeated by many different observers at different times

   C. It can be supported by showing that the measurement is related to other measures of phenomena such as the presence of diseases that are known to cause itching
   D. It can be established by showing that measurement results in a broad range of values
   E. It cannot be established

2.7. A physician or nurse measures a patient's heart rate by feeling the pulse for 10 seconds each time she comes to clinic. The rates might differ from visit to visit because of all the following except:

   A. The patient has a different pulse rate at different times
   B. The measurement may misrepresent the true pulse by chance because of the brief period of observation
   C. The physician and nurse use different techniques (e.g., pressure on the pulse)
   D. The pulse rate varies among patients
   E. An effective treatment was begun between visits.

2.8. "Abnormal" is commonly defined by all of the following except:

   A. The level at which treatment has been shown to be effective
   B. The level at which death rate is increased
   C. Statistically unusual values
   D. Values that do not correspond to a normal distribution
   E. The level at which there is an increased risk of symptoms

Read the following statements and mark each one as True or False.

_____ **2.9.** The normal distribution describes the distribution of most naturally-occurring phenomena

_____ **2.10.** The normal distribution includes 2.5% of people in each tail of the distribution (beyond 2 standard deviations from the mean)

_____ **2.11.** The normal distribution is unimodal and symmetrical

_____ **2.12.** The normal distribution is the best basis for defining abnormal

Read the following scenario and mark each of the statements that follow it as True or False.

A patient is found to have a single serum cholesterol above 200 mg/dL, which is in the 65th percentile for adults in the United States and above a widely-accepted threshold for considering drug treatment.

_____ **2.13.** This patient is likely to have a lower serum cholesterol the next time it is measured

_____ **2.14.** This patient may have been above the threshold by chance

_____ **2.15.** The patient should be treated based on the observation that her cholesterol is higher than her peers.

Answers are in Appendix A.

REFERENCES

1. Feinstein AR. The need for humanized science in evaluating medication. Lancet 1972;2:421–423.
2. Day E, Maddern L, Wood C. Auscultation of foetal heart rate: an assessment of its error and significance. Br Med J 1968;4:422–424.
3. Morganroth J, Michelson EL, Horowitz LN, Josephson ME, et al. Limitations of routine long-term electrocardiographic monitoring to assess ventricular ectopic frequency. Circulation 1978;58:408–414.
4. Elveback LR, Guillier CL, Keating FR. Health, normality, and the ghost of Gauss. JAMA 1970;211:69–75.
5. Prospective Studies Collaboration. Age-specific relevance of usual blood pressure to vascular mortality: A meta-analysis of individual data for one million adults in 61 prospective studies. Lancet 2002;360:1903–13.
6. Manson JE, Willett WC, Stampfer MJ, Colditz GA, Hunter DJ, Hankinson SE, Hennekens CH, Speizer FE. Body weight and mortality among women. N Engl J Med 1995;333:677–685.
7. Epstein KA, Schneiderman LJ, Bush JW, Zettner A. The "abnormal" screening serum thyroxine (T4): Analysis of physician response, outcome, cost, and health and effectiveness. J Chron Dis 1981;34:175–190.

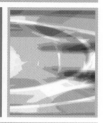

Diagnosis

Diagnostic test
True positive
True negative
False positive
False negative
Gold standard
Criterion standard
Reference standard
Sensitivity
Specificity

Cutoff point
Receiver Operator
   Characteristic (ROC) curve
Positive predictive value
Negative predictive value
Posterior (posttest)
   probability
Accuracy
Prevalence
Prior (pretest) probability

Likelihood ratio
Probability
Odds
Pretest odds
Posttest odds
Parallel testing
Serial testing
Clinical prediction rules
Diagnostic decision-making
   rules

> *Appearances to the mind are of four kinds. Things either are what they appear to be; or they neither are, nor appear to be; or they are, and do not appear to be; or they are not, yet appear to be. Rightly to aim in all these cases is the wise man's task.*
>
> — *Epictetus, 2nd century* A.D.

Doctors spend a great deal of time diagnosing complaints or abnormalities in their patients, generally arriving at a diagnosis after applying various diagnostic tests. Clinicians should be familiar with basic principles when interpreting diagnostic tests. This chapter deals with those principles.

A **diagnostic test** is ordinarily understood to mean a test performed in a laboratory, but the principles discussed in this chapter apply equally well to clinical information obtained from history, physical examination, and imaging procedures. They also apply when a constellation of findings serves as a diagnostic test. Thus, one might speak of the value of prodromal neurologic symptoms, headache, nausea, and vomiting in diagnosing classic migraine; or of hemoptysis and weight loss in a cigarette smoker as indicators of lung cancer.

SIMPLIFYING DATA

In Chapter 2 (Abnormality), we pointed out that clinical measurements, including data from diagnostic tests, are expressed on nominal, ordinal, or interval scales. Regardless of the kind of data produced by diagnostic tests, clinicians generally reduce the data to a simpler form to make them useful in practice. Most ordinal scales are examples of this simplification process. Heart murmurs can vary from very loud to inaudible, but trying to express subtle gradations in the intensity of murmurs is unnecessary for clinical decision making. A simple ordinal scale—grades I to VI—serves just as well. More often, complex data are reduced to a simple dichotomy (for example, present/absent, abnormal/normal, or diseased/well). This is done particularly when test results are used to help determine treatment decisions. For any given test result, therapeutic decisions are either/or decisions; either treatment is begun or it is withheld.

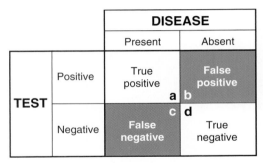

FIGURE 3.1 ■ The relationship between a diagnostic test result and the occurrence of disease. There are two possibilities for the test result to be correct (true positive and true negative) and two possibilities for the result to be incorrect (false positive and false negative).

> ### EXAMPLE
>
> The use of blood pressure data to decide about therapy is an example of how information can be simplified for practical clinical purposes. Blood pressure is ordinarily measured to the nearest 1 mm Hg, i.e., on an interval scale. However, most hypertension treatment guidelines, such as those of the Joint National Committee on the Detection, Evaluation, and Treatment of Hypertension (1), choose a particular level (e.g., 140 mm Hg systolic pressure or 90 mm Hg diastolic pressure) at which to initiate drug treatment. In doing so, they have transformed interval data into dichotomous data. To take the example further which turns the data into an ordinal scale, the Joint National Committee also recommends that physicians choose a treatment plan according to whether the patient's blood pressure is "prehypertension" (systolic 120–139 mm Hg or diastolic 80–89 mm Hg), "Stage 1 hypertension" (systolic 140–159 mm Hg or diastolic 90–99 mm Hg), or "Stage 2 hypertension" (systolic ≥160 mm Hg or diastolic ≥ 100 mm Hg).

between the properties of diagnostic tests and the information they yield in various clinical situations. In many instances, understanding these issues will help the clinician reduce diagnostic uncertainty. In other situations, it may only increase understanding of the degree of uncertainty. Occasionally, it may even convince the clinician to increase his or her level of uncertainty.

A simple way of looking at the relationships between a test's results and the true diagnosis is shown in Figure 3.1. The test is considered to be either positive (abnormal) or negative (normal), and the disease is either present or absent. There are then four possible types of test results, two of which are correct (true) and two, wrong (false). The test has given the correct result when it is positive in the presence of disease (**true positive**) or negative in the absence of the disease (**true negative**). On the other hand, the test has been misleading if it is positive when the disease is absent (**false positive**) or negative when the disease is present (**false negative**).

THE ACCURACY OF A TEST RESULT

Establishing diagnoses is an imperfect process, resulting in a probability rather than a certainty of being right. The doctor's certainty or uncertainty about a diagnosis has been expressed by using terms such as *"rule out"* or *"possible"* before a clinical diagnosis. Increasingly, clinicians express the likelihood that a patient has a disease as a probability. That being the case, it behooves the clinician to become familiar with the mathematical relationships

The Gold Standard

A test's accuracy is considered in relation to some way of knowing whether the disease is truly present or not—a sounder indication of the truth often referred to as the **gold standard** (or **criterion standard** or **reference standard**). Sometimes the standard of accuracy is itself a relatively simple and inexpensive test, such as a throat culture for group A streptococcus to validate the clinical impression of strep throat or an antibody test for human immunodeficiency virus infection. More often, one must turn to relatively elaborate, expensive, or risky tests to be certain whether the disease is present or absent. Among these are biopsy, surgical exploration, radiologic procedures, and of course, autopsy.

For diseases that are not self-limited and ordinarily become overt in a matter of a few years after they are first suspected, the results of follow-up can serve as a gold standard. Screening for most cancers and chronic, degenerative diseases fall into this category. For them, validation is possible even if on-the-spot confirmation of a test's performance is not feasible because the immediately available gold standard is too risky, involved, or expensive. If follow-up is used, the length of the follow-up period must be long enough for the disease to declare itself but not so long that new cases can arise after the original testing.

Because it is almost always more costly, more dangerous, or both to use more accurate ways of establishing the truth, clinicians and patients prefer simpler tests to the rigorous gold standard, at least initially. Chest x-rays and sputum smears are used to determine the cause of pneumonia, rather than lung biopsy with examination of the diseased lung tissue. Electrocardiograms and blood tests are first used to establish the diagnosis of acute myocardial infarction, rather than catheterization or imaging procedures. The simpler tests are used as proxies for more elaborate but more accurate ways of establishing the presence of disease, with the understanding that some risk of misclassification results. This risk is justified by the safety and convenience of the simpler tests. But simpler tests are only useful when the risks of misclassification are known and found to be acceptably low. This requires a sound comparison of their accuracy to an appropriate standard.

Lack of Information on Negative Tests

The goal of all clinical studies aimed at describing the value of diagnostic tests should be to obtain data for all four of the cells shown in Figure 3.1. Without all these data, it is not possible to fully evaluate the accuracy of the test. Most information about the value of a diagnostic test is obtained from clinical, and not research, settings. Under these circumstances, physicians are using the test in the care of patients. Because of ethical concerns, they do not feel justified in proceeding with more exhaustive evaluation when preliminary diagnostic tests are negative. They are naturally reluctant to initiate an aggressive workup,

with its associated risk and expense, unless preliminary tests are positive. As a result, data on the number of true negatives versus false negatives generated by a test (cells c and d in Figure 3.1) tend to be much less complete in the medical literature than data collected about positive test results.

This problem can arise in studies of screening tests because individuals with negative tests usually are not subjected to further testing, especially if the testing involves invasive procedures such as biopsies. One investigation of prostate-specific antigen (PSA) testing for prostate cancer got around the problem by examining stored blood from men who subsequently developed prostate cancer and men who did not develop prostate cancer. (2) The results showed that for a PSA level of 4.0 ng/ml, sensitivity over the subsequent 4 years was 73% and specificity was 91%. The investigators were able to fill in all 4 cells without requiring further testing on people with negative test results. (See below for sensitivity and specificity.)

Lack of Information on Test Results in the Nondiseased

A related problem is that evaluation of a test's performance can be grossly misleading if the test is applied only to patients with the condition or complaint. Test results are also needed for patients thought not to have the condition.

EXAMPLE

Magnetic resonance imaging (MRI) of the lumbar spine is used in the evaluation of patients with low back pain. Many patients with back pain show herniated intervertebral disks on MRI, and the pain is often attributed to the finding. But, how often are herniated disks found in people who do not have back pain? MRIs were performed on 98 asymptomatic volunteers. (3) Radiologists who did not know the symptom status of the patients read the MRIs. Bulging or protruding disks were found in nearly two-thirds of the asymptomatic volunteers, only slightly lower than the frequency of similar abnormality in patients with back pain. The authors concluded that such findings "may frequently be coincidental."

Lack of Objective Standards for Disease

For some conditions, there are simply no hard-and-fast criteria for diagnosis. Angina pectoris is one of these. The clinical manifestations were described nearly a century ago, yet there is still no better way to substantiate the presence of angina pectoris than a carefully taken history. Certainly, a great many objectively measurable phenomena are related to this clinical syndrome, for example, the presence of coronary artery stenosis on angiography, delayed perfusion on a thallium stress test, and characteristic abnormalities on electrocardiograms both at rest and with exercise. All are more commonly found in patients believed to have angina pectoris. But none is so closely tied to the clinical syndrome that it can serve as the standard by which the condition is considered present or absent.

Other examples of medical conditions difficult to diagnose because of the lack of simple gold standard tests include hot flashes, Raynaud's disease, irritable bowel syndrome, and autism. In an effort to standardize practice, expert groups often develop lists of symptoms and other test results that can be used in combination to diagnose the clinical condition. Because there is no gold standard, however, it is possible that these lists are not entirely correct. Circular reasoning should also be avoided, wherein the validity of a laboratory test is established by comparing its results to a clinical diagnosis based on a careful history of symptoms and a physical examination but once established, the test is then used to validate the clinical diagnosis gained from history and physical examination!

Consequences of Imperfect Standards

Because of such difficulties, it is sometimes not possible for physicians in practice to find information on how well the tests they use compare with a thoroughly trustworthy standard. They must choose as their standard of validity another test that admittedly is imperfect, but is considered the best available. This may force them into comparing one imperfect test against another, with one being taken as a standard of validity because it has had longer use or is considered superior by a consensus of experts. In doing so, a paradox may arise. If a new test is compared with an old (but imperfect) standard test, the new test may seem worse even though it is actually better. For example, if the new test were more sensitive than the standard test, the additional patients identified by the new test would be considered false positives in relation to the old test. Similarly, if the new test is more often negative in patients who

really do not have the disease, results for those patients would be considered false negatives compared with the old test. Thus, a new test can perform no better than an established gold standard test, and it will seem inferior when it approximates the truth more closely unless special strategies are used.

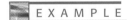

E X A M P L E

Computed tomographic ("virtual") colonoscopy was compared to traditional (optical) colonoscopy in screening for colon cancer. (4) Both tests were performed on every patient without the clinician interpreting each test knowing the results of the other test. Traditional colonoscopy is usually considered the gold standard for identifying colon cancer or polyps in asymptomatic adults. However, virtual colonoscopy identified a colon cancer missed by the traditional colonoscopy. In order not to penalize the new test in comparison to the old, the investigators ingeniously created a new gold standard—a repeat optical colonoscopy after reviewing the results of both testing procedures—whenever there was disagreement between the tests.

SENSITIVITY AND SPECIFICITY

Figure 3.2 summarizes some relationships between a diagnostic test and the actual presence of disease. It is an expansion of Figure 3.1, with the addition of some useful definitions. Most of the rest of this chapter deals with these relationships in detail.

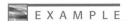

E X A M P L E

Figure 3.3 illustrates these relationships with an actual study. (5) Deep venous thrombosis in the lower extremities (DVT) is a serious condition that can lead to pulmonary embolism; patients with DVT should receive anticoagulation. However, because anticoagulation is not without risks, it is important to differentiate between patients with and without DVT. Compression ultrasonography is highly sensitive and specific for proximal thrombosis and has been used to confirm or rule out DVT. However, compression ultrasonography is expensive and dependent on highly trained personnel, so a search for a simpler diagnostic test was undertaken. Markers of endogenous fibrinolysis, D-dimer assays, were developed as blood tests and evaluated in DVT diagnosis. Figure 3.3 shows the performance of a D-dimer assay in the diagnosis of DVT. The gold standard in the study was the result of compression ultrasonography, and/or a 3-month follow-up.

		DISEASE	
		Present	Absent
TEST	Positive	**a**	**b**
	Negative	**c**	**d**

$$+PV = \frac{a}{a+b}$$

$$-PV = \frac{d}{c+d}$$

$$Se = \frac{a}{a+c} \qquad Sp = \frac{d}{b+d} \qquad P = \frac{a+c}{a+b+c+d}$$

FIGURE 3.2 ■ Diagnostic test characteristics and definitions. Se = sensitivity; Sp = specificity; P = prevalence; PV = predictive value; LR = likelihood ratio. Note that LR+ calculations are the same as Se/(1-Sp) and calculations for LR- are the same as (1-Se)/Sp.

$$LR+ = \frac{\dfrac{a}{a+c}}{\dfrac{b}{b+d}} \qquad LR- = \frac{\dfrac{c}{a+c}}{\dfrac{d}{b+d}}$$

		DISEASE DVT according to gold standard (Compression ultrasonography and/or 3 month follow up)	
		Present	Absent
TEST D-dimer assay for diagnosis of DVT	Positive	**34**	**168**
	Negative	**1**	**282**

$$+PV = \frac{34}{202} = 17\%$$

$$-PV = \frac{282}{283} = 100\%$$

$$Se = \frac{34}{35} = 97\% \quad Sp = \frac{282}{450} = 63\% \quad P = \frac{35}{485} = 7\%$$

FIGURE 3.3 ■ Diagnostic characteristics of a D-dimer assay in diagnosing deep venous thrombosis (DVT). (Source: Bates SM, Kearon C, Crowther M, Linkins L, O'Donnell M, Douketis J, et al. A diagnostic strategy involving a quantitative latex D-dimer assay reliably excludes deep venous thrombosis. Ann Intern Med 2003;138:787–794.)

$$LR+ = \frac{\dfrac{34}{34+1}}{\dfrac{168}{168+282}} = 2.6 \qquad LR- = \frac{\dfrac{1}{1+34}}{\dfrac{282}{282+168}} = 0.05$$

Se = Sensitivity
Sp = Specificity
PV = Predictive value
LR = Likelihood ratio
P = Prevalence

Definitions

As can be seen in Figure 3.2, **sensitivity** is defined as the proportion of people with the disease who have a positive test for the disease. A sensitive test will rarely miss people with the disease. **Specificity** is the proportion of people without the disease who have a negative test. A specific test will rarely misclassify people as having the disease when they do not.

Applying these definitions to the DVT example (Figure 3.3), we see that 34 of the 35 patients with DVT had positive D-dimer results—for a sensitivity of 97%. On the other hand, of the 450 patients who did not have DVT, D-dimer results were correctly negative for only 282, for a specificity of 63%.

Use of Sensitive Tests

Clinicians should take the sensitivity and specificity of a diagnostic test into account when a test is selected. A sensitive test (i.e., one that is usually positive in the presence of disease) should be chosen when there is an important penalty for missing a disease. This would be so, for example, when there is reason to suspect a dangerous but treatable condition, such as tuberculosis, syphilis, or Hodgkin's disease, or in a patient suspected of having DVT. Sensitive tests are also helpful during the early stages of a diagnostic workup, when a great many possibilities are being considered, to reduce the number of possibilities. Diagnostic tests are used in these situations to rule out diseases with a negative result of a highly sensitive test (as in the DVT example). In another example, one might choose the highly sensitive HIV antibody test early in the evaluation of lung infiltrates and weight loss to rule out an AIDS-related infection in certain patients. In sum, a highly sensitive test is most helpful to the clinician when the test result is negative.

Use of Specific Tests

Specific tests are useful to confirm (or "rule in") a diagnosis that has been suggested by other data. This is because a highly specific test is rarely positive in the absence of disease; it gives few false-positive results. (Note that in the DVT example, the D-dimer test was not specific enough [63%] to initiate treatment after a positive test. All patients with positive results underwent compression ultrasonography, a much more specific test.) Highly specific tests are particularly needed when false-positive

results can harm the patient physically, emotionally, or financially. Thus, before patients are subjected to cancer chemotherapy (with all its attendant risks, emotional trauma, and financial costs) tissue diagnosis (a highly specific test) is generally required. In sum, a highly specific test is most helpful when the test result is positive.

Trade-Offs Between Sensitivity and Specificity

It is obviously desirable to have a test that is both highly sensitive and highly specific. Unfortunately, this is usually not possible. Instead, there is a trade-off between the sensitivity and specificity of a diagnostic test. This is true whenever clinical data take on a range of values. In those situations, the location of a **cutoff point**, the point on the continuum between normal and abnormal, is an arbitrary decision. As a consequence, for any given test result expressed on a continuous scale, one characteristic, such as sensitivity, can be increased only at the expense of the other (e.g., specificity). Table 3.1 demonstrates this interrelationship for prostate-specific antigen (PSA) levels in screening African American men in their 70s for prostate cancer. (6) If the cutoff level of the test were set too low (3.0 ng per milliliter and above), sensitivity is high (100%), but the trade-off is low specificity (60%), which would require many men without prostate cancer to undergo further testing. On the other hand, if the cutoff level were set too high, more men with prostate cancer would be missed. The authors suggested that an acceptable compromise would be a cutoff level of 5.5 ng per milliliter, with a sensitivity of 95% and a specificity of 78%. There is no way, using a PSA test alone, that one can improve both the sensitivity and specificity of the test at the same time.

The ROC Curve

Another way to express the relationship between sensitivity and specificity for a given test is to construct a curve, called a **receiver operator characteristic (ROC) curve.** An ROC curve for the PSA levels in Table 3.1 is illustrated in Figure 3.4. It is constructed by plotting the true-positive rate (sensitivity) against the false-positive rate (1-specificity) over a range of cutoff values. The values on the axes run from a probability of 0 to 1.0 (or, alternatively, from 0 to 100%). Figure 3.4 illustrates visually the trade-off between sensitivity and specificity.

TABLE 3.1 ■ Trade-Off Between Sensitivity and Specificity When Using PSA Levels to Detect Prostate Cancer in Black Men Ages 70–79

PSA Level (ng/ml)	Sensitivity	Specificity
1.0	100	21
2.0	100	48
3.0	100	60
4.0	99	73
5.0	96	76
6.0	94	79
7.0	90	83
8.0	90	88
9.0	68	90
10.0	54	93
11.0	47	94
12.0	30	95
13.0	23	96
14.0	17	97
15.0	11	97

Source: Morgan TO, Jacobsen SJ, McCarthy WF, Jacobson DJ, McLeod DG, Moul JW. Age-specific reference ranges for serum prostate-specific antigen in black men. N Eng J Med 1996;335:304–310.

Tests that discriminate well crowd toward the upper left corner of the ROC curve; for them, as the sensitivity is progressively increased (the cutoff point is lowered) there is little or no loss in specificity until very high levels of sensitivity are achieved. Tests that perform less well have curves that fall closer to the diagonal running from lower left to upper right. The diagonal shows the relationship between true-positive and false-positive rates that would occur for a test yielding no information—as if the clinician merely flipped a coin, for example.

The ROC curve shows how severe the trade-off between sensitivity and specificity is for a test and can be used to help decide where the best cutoff point should be. Generally, the best cutoff point is at or near the "shoulder" of the ROC curve, unless there are clinical reasons for minimizing either false negatives or false positives.

ROC curves are particularly valuable ways of comparing alternative tests for the same diagnosis. The overall accuracy of a test can be described as the area under the ROC curve; the larger the area, the better the test. Figure 3.5 compares the ROC curves for two questionnaires used to screen for alcoholism in elderly patients. These are the CAGE and the

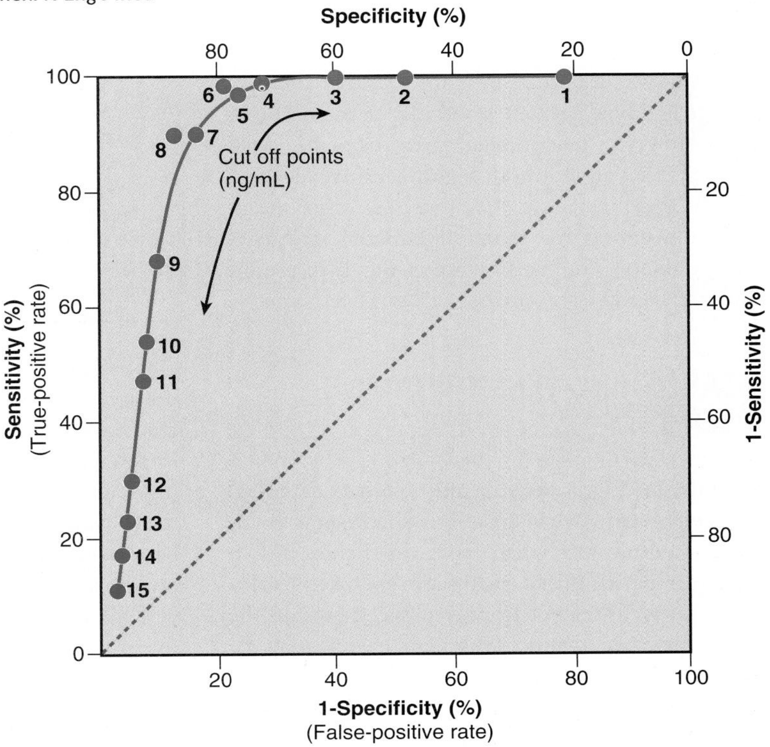

FIGURE 3.4 ■ A receiver operator characteristic (ROC) curve. The accuracy of prostate-specific antigen (PSA) in screening for prostate cancer according to cut-off points between normal and abnormal. (Source: Morgan TO, Jacobsen SJ, McCarthy WF, Jacobson DJ, McLeod DG, Moul JW. Age-specific reference ranges for serum prostate-specific antigen in black men. N Eng J Med 1996;335:304–310.)

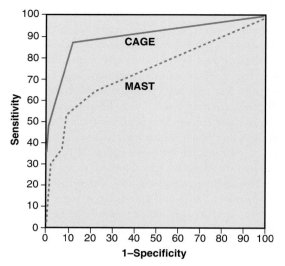

FIGURE 3.5 ■ ROC curves for the CAGE and MAST questionnaires in elderly patients with and without alcoholism. CAGE is more sensitive and more specific than MAST, resulting in more area under the curve. (Redrawn from Jones TV, Lindsey BA, Yount P, Soltys R, Farani-Enayat B. Alcoholism screening questionnaires: Are they valid in elderly medical outpatients? J Gen Intern Med 1993;8:674–678.)

MAST (Michigan Alcoholism Screening Test). (7) The CAGE is both more sensitive and more specific than the MAST and includes a much larger area under its curve.

Obviously, tests that are both sensitive and specific are highly sought after and can be of enormous value. However, practitioners must frequently work with tests that are not both highly sensitive and specific. In these instances, they must use other means of circumventing the trade-off between sensitivity and specificity. The most common way is to use the results of several tests together, as discussed below.

ESTABLISHING SENSITIVITY AND SPECIFICITY

Not infrequently, a new diagnostic test is described in glowing terms when first introduced, only to be found wanting later when more experience with it has accumulated. Initial enthusiasm followed by disappointment arises not from any dishonesty on the part of early investigators or unfair skepticism by the medical community later. Rather, it is related to limitations in the methods by which the properties of the test were established in the first place. At the

crudest level, sensitivity and specificity may be inaccurately described because an improper gold standard has been chosen, as discussed earlier in this chapter. However, two other issues related to the selection of diseased and nondiseased patients can profoundly affect the determination of sensitivity and specificity as well. They are the *spectrum* of patients to which the test is applied and *bias* in judging the test's performance. Statistical uncertainty, related to studying a relatively small number of patients, also can lead to inaccurate estimates of sensitivity and specificity.

Spectrum of Patients

Difficulties may arise when the patients used to describe the test's properties are somehow different from those to whom the test will be applied in clinical practice. Early reports often assess the test's value among people who are clearly diseased compared with people who are clearly not diseased, such as medical student volunteers for example. The test may be able to distinguish between these extremes very well, but perform more poorly when differences are subtler. Also, patients with disease often differ in severity, stage, or duration of the disease, and a test's sensitivity will tend to be higher in more severely affected patients.

EXAMPLE

Figure 3.6 illustrates how the performance of carcinoembryonic antigen (CEA) in diagnosing colorectal cancer varies with the stage of the tumor. CEA performs well for metastatic disease and poorly for localized cancer. Thus, the sensitivity for "colorectal cancer" depends on the particular mix of stages of patients with disease used to describe the test. (8)

Similarly, some kinds of people without a given disease, such as those in whom disease is suspected, may have other conditions that cause a positive test, thereby increasing the false-positive rate and decreasing specificity. For example, CEA is also elevated in many patients with ulcerative colitis or cirrhosis. If patients with these diseases were included in the nondiseased group when studying the performance of CEA for diagnosing colorectal cancer, false positives would increase and the specificity of the test for cancer would fall.

In theory, the sensitivity and specificity of a test are independent of the prevalence of diseased indi-

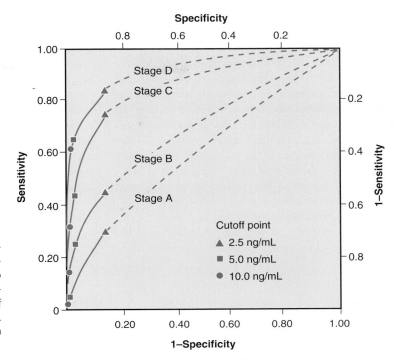

FIGURE 3.6 ▨ ROC curves for carcinoembryonic antigen (CEA) as a diagnostic test for colorectal cancer, according to stage of disease. The sensitivity and specificity of the test varies with the stage of disease. (Redrawn from Fletcher RH. Carcinoembryonic antigen. Ann Intern Med 1986;104:66–73.)

viduals in the sample in which the test is being evaluated. (Work with Figure 3.2 to confirm this for yourself.) In practice, however, several characteristics of patients, such as stage and severity of disease, may be related both to the sensitivity and specificity of a test and to the prevalence, because different kinds of patients are found in high- and low-prevalence situations. Using a test to screen for disease illustrates this point. Screening involves the use of the test in an asymptomatic population in which the prevalence of the disease is generally low and the spectrum of disease favors earlier and less severe cases (see Chapter 9 for a more detailed discussion of screening). In such situations, sensitivity tends to be lower and specificity higher than when the same test is applied to patients suspected of having the disease, more of whom have advanced disease.

E X A M P L E

A study was made of the sensitivity and specificity of the clinical breast examination in about 750,000 women. (9) When the clinical breast examination was used as a *diagnostic* test on women with breast complaints, the sensitivity and specificity for breast cancer were 85% and 73%, respectively. However, when the examination was used as a *screening* test on women who had no breast symptoms, sensitivity fell to 36% and specificity rose to 96%.

Bias

The sensitivity and specificity of a test should be established independently of the means by which the true diagnosis is established. Otherwise, there could be a biased assessment of the test's properties. This can occur in several ways. As already pointed out, if the test is evaluated using data obtained during the course of a clinical evaluation of patients suspected of having the disease in question, a positive test may prompt the clinician to continue pursuing the diagnosis, increasing the likelihood that the disease will be found. On the other hand, a negative test may cause the clinician to abandon further testing, making it more likely that the disease, if present, will be missed.

When the sensitivity and specificity of a test is being assessed, the test result should not be part of the information used to establish the diagnosis. In the original study of deep venous thrombosis diagnosis by D-dimer assay, the investigators made sure that the physicians performing the gold standard tests were unaware of the results of the D-dimer assays so that the results would not influence their interpretations of the gold standard tests. (10)

In the course of routine clinical care, this kind of bias can be used to advantage if recognized. Sometimes, the test is interpreted while taking other clinical information into account, especially if the test result is subjectively interpreted. Many x-ray interpretations are subjective, and it is easy to be influenced by the clinical information provided. All clinicians have experienced having x-rays over-read because of a clinical impression, or conversely, of going back over old x-rays in which a finding was missed because a clinical fact was not communicated at the time, and therefore, attention was not directed to the particular area in the x-ray. Both to minimize and to take advantage of these biases, some radiologists prefer to read x-rays twice, first without, then with the clinical information.

All the biases discussed tend to increase the agreement between the test and the gold standard. That is, they tend to make the test seem more useful than it actually is.

values, typically characterized by the "95% confidence intervals" (see Chapter 10).[1] The width of this range of values defines the degree of precision of the estimates of sensitivity and specificity. Therefore, reported values for sensitivity and specificity should not be taken too literally if a small number of patients is studied.

Figure 3.7 shows how the precision of estimates of sensitivity increases as the number of people on which the estimate is based increases. In this particular example, the observed sensitivity of the diagnostic test is 75%. Figure 3.7 shows that if this estimate is based on only 10 patients, by chance alone the true sensitivity could be as low as 45% and as high as nearly 100%. When more patients are studied, the 95% confidence interval narrows and the precision of the estimate increases.

Chance

Values for sensitivity and specificity are usually estimated from observations on relatively small samples of people with and without the disease of interest. Because of chance (random variation) in any one sample, particularly if it is small, the true sensitivity and specificity of the test can be misrepresented, even if there is no bias in the study. The particular values observed are compatible with a range of true

---

[1]The 95% confidence interval of a proportion is easily estimated by the following formula, based on the binomial theorem:

$$p \pm 2 \sqrt{\frac{p(1-p)}{N}}$$

where p is the observed proportion and N is the number of people observed. To be more nearly exact, multiply by 1.96.

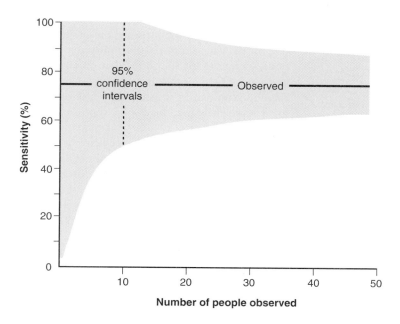

FIGURE 3.7 ■ The precision of an estimate of sensitivity. The 95% confidence interval for an observed sensitivity of 75%, according to the number of people observed.

PREDICTIVE VALUE

Sensitivity and specificity are properties of a test that should be taken into account when deciding whether or not to use the test. However, once the results of a diagnostic test are available, whether positive or negative, the sensitivity and specificity of the test are no longer relevant because these values are obtained in persons known to have or not to have the disease. But if one knew the disease status of the patient, it would not be necessary to order the test! For the clinician, the dilemma is to determine whether or not the patient has the disease, given the results of a test. (In fact, clinicians are usually more concerned with this question than the sensitivity and specificity of the test.)

Definitions

The probability of disease, given the results of a test, is called the *predictive value* of the test (see Figure 3.2). **Positive predictive value** is the probability of disease in a patient with a positive (abnormal) test result. **Negative predictive value** is the probability of *not* having the disease when the test result is negative (normal). Predictive value answers the question, "If my patient's test result is positive (negative), what are the chances that my patient does (does not) have the disease?" Predictive value is sometimes called **posterior (or posttest) probability**, the probability of disease *after* the test result is known. Figure 3.3 illustrates these concepts. Of the 202 patients with positive D-dimer assays, only 17% had DVT (positive predictive value). The negative predictive value of the test was much better, almost 100%.

The term **accuracy** is sometimes used to summarize the overall value of a test. Accuracy is the proportion of all test results, both positive and negative, that are correct. For the DVT example in Figure 3.3, the accuracy of D-dimer assays was 65%. (Calculate this for yourself.) The area under the ROC curve is another useful summary measure of the information provided by a test result. However, these summary measures usually are too crude to be useful clinically because specific information about the component parts—sensitivity, specificity, and predictive value at specific cutoff points—is lost when they are aggregated into a single number.

Determinants of Predictive Value

The predictive value of a test is not a property of the test alone. It is determined by the sensitivity and specificity of the test and the prevalence of disease in the population being tested, when **prevalence** has its customary meaning, the proportion of persons in a defined population at a given point in time having the condition in question. Prevalence is also called **prior (or pretest) probability**, the probability of disease before the test result is known. (For a full discussion of prevalence, see Chapter 4.)

The mathematical formula relating sensitivity, specificity, and prevalence to positive predictive value is derived from Bayes's theorem of conditional probabilities:

$$\text{Positive predictive value} = \frac{\text{Sensitivity} \times \text{Prevalence}}{(\text{Sensitivity} \times \text{Prevalence}) + (1\text{-Specificity}) \times (1\text{-Prevalence})}$$

The more sensitive a test is, the better will be its negative predictive value (the more confident the clinician can be that a negative test result rules out the disease being sought). Conversely, the more specific the test is, the better will be its positive predictive value (the more confident the clinician can be that a positive test confirms or rules in the diagnosis being sought). Because predictive value is also influenced by prevalence, it is not independent of the setting in which the test is used. Positive results, even for a very specific test, when applied to patients with a low likelihood of having the disease, will be largely false positives. Similarly, negative results, even for a very sensitive test, when applied to patients with a high chance of having the disease, are likely to be false negatives. In sum, the interpretation of a positive or negative diagnostic test result varies from setting to setting, according to the prevalence of disease in the particular setting.

It is not intuitively obvious why prevalence should affect interpretation of a test result. For those who are skeptical, it might help to consider how a test would perform at the extremes of prevalence. Remember that no matter how sensitive and specific a test might be (short of perfection), there will still be a small proportion of patients who are misclassified by it. Imagine a population in which no one has the disease. In such a group all positive results, even for a very specific test, will be false positives. Therefore, as the prevalence of disease in a population approaches zero, the positive predictive value of a test also approaches zero. Conversely, if everyone in a population tested has the disease, all negative results will be false negatives, even for a very sensitive test. As prevalence approaches 100%, negative predictive value approaches zero. Another way for the skeptic to convince himself or herself of these relationships is to work with Figure 3.2, holding sensitivity and specificity constant, changing prevalence, and calculating the resulting predictive values.

The effect of prevalence on positive predictive value, for a test at different but generally high levels of sensitivity and specificity, is illustrated in Figure 3.8. When the prevalence of disease in the population tested is relatively high—more than several percent—the test performs well. But at lower prevalences, the positive predictive value drops to nearly zero, and the test is virtually useless. As sensitivity and specificity fall, the influence of prevalence on predictive value becomes more pronounced.

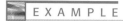
E X A M P L E

In a study of the accuracy of a D-dimer assay for diagnosing deep venous thrombosis (DVT), investigators found that among all patients with suspected DVT, the prevalence of DVT was 19% and the positive predictive value was 29%. However, among patients with suspected DVT and known to have cancer (a risk factor for DVT), the prevalence of DVT rose to 44% and the positive predictive value was 58%. These differences occurred even though the sensitivity of the D-dimer assay was almost identical in the two groups (96% and 97%), as was specificity (45% and 46%) (10).

Screening for acquired immunodeficiency syndrome (AIDS) is another example of the effect of disease prevalence on positive predictive value.

E X A M P L E

The usual screening test for HIV-1 is an enzyme immunoassay that is both highly sensitive and specific (>99%). Most expert groups making recommendations for HIV testing recommend that clinicians offer HIV testing to people at high risk (such as intravenous drug users, in whom the prevalence of HIV is about 15%). (11) When used in these groups, relatively few false positive results occur. However, prevalence of HIV in the general U.S. population is much lower, .01 − .05%. Because of this low prevalence, most positive tests would be false positive. (Calculate this for yourself.) Therefore, most expert groups recommend concentrating on high-risk groups rather than screening the general population. (An exception is that many groups suggest testing all pregnant women because treatment of sero-positive women can prevent perinatal HIV infection in newborns.)

In general, prevalence is more important than sensitivity and specificity in determining predictive value (Figure 3.8). One reason why this is so is that prevalence can vary over a much wider range than sensitivity and specificity can. Prevalence of disease can vary from a fraction of a percent to near certainty in clinical settings, depending on the age, gender, risk factors, and clinical findings of the patient. Consider the difference in prevalence of liver disease in healthy, young adults who use no drugs, are not sexually promiscuous, and consume only occasional alcohol with that of jaundiced intravenous drug users having multiple sex partners. In contrast, sensitivity and specificity of diagnostic tests vary over a much narrower range, from about 50% to 99%.

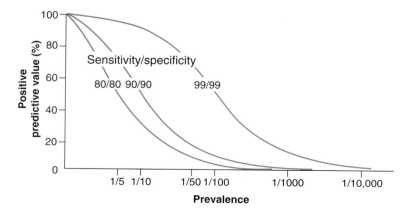

FIGURE 3.8 ■ Positive predictive value according to sensitivity, specificity, and prevalence of disease

Estimating Prevalence

Because prevalence of disease is such a powerful determinant of how useful a diagnostic test will be, clinicians must consider the probability of disease before ordering a test. But how can a doctor estimate the prevalence or probability of a particular disease in his or her patients? Until recently, clinicians relied on clinical observations and their experience to estimate the pretest probability of a disease. Studies have shown that these estimates are often inaccurate (perhaps because doctors tend to remember recent or remarkable patients and, consequently, give them too much weight when making estimates).

The medical literature is another source for estimating prevalence. In one study of patients in a Veterans' Administration hospital, investigators searched MEDLINE and found prevalence (or pretest) information for 78% of the clinical problems encountered. (12) Large clinical computer data banks also provide quantitative estimates of the probability of disease, given various combinations of clinical findings. (13) Although the resulting estimates of prevalence are not likely to be very precise, using estimates from the medical literature is bound to be more accurate than implicit judgment alone. Also, any inaccuracies are not likely to be so great as to change clinical judgments that are based on the estimates.

Increasing the Prevalence of Disease Before Testing

Considering the relationship between the predictive value of a test and prevalence, it is obviously to the physician's advantage to apply diagnostic tests to patients with an increased likelihood of having the disease being sought. In fact, as Figure 3.8 shows, diagnostic tests are most helpful when the presence of disease is neither very likely nor very unlikely.

There are several ways in which the probability of a disease can be increased before using a diagnostic test.

Referral Process

Referral to teaching hospital wards, clinics, and emergency departments increases the chance that significant disease will underlie patients' complaints. Therefore, relatively more aggressive use of diagnostic tests might be justified in these settings. In primary care practice, on the other hand, and particularly among patients without complaints, the chance of finding disease is considerably smaller, and tests should be used more sparingly.

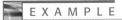

> **EXAMPLE**
>
> While practicing in a military clinic, one of us saw hundreds of people with headache, rarely ordered diagnostic tests, and never encountered a patient with a severe underlying cause of headache. (It is unlikely that important conditions were missed, because the clinic was virtually the only source of medical care for these patients, and the soldiers remained in the military community for many months.) However, during the first week back in a medical residency, a patient visiting the hospital's emergency department because of a headache similar to the ones managed in the military was found to have a cerebellar abscess!

Because clinicians may work at different extremes of the prevalence spectrum at various times in their clinical practices, they should bear in mind that the intensity of their diagnostic evaluations may need to be adjusted to suit the specific situation.

Selected Demographic Groups

In a given setting, physicians can increase the yield of diagnostic tests by applying them to demographic groups known to be at higher risk for a disease. A man of 65 is 15 times more likely to have coronary artery disease as the cause of atypical chest pain than a woman of 30; thus the electrocardiographic stress test, a diagnostic test for coronary disease, is more useful in confirming the diagnosis in the older man than in the younger woman. (14) Similarly, a sickle-cell test would obviously have a higher positive predictive value among African Americans than among whites of Norwegian descent.

Specifics of the Clinical Situation

The specifics of the clinical situation are clearly the strongest influence on the decision to order tests. Symptoms, signs, and disease risk factors all raise or lower the probability of finding a disease. For example, a woman with chest pain is more likely to have coronary disease if she has typical angina and hypertension and she smokes. As a result, an abnormal electrocardiographic stress test is more likely to represent coronary disease in such a woman than in persons with nonspecific chest pain and no coronary risk factors.

The value of applying diagnostic tests to persons more likely to have a particular illness is intuitively obvious to most doctors. Nevertheless, with the increasing availability of diagnostic tests, it is easy to adopt a less selective approach when ordering tests. However, the less selective the approach, the lower the prevalence of the disease is likely to be and the lower will be the positive predictive value of the test. The magnitude of this effect can be large.

EXAMPLE

Factors that influence the interpretation of an abnormal electrocardiographic stress test are illustrated in Figure 3.9. It shows that the positive predictive value for coronary artery disease (CAD) associated with an abnormal test can vary from 1.7% to 99.8%, depending on age, symptoms, and the degree of abnormality of the test. Thus, an exercise test in an asymptomatic, 35-year-old man showing 1 mm ST segment depression will be a false-positive test in more than 98% of cases. The same test result in a 60-year-old man with typical angina by history will be associated with coronary artery disease in more than 90% of cases. (14)

Because of this effect, physicians must interpret similar test results differently in different clinical situations. A negative stress test in an asymptomatic,

35-year-old man merely confirms the already low probability of coronary artery disease. But a positive test usually will be misleading if it is used to search for unsuspected disease, as sometimes has been done among joggers and on "executive physicals" for airline pilots and business executives. The opposite applies to the 65-year-old man with typical angina. In this case, the test may be helpful in confirming disease but not in excluding disease.

A diagnostic test is most useful in intermediate situations, in which prevalence is neither very high nor very low. For example, a 60-year-old man with atypical chest pain has a 67% chance of having coronary artery disease before stress testing (Figure 3.9); but afterward, with greater than 2.5 mm ST segment depression, he has a 99% probability of coronary artery disease.

Implications for Interpreting the Medical Literature

Published descriptions of diagnostic tests often include, in addition to sensitivity and specificity, some

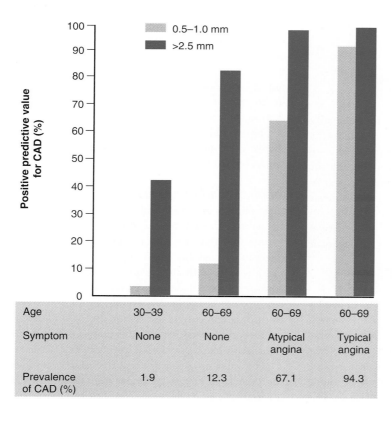

Age	30–39	60–69	60–69	60–69
Symptom	None	None	Atypical angina	Typical angina
Prevalence of CAD (%)	1.9	12.3	67.1	94.3

FIGURE 3.9 ■ Effect of disease prevalence on positive predictive value of a diagnostic test. Probability of coronary artery disease in men according to age, symptoms, and depression of ST segment on electrocardiogram. (Source: Diamond GA, Forrester JS. Analysis of probability as an aid in the clinical diagnosis of coronary artery disease. N Engl J Med 1979;300:1350–1358.)

conclusions about the interpretation of a positive or negative test (its predictive value). This is done, quite rightly, to provide information directly useful to clinicians. But the data for these publications are often gathered in university teaching hospitals where the prevalence of serious disease is relatively high. As a result, statements about predictive value in the medical literature may be misleading when the test is applied in less highly selected settings. What is worse, occasionally authors compare the performance of a test in a number of patients known to have the disease and an equal number of patients without the disease. This is an efficient way to describe sensitivity and specificity. However, any reported positive predictive value from such studies means little because it has been determined for a group of patients in which the investigators artificially set the prevalence of disease at 50%.

LIKELIHOOD RATIOS

Likelihood ratios are an alternative way of describing the performance of a diagnostic test. They summarize the same kind of information as sensitivity and specificity and can be used to calculate the probability of disease after a positive or negative test (positive or negative predictive value). An advantage of likelihood ratios is that they can be used at multiple levels of test results.

Odds

Because the use of likelihood ratios depends on odds, to understand them it is first necessary to distinguish odds from probability. **Probability**—used to express sensitivity, specificity, and predictive value—is the proportion of people in whom a particular characteristic, such as a positive test, is present. **Odds**, on the other hand, is the ratio of two probabilities, the probability of an event to that of 1—the probability of the event. Odds and probability contain the same information, but they express it differently. The two can be interconverted using simple formulas:

Odds = Probability of event ÷ (1 − Probability of event)

Probability = Odds ÷ (1 + Odds)

These terms should be familiar to most readers because they are used in everyday conversation. For example, we may say that the odds are 4:1 that the New England Patriots will win tonight or that they have an 80% probability of winning.

Definitions

The likelihood ratio for a particular value of a diagnostic test is defined as the probability of that test result in people with the disease divided by the probability of the result in people without disease (see Figure 3.2). Likelihood ratios express how many times more (or less) likely a test result is to be found in diseased, compared with nondiseased, people. If a test yields dichotomous results (both positive and negative), two types of likelihood ratios describe its ability to discriminate between diseased and nondiseased people. In the case of a test's positive likelihood ratio (LR+), it is the ratio of the proportion of diseased people with a positive test result (sensitivity) to the proportion of nondiseased people with a positive result (1–specificity). A test's negative likelihood ratio (LR-) is calculated when the test result is negative. In that case, it is the proportion of diseased people with a negative test result (1- sensitivity) divided by the proportion of nondiseased people with a negative test result (specificity) (see Figure 3.2).

In the example of deep venous thrombosis (see Figure 3.3), the data can be used to calculate likelihood ratios for DVT in the presence of a positive or negative test (D-dimer assay). A positive test is about 2.6 times more likely to be found in the presence of DVT than in the absence of it. If the D-dimer assay was negative, the likelihood ratio for this negative test is 0.05.

Use of Likelihood Ratios

Likelihood ratios must be used with odds, not probability. Therefore, the first step is to convert pretest probability (prevalence) to **pretest odds**, as outlined above:

Odds = Probability of event ÷ (1 − Probability of event)

Likelihood ratios can then be used to convert pretest odds to **posttest odds**, by means of the following formula:

Pretest odds × Likelihood ratio = Posttest odds

Posttest odds can, in turn, be converted back to a probability, using the formula:

Probability = Odds ÷ (1 + Odds)

In these relationships, pretest odds contain the same information as prior or pretest probability (prevalence), likelihood ratios the same as sensitivity/specificity, and posttest odds the same as positive predictive value (posttest probability).

Why master the concept of likelihood ratios when they are much more difficult to understand than prevalence, sensitivity, specificity and predictive value? The main advantage of likelihood ratios is that they make it possible to go beyond the simple and clumsy classification of a test result as either abnormal or normal, as is usually done when describing the accuracy of a diagnostic test only in terms of sensitivity and specificity at a single cutoff point. Obviously, disease is more likely in the presence of an extremely abnormal test result than it is for a marginal one. With likelihood ratios, it is possible to summarize the information contained in a test result at different levels. One can define likelihood ratios for each of an entire range of possible values. In this way, information represented by the degree of abnormality is not discarded in favor of just the crude presence of absence of it.

In computing likelihood ratios across a range of test results, a limitation of sensitivity and specificity is overcome. Instead of referring to the ability of the test to identify all individuals with a given result or worse, it refers to the ability of a particular test result to identify people with the disease. The same is true for the calculation of specificity. Thus, for tests with a range of results, LRs can report information at each level.

In sum, likelihood ratios can accommodate the common and reasonable clinical practice of putting more weight on extremely high (or low) test results than on borderline ones when estimating the probability (or odds) that a particular disease is present.

E X A M P L E

How accurate is serum thyroxine (T$_4$) alone as a test for hypothyroidism? This question was addressed in a study of 120 ambulatory general medical patients suspected of having hypothyroidism. (15) Patients were diagnosed as being hypothyroid if serum thyrotropin (TSH) was elevated and if subsequent evaluations, including other thyroid tests and response to treatment, were consistent with hypothyroidism. The authors studied the initial T$_4$ level in 27 patients with hypothyroidism and 93 patients who were found not to have it to determine how accurately the simple test alone might have diagnosed hypothyroidism.

As expected, likelihood ratios for hypothyroidism were highest for low levels of T4 and lowest for high levels (Table 3.2). The lowest values in the distribution of T$_4$ (<4.0 µg/dL) were only seen in patients with hypothyroidism (these levels ruled in the diagnosis). The highest levels (>8.0 µg/dL) were not seen in patients with hypothyroidism (the presence of these levels ruled out the disease).

The authors concluded "it may be possible to achieve cost savings without loss of diagnostic accuracy by using a single total T$_4$ measurement for the initial evaluation of suspected hypothyroidism in selected patients."

The likelihood ratio has several other advantages over sensitivity and specificity as a description of test performance. The information contributed by the test is summarized in one number corresponding to each level of test result. Also, likelihood ratios are particularly well suited for describing the overall odds of disease when a series of diagnostic tests is used (see below).

Techniques for Using Likelihood Ratios

Figures 3.10 and 3.11 on pages 52–53 demonstrate two ways of arriving at posttest probability: by calculation and with a nomogram. Figure 3.11 makes the calculations using the deep venous thrombosis example in Figure 3.3 and shows that the calculated posttest probability (16%) is close to the 17% positive predictive value calculated in Figure 3.3. Although the process is conceptually simple and each individual calculation is easy, the overall effort is a bit daunting. The nomogram simplifies the process, but it requires having the nomogram available.

These calculations demonstrate a disadvantage of likelihood ratios. One must use odds, not probabilities, and most of us find thinking in terms of odds more difficult than probabilities. Also, the conversion from probability to odds and back requires math or the use of a nomogram, which can complicate calculating posttest odds and predictive value during the routine course of patient care.

Table 3.3 displays an easier way. It shows a way of using likelihood ratios to provide a rough approximation of the effect of a test result on the probability a patient with a given test result has the disease (predictive value). (16) Likelihood ratios of 2, 5, and 10 increase the probability of disease approximately 15%, 30%, and 45%, respectively, and the inverse of these (likelihood ratios of 0.5, 0.2, and 0.1) decrease the proba-

TABLE 3.2 ▓ **Distribution of Values for Serum Thyroxine in Hypothyroid and Normal Patients, With Calculation of Likelihood Ratios**[a]

Total Serum Thyroxine (µg/dL)	Patients with Test Result		Likelihood Ratio
	Hypothyroid number (percent)	Normal number (percent)	
<1.1	2 (7.4)		↑
1.1–2.0	3 (11.1)		Ruled in
2.1–3.0	1 (3.7)		
3.1–4.0	8 (29.6)		↓
4.1–5.0	4 (14.8)	1 (1.1)	13.8
5.1–6.0	4 (14.8)	6 (6.5)	2.3
6.1–7.0	3 (11.1)	11 (11.8)	.9
7.1–8.0	2 (7.4)	19 (20.4)	.4
8.1–9.0		17 (18.3)	↑
9.1–10		20 (21.5)	
10.1–11		11 (11.8)	Ruled out
11.1–12		4 (4.3)	
>12		4 (4.3)	↓
Total	27 (100)	93 (100)	

[a] Source: Goldstein BJ, Mushlin AI. Use of a single thyroxine test to evaluate ambulatory medical patients for suspected hypothyroidism. J Gen Intern Med 1987;2:20–24.

bility of disease similarly 15%, 30%, and 45%. Bedside use of likelihood ratios is easier when the three specific likelihood ratios and their effect (multiples of 15) on posttest probability are remembered, especially when the clinician can estimate the probability of disease in the patient before the test is done. Using this algorithm in the deep venous thrombosis example (Figure 3.3), the probability of disease with a LR+ of 2.6 would be approximately 22% (the underlying 7% prevalence plus about 15%). This is a somewhat higher estimate than that obtained with the mathematical calculation, but it is close enough to conclude that a patient with a positive D-dimer assay needs some other test before the presence of deep venous thrombosis can be confirmed.

MULTIPLE TESTS

Because clinicians commonly use imperfect diagnostic tests with less than 100% sensitivity and specificity and intermediate likelihood ratios, a single test frequently results in a probability of disease that is neither very high nor very low (somewhere between 10% and 90%, for example). Usually, it is not acceptable to stop the diagnostic process at such a point. Would a physician or patient be satisfied with the conclusion that the patient has even a 20% chance of having carcinoma of the colon? Or that an asymptomatic, 35-year-old man with 2.5 mm ST segment depression on a stress test has a 42% chance of coronary artery disease (see Figure 3.9)? Even for less deadly diseases, such as hypothyroidism, tests resulting in intermediate posttest probabilities are of little help. The physician is ordinarily bound to raise or lower the probability of disease substantially in such situations—unless, of course, the diagnostic possibilities are all trivial, nothing could be done about the result, or the risk of proceeding further is prohibitive. When these exceptions do not apply, the doctor will want to find a way to rule in or rule out the disease more decisively.

When multiple different tests are performed and all are positive or all are negative, the interpretation is straightforward. All too often, however, some are positive and others are negative. Interpretation is

A) Mathematical approach

1) Convert pretest probability (prevalence) to pretest odds
      Pretest odds = prevalence/(1–prevalence)
2) Multiply pretest odds by likelihood ratio to obtain posttest odds
      Pretest odds x likelihood ratio = posttest odds
3) Convert posttest odds to posttest probability (predictive value)
      Posttest probability = posttest odds/(1+posttest odds)

B) Using a likelihood ratio nomogram

Place a straight edge at the correct prevalence and likelihood ratio values
and read off the posttest probability where the straight edge crosses the line.

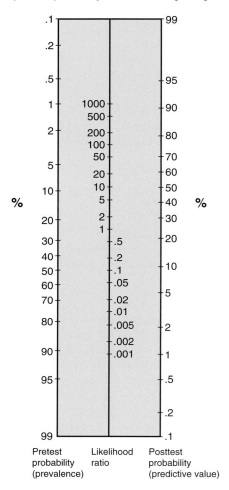

Pretest probability (prevalence)   Likelihood ratio   Posttest probability (predictive value)

FIGURE 3.10 ▨ Formula and nomogram using test likelihood ratios to determine posttest probability of disease. (Corrected from Fagan TJ. Nomogram for Bayes's theorem. N Eng J Med 1975;293:257.)

then more complicated. This section discusses the principles by which multiple tests are applied and interpreted.

Multiple diagnostic tests can be applied in two basic ways (Figure 3.12). They can be used in **parallel testing** (i.e., all at once), and a positive result of any test is considered evidence for disease. Or they can be done in **serial** (i.e., consecutive) **testing**, with the decision to order the next test in the series based on the results of the previous test. For serial testing, all tests must give a positive result in order for the diagnosis to be made because the diagnostic process is stopped with a negative result.

Parallel Testing

Physicians usually order tests in parallel when rapid assessment is necessary, as in hospitalized or emer-

A) Mathematical approach
　1) Convert pretest probability (prevalence) to pretest odds
　　　.07/(1-.07) = .075
　2) Multiply pretest odds by likelihood ratio of positive test
　　　.075 x 2.6 = 0.195
　3) Convert posttest odds to posttest probability (positive predictive value)
　　　0.195/(1 + 0.195) = .16 = 16%

B) Using a likelihood ratio nomogram
The pretest probability is 7% and the LR + is 2.6. Place a ruler to intersect these 2 values and it crosses the posttest probability line at ~ 16% –17%.

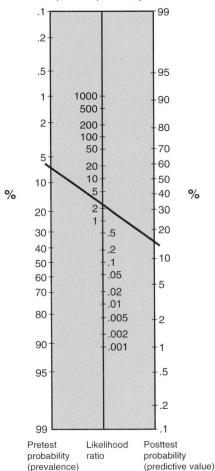

FIGURE 3.11 ▨ Calculating the posttest probability of a positive D-dimer assay test for deep venous thrombosis (See Figure 3.3).

gency patients, or for ambulatory patients who cannot return easily because they have come from a long distance for evaluation.

　Multiple tests in parallel generally increase the sensitivity and, therefore, the negative predictive value for a given disease prevalence, above those of each individual test. On the other hand, specificity and positive predictive value are lower than for each individual test. That is, disease is less likely to be missed (parallel testing is probably one reason why referral centers seem to diagnose disease that local physicians miss). But false-positive diagnoses are also more likely to be made (thus the propensity for over-diagnosing in such centers as well). In sum, parallel testing is particularly useful when the clinician is faced with the need for a very sensitive testing strategy but has available only two or more relatively insensitive tests that measure different clinical

TABLE 3.3	Simple "Rule of Thumb" for Determining Effect of Likelihood Ratios on Disease Probability

Likelihood Ratio	Approximate Change in Disease Probability (%)
10	+45
9	+40
8	
7	
6	+35
5	+30
4	+25
3	+20
2	+15
1	No Change
0.5	−15
0.4	−20
0.3	−25
0.2	−30
0.1	−45

Adapted from McGee S. Simplifying likelihood ratios. J Gen Intern Med 2002;17:646–649.

phenomena. By using the tests in parallel, the net effect is a more sensitive diagnostic strategy. The price, however, is further evaluation or treatment of some patients without the disease.

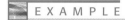

E X A M P L E

Neither PSA nor digital rectal exam is a very sensitive test for the diagnosis of prostate cancer. Table 3.4 shows their sensitivity, specificity, and predictive values in the screening setting (men without symptoms). When the two tests are used in parallel, the sensitivity increases but the specificity falls. The positive predictive value is lower than for PSA testing alone. (17)

The degree to which sensitivity and negative predictive value increases with parallel testing depends on the extent to which each test contributes information that is independent of the others; that is, each test identifies patients with the disease that were missed by the other tests. For example, if two tests are used in parallel with 60 and 80% sensitivities, the sensitivity of the parallel testing will be only 80% if the better test identifies all the cases found by the less sensitive test. If the two tests each detect all the cases missed by the other, the sensitivity of parallel testing is, of course, 100%. If the two tests

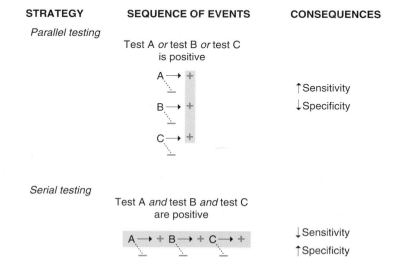

FIGURE 3.12 Parallel and serial testing. In parallel testing, all tests are done at the same time. In serial testing, each subsequent test is done only when the previous test result is positive.

TABLE 3.4 ■ **Test Characteristics of PSA and Digital Rectal Examination (DRE)**[a]

Test	Sensitivity	Specificity	Positive Predictive Value
PSA 4.0 μg/mL	0.67	0.97	0.43
Abnormal DRE	0.50	0.94	0.24
Abnormal PSA or DRE	0.84	0.92	0.28
Abnormal PSA and DRE	0.34	0.995	0.49

[a] PSA and DRE alone and in combination (parallel and serial testing) in the diagnosis of prostate cancer.
Adapted from Kramer BS, Brown ML, Prorock PC, Potosky AL, Gohagen JK. Prostate cancer screening: What we know and what we need to know. Ann Int Med 1993;119:914–923.

were completely independent of each other (see discussion of test independence below), then the sensitivity of parallel testing would be 92%.

Clinical Prediction Rules

A modification of parallel testing occurs when clinicians use the combination of multiple tests, some with positive and some with negative results, to arrive at a diagnosis. Usually, they start by taking a history and conducting a physical examination, searching for certain answers and findings. They may also order certain laboratory tests. The results of the combined testing from history, physical examination, and laboratory tests are then used to make a diagnosis. This process, long an implicit part of clinical medicine, has been examined systematically for an increasing number of diagnoses. For some medical conditions certain history items, physical findings, and laboratory results are particularly important in their predictive power for making a diagnosis. The resulting test combinations are called **clinical prediction rules** or **diagnostic decision-making rules**; sensitivity, specificity, and likelihood ratios are then calculated for these rules.

EXAMPLE

"Sinus trouble" is among the most common complaints in office practice, but the list of possible causes is long. Because acute bacterial sinusitis should be treated with antibiotics, it is important to diagnose the condition correctly but it is difficult to do so. Radiographic examination, the most accurate diagnostic test, is expensive and not always easily available. A study was undertaken to determine if a combination of history and physical examination tests could be used instead. In 111 patients presenting with nasal complaints, 3 history and 2 physical examination tests independently predicted sinusitis (Table 3.5). However, none did so very well. But, when the results of

these 5 tests were combined, a more useful prediction rule emerged. In a patient with at least 4 positive results, the likelihood ratio was 6.4, and the positive predictive value in this group of patients was 80%, while when all test results were negative, the likelihood ratio was 0.1, with a positive predictive of 6%. (18)

Serial Testing

Serial testing maximizes specificity and positive predictive value, but lowers sensitivity and the negative

TABLE 3.5 ■ **An Example of a Diagnostic Decision-Making Rule: Predictors of Sinusitis**

Independent Predictors	Positive Likelihood Ratio
Individual positive symptoms and signs	
Maxillary toothache	2.5
Purulent nasal secretion	2.1
Poor response to decongestants	2.1
Abnormal transillumination	1.6
History of colored nasal discharge	1.5
Combined number of positive symptoms and signs	
4 or 5	6.4
3	2.6
2	1.1
1	0.5
0	0.1

Source: Williams J, Simel DL. Does this patient have sinusitis? Diagnosing acute sinusitis by history and physical examination. JAMA 1993;270:1242–1246.

predictive value (see Table 3.4). One ends up surer that positive test results represent disease, but runs an increased risk that disease will be missed. Serial testing is particularly useful when none of the individual tests available to a clinician is highly specific.

Physicians most often use serial testing strategies in clinical situations where rapid assessment of patients is not required, such as in office practices and hospital clinics in which ambulatory patients are followed over time. Serial testing is also used when some of the tests are expensive or risky, these tests being employed only after simpler and safer tests suggest the presence of disease. For example, maternal age and blood tests (α-fetoprotein, chorionic gonadotropin and estriol) are used to identify pregnancies at higher risk of delivering a baby with Down syndrome. Mothers found to be at high risk by those tests are then offered amniocentesis. (19) Serial testing leads to less laboratory use than parallel testing because additional evaluation is contingent on prior test results. However, serial testing takes more time because additional tests are ordered only after the results of previous ones become available. Usually the test that is less risky, less invasive, easier to do, and cheaper should be done first. If these factors are not in play, performing the test with the highest specificity is usually more efficient, requiring fewer patients to undergo both tests.

Serial Likelihood Ratios

When a series of tests is used, an overall probability can be calculated, using the likelihood ratio for each test result, as shown in Figure 3.13. The prevalence of disease before testing is first converted to pretest odds. As each test is done, the posttest odds of one become the pretest odds for the next. In the end, a new probability of disease is found that takes into account the information contributed by all the tests in the series.

Assumption of Independence

When multiple tests are used, the accuracy of the final result depends on whether the additional information contributed by each test is somewhat independent of that already available from the preceding ones, such as when the next test does not simply duplicate known information. For example, in the diagnosis of endocarditis, it is likely that fever (an indication of inflammation), a new heart murmur (an indication of valve destruction), and Osler nodes (an indication of emboli) each add independent, useful information. In the example of acute bacterial sinusitis, the investigators used statistical techniques to ensure that each diagnostic test included in the decision rule contributed independently to the diagnosis. The premise of independence underlies the entire approach to the use of multiple tests. However, it seems unlikely that tests for most diseases are fully independent of one another. If the assumption that the tests are completely independent is wrong, calculation of the probability of disease from several tests would tend to overestimate the tests' value.

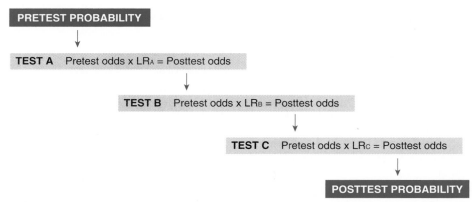

FIGURE 3.13 ■ Use of likelihood ratios in serial testing. As each test is completed, its posttest odds become the pretest odds for the subsequent test.

REVIEW QUESTIONS

A study was made of clinicians' ability to diagnose streptococcal infection in 149 patients coming to the emergency department with sore throats. (20) Doctors' clinical impressions were compared to results of throat cultures for group A streptococcus. *Thirty-seven patients had positive throat cultures, and 27 of these were diagnosed by doctors as having strep throat. One hundred twelve patients had negative cultures, and doctors diagnosed 35 of these as having strep throat.*

3.1. What is the sensitivity of the doctors' clinical impression of strep throat in this study?

3.2. What is the specificity?

3.3. If the doctor thought the patient had strep throat, for what percent of patients was she correct?

3.4. If the doctor thought the patient did not have strep throat, for what percent of the patients was he correct?

3.5. How common was strep throat in patients coming to the emergency department?

3.6. Calculate the posttest probability of a clinical impression of strep throat in this study.

Read the following statements and mark each one as True or False.

Overall, clinical impression of doctors about whether a patient has a strep throat

_____ **3.7** Is about the same as flipping a coin to decide whether a patient has strep throat.

_____ **3.8** Could be affected if doctors knew results of the throat cultures when recording their clinical impressions.

_____ **3.9** Could be affected if only some patients with sore throats got throat cultures.

_____ **3.10** Is sufficiently accurate that no other testing is necessary.

Answers are in Appendix A.

REFERENCES

1. Chobanian AV, Bakris GL, Black HR, Cushman WC, Green LA, Izzo JL, Jones DW, Materson BJ, Oparil S, Wright JT, Roccella EJ. The Seventh Report of the Joint National Committee on Prevention, Detection, Evaluation, and Treatment of High Blood Pressure: The JNC 7 Report. JAMA 2003: 289:2560–2571.

2. Gann PH, Hennekens CH, Stampfer MJ. A prospective evaluation of plasma prostate-specific antigen for detection of prostatic cancer. JAMA 1995;273: 289–294.

3. Jensen MC, Brant-Zawadzki MN, Obuchowski N, Modic MT, Malkasian D, Ross JS. Magnetic resonance imaging of the lumbar spine in people without back pain. N Engl J Med 1994;331:69–73.

4. Pickhardt PJ, Choi JR, Hwang I, Butler JA, Puckett ML, Hildebrandt HA, Wong RK, Nugent PA, Mysliwiec PA, Schindler WR. Computed tomographic virtual colonoscopy to screen for colorectal neoplasia in aymptomatic adults. N Engl J Med 2003;349:2191–2200.

5. Bates SM, Kearon C, Crowther M, Linkins L, O'Donnell M, Douketis J, Lee AYY, Weitz JI, Johnston M, Ginsberg JS. A diagnostic strategy involving a quantitative latex D-dimer assay reliably excludes deep venous thrombosis. Ann Intern Med 2003;138: 787–794.

6. Morgan TO, Jacobsen SJ, McCarthy WF, Jacobson DJ, McLeod DG, Moul JW. Age-specific reference ranges for serum prostate-specific antigen in black men. N Eng J Med 1996;335:304–310.

7. Jones TV, Lindsey BA, Yount P, Soltys R, Farani-Enayat B. Alcoholism screening questionnaires: Are they valid in elderly medical outpatients? J Gen Intern Med 1993;8:674–678.

8. Fletcher RH. Carcinoembryonic antigen. Ann Intern Med 1986;104:66–73.

9. Bobo JK, Lee NC, Thames SF. Findings from 752,081 clinical breast examinations reported to a national screening program from 1995 through 1998. J Natl Cancer Inst 2000;92:971–976.

10. Bates SM, Grand'Maison A, Johnston M, Naguit I, Kovacs MJ, Ginsberg JS. A latex D-dimer reliably excludes venous thromboembolism. Arch Intern Med 2001;161:447–453.

11. Centers for Disease Control and Prevention. National HIV prevalence surveys, 1997 summary. Atlanta, GA: Centers for Disease Control and Prevention, 1998: 1–25.

12. Richardson WS, Polashenski WA, Robbins BW. Could our pretest probabilities become evidence based? A prospective survey of hospital practice. J Gen Intern Med 2003;18:203–208.

13. Tierney WM, McDonald CJ. Practice databases and their uses in clinical research. Stat Med 1991; 10:541–557.

14. Diamond GA, Forrester JS. Analysis of probability as an aid in the clinical diagnosis of coronary artery disease. N Engl J Med 1979;300:1350–1358.

15. Goldstein BJ, Mushlin AI. Use of a single thyroxine test to evaluate ambulatory medical patients for suspected hypothyroidism. J Gen Intern Med 1987;2: 20–24.

16. McGee S. Simplifying likelihood ratios. J Gen Intern Med 2002;17:646–649.

17. Kramer BS, Brown ML, Prorock PC, Potosky AL, Gohagen K. Prostate cancer screening: What we know and what we need to know. Ann Intern Med 1993;119:914–923.

18. Williams J, Simel DL. Does this patient have sinusitis?: Diagnosing acute sinusitis by history and physical examination. JAMA 1993;270:1242–1246.

19. Haddow JE, Palomaki GE, Knight GJ, Williams J, Pulkkinen A, Canick JA, Saller DN Jr, Bowers GB. Prenatal screening for Down's syndrome with use of maternal serum markers. N Engl J Med 1992;327: 588–593.

20. Fletcher SW, Hamann C. Emergency room management of patients with sore throats in a teaching hospital: Influence of non-physician factors. J Comm Health 1976;1:196–204.

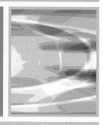

CHAPTER **4**

Frequency

KEY WORDS

Numerator	Perinatal mortality rate	Population at risk
Denominator	Prevalence studies	Random sample
Prevalence	Cross-sectional studies	Probability sample
Point prevalence	Cohort	Sampling fraction
Period prevalence	Incidence studies	Oversample
Incidence	Cohort studies	Convenience samples
Duration of disease	Cumulative incidence	Grab samples
Case fatality rate	Incidence density	Epidemic
Complication rate	Person-time	Pandemic
Infant mortality rate	Dynamic population	Epidemic curve

Medicine is the science of uncertainty and the art of probability.

— E. Mumford

In Chapter 1, we outlined the questions that clinicians need to answer as they care for patients. We noted that answers were usually in the form of probabilities and only rarely as certainties. We mentioned that frequencies obtained from clinical research are the basis for probability estimates during patient care. In this chapter, we describe basic expressions of frequency, how they are obtained from clinical research, and how to recognize threats to their validity. We introduce these topics with the following patient.

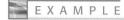 E X A M P L E

A 72-year-old man presents with slowly progressive urinary frequency, hesitancy, and dribbling. Digital rectal examination reveals a symmetrically enlarged prostate gland. Urinary flow measurements show reduction in flow rate, and serum PSA is not elevated. The clinician diagnoses benign prostatic hyperplasia (BPH). In deciding on treatment, the clinician and patient must weigh the benefits and hazards of various therapeutic options. To simplify, let us say the options are medical therapy with drugs or surgery. The patient might choose medical treatment but runs the risk of worsening symptoms or obstructive renal disease because the treatment is less immediately effective than surgery. Or he might choose surgery, gaining immediate relief of symptoms but at the risk of operative mortality and urinary incontinence.

59

Decisions such as the one this patient and clinician must make traditionally have been called "clinical judgment" and are based on experience at the bedside and in the clinics. In modern times, clinical research has become sufficiently strong and extensive that it has become possible to ground clinical judgment in research-based probabilities—or frequencies—as well. Probabilities of disease, improvement, deterioration, cure, side effects, and death form the basis for answering most clinical questions. For this patient, sound clinical judgment requires accurate information about how his symptoms will change over time. On the one hand is the likelihood of acute urinary retention or renal damage with medical treatment; on the other is symptom relief, mortality, and urinary incontinence with surgery.

ARE WORDS SUITABLE SUBSTITUTES FOR NUMBERS?

Physicians often communicate probabilities as words, such as usually, sometimes, rarely, and the like, rather than as numbers. Substituting words for numbers is convenient and avoids making a precise statement when one is uncertain about a probability. However, words are a poor substitute for numbers because there is little agreement about the meanings of commonly used adjectives describing probability.

EXAMPLE

Physicians were asked to estimate the likelihood of disease for each of 30 expressions of probability found by reviewing radiology and laboratory reports. There was great difference of opinion for each expression. Probabilities for "consistent with" ranged from 0.18 to 0.98; for "unlikely" the range was 0.01 to 0.93. These data support the authors' assertion that "difference of opinion among physicians regarding the management of a problem may reflect differences in the meaning ascribed to words used to define probability." (1)

Patients also assign widely varying probabilities to word descriptions. In another study, highly skilled and professional workers thought "usually" referred to probabilities of 0.35 to 1.0; "rarely" meant to them a probability of 0 to 0.15. (2)

Thus, substituting words for numbers diminishes the information conveyed. We advocate using numbers whenever possible.

PREVALENCE AND INCIDENCE

In general, clinically relevant measures of the frequency of events are fractions in which the **numerator** is the number of patients experiencing the outcome (cases) and the **denominator** is the number of people in whom the outcome could have occurred (population).

The two basic measures of frequency are prevalence and incidence.

Prevalence

Prevalence (sometimes referred to as prevalence rate) is the fraction (proportion or percent) of a group of people possessing a clinical condition or outcome at a given point in time (see Chapter 3). Prevalence is measured by surveying a defined population comprised of people with and without the condition of interest. **Point prevalence** is measured at a single point in time for each patient (although actual measurements need not necessarily be made at the same point in calendar time for all the people in the population). **Period prevalence** describes cases that were present at any time during a specified period of time.

Incidence

Incidence, on the other hand, is the fraction or proportion of a group of people initially free of the outcome of interest that develops the condition over a given period of time. Incidence refers then to *new* cases of disease occurring in a population initially free of the disease or new outcomes such as symptoms, disability or death occurring in patients with a disease.

EXAMPLE

Figure 4.1 illustrates the differences between incidence and prevalence. It shows the occurrence of disease in a population of 100 people over the course of 3 years (2002–2004). As time passes, individuals in the population develop the disease. They remain in this state until they either recover or die. In the 3 years, 16 people suffer the onset of disease, and 4 already had it before the period of observation. The remaining 80 people do not develop disease, and do not appear in the figure.

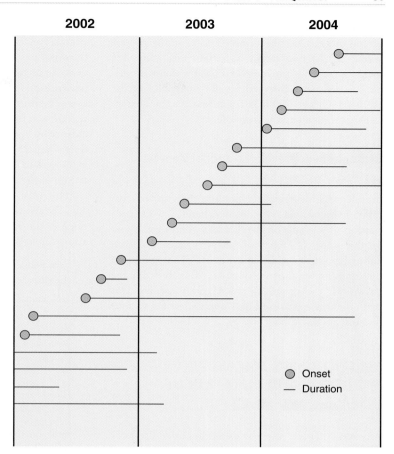

FIGURE 4.1 ▧ Incidence and Prevalence. Occurrence of disease in 100 people at risk from 2002 to 2004.

At the beginning of 2002, there already existed four cases, so the prevalence at that point in time is 4/100. If all 100 people, including prior cases, are examined at the beginning of each year, one can compute the prevalence at those points in time. At the beginning of 2003, the prevalence is 5/100 because two of the pre-2002 cases lingered on into 2003, and two of the new cases developing in 2002 terminated (hopefully in a cure) before the examination at the start of 2003. Prevalences can be computed for each of the other two annual examinations and, assuming that none of the original 100 people died, moved away, or refused examination, these prevalences are 7/100 at the beginning of 2004 and 5/100 at the beginning of 2005.

To calculate the incidence of new cases developing in the population, we consider only the 96 individuals free of the disease at the beginning of 2002 and what happens to them over the next 3 years.

Five new cases developed in 2002; six new cases developed in 2003, and five additional new cases developed in 2004. The 3-year incidence of the disease is all new cases developing in the 3 years (16) divided by the number of susceptible individuals at the beginning of the follow-up period (96), or 16/96 in 3 years. What are the annual incidences for 2002, 2003, and 2004, respectively? Remembering to remove the previous cases from the denominator, we would calculate the annual incidences as 5/96 for 2002, 6/91 for 2003, and 5/85 for 2004.

Prevalence and Incidence in Relation to Time

Every measure of disease frequency necessarily contains some indication of time. With measures of prevalence, time is assumed to be instantaneous, as in a single frame from a motion picture. Prevalence depicts the situation at that point in time for each patient, even though it may, in reality, have taken several months to collect observations on the various people in the population. On the other hand, for incidence, time is the interval during which susceptible subjects were observed for the emergence of the event of interest. Table 4.1 summarizes the characteristics of incidence and prevalence.

Distinguishing Prevalence and Incidence

Why is it important to know the difference between prevalence and incidence? Because they answer two different questions: On the one hand, "What proportion of a group of people has a condition?"; and on the other, "At what rate do new cases arise in a defined population as time passes?" The answer to one question cannot be obtained directly from the answer to the other. Prevalent cases are incident cases that have persisted in a population for various reasons, good and bad.

RELATIONSHIPS AMONG PREVALENCE, INCIDENCE, AND DURATION OF DISEASE

Anything that increases the duration of the disease or clinical finding in a patient will increase the chance that that patient will be identified in a prevalence study. Another look at Figure 4.1 will confirm this. Prevalent cases are those that remain affected—to the extent that patients are either cured, die of their disease, or leave the population under study, they are no longer a case in a prevalence survey. Disease of brief duration will be more likely to be missed by a preva-

lence study. For example, 25%–40% of all deaths from coronary heart disease occur within 24 hours of the onset of symptoms in people having no prior evidence of disease. A prevalence study would, therefore, underestimate the true burden of coronary heart disease. In contrast, diseases of long duration are well represented in prevalence surveys, even when their incidence is low. The incidence of Crohn's disease is only about 2 to 7 per 100,000/year, but its prevalence is more than 100 per 100,000, reflecting the chronic nature of the disease. (3)

The relationship among incidence, prevalence and **duration of disease** in a steady state, in which none of the variables is changing much over time, is approximated by the following expression:

Prevalence = Incidence × Average duration of the disease

EXAMPLE

Table 4.2 shows the approximate annual incidence and prevalence rates for asthma. Incidence falls with increasing age, illustrating the fact that the disease arises primarily in childhood. But prevalence stays fairly stable over the entire age span, indicating that asthma tends to be chronic and is especially chronic among older individuals. Also, because the pool of prevalent cases does not increase in size, with increasing age, approximately the same number of patients is recovering from asthma as new patients are developing it.

The rearranged formula [average duration = prevalence ÷ incidence] shows that asthma has an average duration of 10 years. When the duration of asthma is determined for each age category (by dividing the prevalences by the incidences), it is apparent that the duration of asthma increases with

---

TABLE 4.1 ■ Characteristics of Incidence and Prevalence

Characteristic	Incidence	Prevalence
Numerator	New cases occurring during a period of time among a group initially free of disease	All cases counted on a single survey or examination of a group
Denominator	All susceptible people without disease at the beginning of the period	All people examined, including cases and noncases
Time	Duration of the period	Single point or period
How measured	Cohort study (see Chapter 5)	Prevalence (cross-sectional) study

TABLE 4.2 ■ The Relationships Among Incidence, Prevalence, and Duration of Disease: Asthma in the United States[a]

Age	Annual Incidence	Prevalence	Duration = Prevalence/ Annual Incidence
0–5	6/1,000	29/1,000	4.8 years
6–16	3/1,000	32/1,000	10.7 years
17–44	2/1,000	26/1,000	13.0 years
45–64	1/1,000	33/1,000	33.0 years
65+	0	36/1,000	33.0 years
Total	3/1,000	30/1,000	10.0 years

[a] Approximated from several sources.

increasing age. This reflects the clinical observation that childhood asthma often clears with time, whereas adult asthma tends to persist.

SOME OTHER RATES

Some rates are expressions of events over time, but the period of follow-up is implicit. For example, a **case fatality rate** is the proportion of people having a disease who die of it, with the implication being that deaths are counted over a long enough period of time for all deaths that might occur to have occurred. Similarly, **complication rate**, the proportion of people with a disease or treatment who experience complications, assumes that enough time has passed for the complications to have occurred. These kinds of measures can be underestimations if follow-up is not really long enough. For example, surgical site infection rates have been under-reported because they have been counted up to the time of hospital

discharge, whereas some wound infections are first apparent after discharge, (4) Other rates, such as **infant mortality rate** and **perinatal mortality rate** (defined in Table 4.3) are approximations of incidence because the children in the numerator are not necessarily those in the denominator. In the case of infant mortality rate for a given year, some of the children who die in that year were born in the previous year; similarly, the last children to be born in that year may die in the following year. These rates are constructed in this way to make measurement more feasible, while providing a good approximation of a true rate. Table 4.3 summarizes some rates used in health care.

STUDIES OF PREVALENCE AND INCIDENCE

Prevalence and incidence are measured by entirely different kinds of studies.

TABLE 4.3 ■ Some Commonly Used Rates

Case Fatality Rates	Proportion of patients who die of a disease
Complication Rate	Proportion of patients who suffer a complication of a disease or its treatment
Infant Mortality Rate	$\dfrac{\text{Number of deaths in a year of children} < 1 \text{ year of age}}{\text{Number of live births in the same year}}$
Perinatal Mortality Rate (Per thousand)	$\dfrac{\text{Fetal deaths (28 + weeks to gestation) + neonatal deaths (first week)} \times 1,000}{\text{fetal deaths (28 weeks + of gestation) + Live births}}$

Prevalence Studies

In **prevalence studies**, people in a population are examined for the presence of the condition of interest. Some members of the population have the condition at that point in time, while others do not (Figure 4.2). The fraction or proportion of the population that has the condition (i.e., cases) constitutes the prevalence of the disease.

Another term is **cross-sectional studies** because people are studied at a cross-section of time. Prevalence is given more attention than incidence in this chapter because incidence will be taken up in greater detail in the following chapter.

The following is an example of a typical prevalence study:

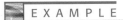

> E X A M P L E
>
> What is the prevalence of major depressive disorder among adults in the United States? To answer this question, investigators surveyed a representative sample of all households in the 48 contiguous states and interviewed residents ages 18 years or older. Depression was measured by a scale developed by the World Health Organization for use by trained interviewers who do not have clinical experience. Results from this scale had been shown to agree with clinical examination. A total of 9,090 people responded to the survey. The 12-month prevalence was 6.6%. (5) Other studies had shown that the point prevalence in the adult population is comparable to the 12-month prevalence and that the prevalence of minor depression is about twice that of major depression.

Incidence Studies

The population under examination in an incidence study is a **cohort**, which is defined as a group of people having something in common when they are first assembled and are then followed over time for the development of outcome events. For this reason, **incidence studies** are also called **cohort studies**. First, a sample of people free of the outcome of interest is identified and observed over time to see whether an outcome event occurs. Members of the cohort may be healthy at first, then followed for the emergence of disease. Or, all of them may have a disease, then be followed for outcomes of that disease, such as symptoms or death. Incidence studies will be discussed in greater detail in Chapter 5.

Cumulative Incidence

To this point, the term "incidence" has been used to describe the rate of new events in a group of people of fixed size, all members of which are observed over a period of time. This is called **cumulative incidence** because new cases are accumulated over time.

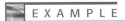

> E X A M P L E
>
> To study the incidence of dementia, investigators identified a cohort of older people who did not at the time have dementia. (6) Of 1,778 people followed over time, 305 died, 190 refused further testing, and 88 could not be found or were too ill to be examined. The remaining 1,195 were reexamined for an average of 2.5 years after the original examination. Overall, the incidence rate of dementia in this cohort was 4.3% per year and exceeded 8% per year for those who were over age 85 at the time of the first examination.

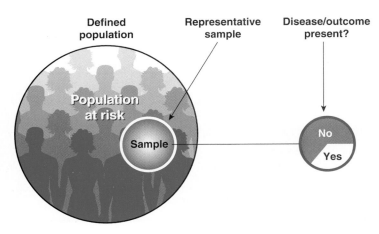

FIGURE 4.2 ■ The design of a prevalence study.

Incidence Density (Person-Years)

Another approach to studying incidence is to measure the number of new cases emerging in an ever-changing population, one in which people are under study and susceptible for varying lengths of time. The incidence derived from studies of this type is called **incidence density** because it is, figuratively speaking, the density of new cases in time and place. Typical examples are clinical trials in which eligible patients are enrolled over several years so that early enrollees are treated and followed for longer periods than late enrollees. In an effort to keep the contribution of individual patients commensurate with their follow-up interval, the denominator of an incidence density measure is not persons at risk for a specific time period but **person-time** at risk for the outcome event. A patient followed for 10 years without an outcome event contributes 10 person-years, whereas one followed for 1 year contributes only one person-year to the denominator. Incidence density is expressed as the number of new cases per total number of person-years at risk.

The person-years approach is also useful for estimating the incidence of disease in large populations when an accurate count of new cases is available along with an estimate of the population at risk, even though the population, called a **dynamic population,** is continually changing. Most sizes and compositions of populations are relatively stable over short periods of time, even though individual members of the population are continually changing (Figure 4.3). For example, cancer registries have an accurate count of new cases of cancer in their region, but they have only a relatively good estimate of population size and makeup

because people are entering and leaving the region continually.

A disadvantage of the person-years approach is that it lumps together different lengths of follow-up. A small number of patients followed for a long time can contribute as many person-years as a large number of patients followed for a short time. If patients with long follow-up are systematically different from those with short follow-up—perhaps because outcome events take a long time to develop or because patients with especially bad prospects tend to leave the population—the resulting incidence density will depend on the particular combination of number of patients and follow-up time.

E X A M P L E

Under what conditions could a potential carcinogen be identified, given that the latency period between exposure and onset of cancer is at least 10 years for most cancers? It might be possible to see an increase in cancer rate in a study of 1,000 people exposed to a carcinogen and followed up for 10 years. On the other hand, a study of 10,000 people for one year would not, even though it involves the same number of person-years (10,000) because the follow-up time is too short.

INTERPRETING MEASURES OF FREQUENCY

To make sense of a prevalence or incidence rate, the first steps involve careful definition of both the numerator and the denominator.

What Is a Case?: Defining the Numerator

Cases might be people in the general population who develop a disease or patients in clinical settings with disease who develop an outcome event such as recurrence, complication of treatment, or death. In either situation, the way in which a case is defined affects rates.

The definition of a case may change from time to time, changing the resulting rate.

E X A M P L E

The prevalence of hypertension in adults depends on the cutoff value chosen to divide normal from abnormal. In 1997, the Joint Committee on High Blood Pressure changed its definition of hypertension; the old definition

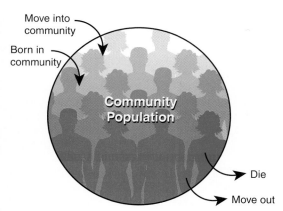

FIGURE 4.3 ■ A dynamic population

called for treatment of people with systolic blood pressure ≥ 160, while the new definition would treat people with systolic blood pressure ≥ 140. Figure 4.4 shows the distribution of systolic blood pressure in the U.S. population and where the old and new definitions fall on this curve. Changing the definition resulted in an increase in prevalence of hypertension from 21% to 29% and an additional 13 million people in the United States meeting criteria for antihypertensive therapy. (7)

Rates may also be affected by how aggressively one looks for cases.

> **E X A M P L E**
>
> Aspirin can induce asthma in some people. How often does this occur? It depends on the definition of a case. When people are simply asked whether they have a breathing problem after taking aspirin, rates are relatively low, about 2%–4% in adults. When a case is defined more rigorously, by giving aspirin and measuring whether this was followed by bronchoconstriction, the prevalence of aspirin-induced asthma is much higher, about 21% in adults. (8) The lower rate pertains to clinical situations, while the higher rate tells us something about the biology of this disease.

Incidence can also change in relation to better ways of detecting disease.

> **E X A M P L E**
>
> Many cases of prostate cancer remain indolent and are not detected during life. With use of prostate-specific antigen (PSA), a blood test for prostate cancer, many of

these indolent cases are now found. The test is relatively sensitive and leads to prostate biopsies that discover otherwise undetected cancers. The result of widespread use of PSA testing has been a rapid rise in the reported incidence of prostate cancer (Figure 4.5). The rise in incidence probably does not correspond to an increase in the true incidence in the population because it has occurred so fast and because similar increases have not been seen in countries, such as England and Wales, where PSA testing is less common. Note that incidence has subsequently fallen somewhat, presumably because the reservoir of prevalent cases, brought to attention by this new test, has been exhausted. (9)

What Is the Population?: Defining the Denominator

A rate is useful only to the extent that the population in which it is measured—the denominator of the rate—is clearly defined and right for the question. Four characteristics of the denominator are especially important.

First, all members of the population should be susceptible to the outcome of interest; that is, they should comprise a **population at risk.** If members of the population cannot experience the event or condition counted in the numerator, they do not belong in the denominator. For example, rates of cervical cancer should be assessed in women who still have a cervix; to the extent that cervical cancer rates are based on populations that include women who have had hysterectomies (or for that matter, men), true rates will be underestimated.

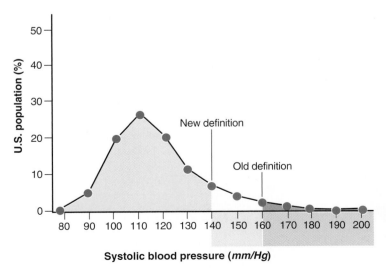

FIGURE 4.4 ■ Prevalence depends on the definition of a case. Distribution of systolic blood pressure for the U.S. adult population and two definitions of hypertension. (Redrawn from Schwartz LM, Woloshin S. Changing disease definitions: Implications for disease prevalence. Analysis of the Third National Health and Nutrition Examination Survey, 1988–1994. Effective Clinical Practice 1999;2:76–85.)

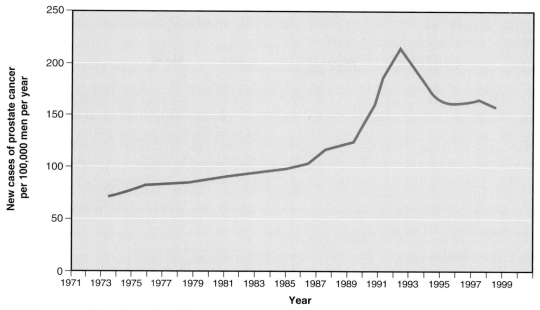

FIGURE 4.5 ■ Incidence depends on the intensity of efforts to find cases. Incidence of prostate cancer in the United States during the widespread use of screening with prostate-specific antigen (PSA). (Source: Quinn MJ. Cancer trends in the United States—A view from Europe. J National Cancer Institute 2003;95:1258–1261.)

Second, the population should be relevant to the question being asked. For example, if we wanted to know the prevalence of rheumatoid arthritis in the U.S. population, we would prefer to include in the denominator a random sample of all people in the United States. But if we wanted to know the prevalence of rheumatoid arthritis in a medical practice, perhaps to estimate a pretest probability for diagnostic testing or to plan services, the relevant denominator would be patients seen in the practice, not people in the population at large.

Third, the population should be described in sufficient detail so that it is a useful basis for judging to whom it applies. What is at issue here is the generalizability of rates—deciding whether a reported rate applies to the kind of patients in your setting. A huge gradient in rates of disease exists across practice settings, from the general population to primary care practice to referral centers. Clinicians need to locate the reported rates on that spectrum if they are to use the information effectively.

Finally, the samples on which actual measurement of rates are made should be representative of the population from which they are derived.

Sampling

As we mentioned briefly in Chapter 1, it is rarely possible to study all the people who have or might develop the condition of interest. Usually, one takes a sample so that the number studied is of manageable size. This leads to a central question: Does the sample accurately represent the parent population? In general, there are two basic ways of obtaining a sample, random and nonrandom, with different consequences.

Random samples are intended to produce representative samples of the population. In a simple **random sample**, every individual in the population has an equal probability of being selected. A more general term, **probability sample,** is used when every person has a known (not necessarily equal) probability of being selected. Probability samples are useful because it is often more informative to include in the sample a sufficient number of people in particular subgroups of interest, such as ethnic minorities or the elderly. If members of these subgroups comprise only a small proportion of the population, a simple random sample of the entire population might not include enough of them.

To remedy this, the investigators can vary the **sampling fraction**, which is the fraction of all members of each subgroup included in the sample. Investigators can **oversample** low frequency groups relative to the rest; that is, a larger percentage of them is selected at random. The final sample will still be representative of the entire population if the different sampling fractions are taken into account in the analysis.

On average, the characteristics of people in probability samples are similar to those of the population from which they were selected, particularly when the sample is large. To the extent that the sample differs from the parent population, it is by chance and not because of systematic error.

Nonrandom samples are common in clinical research for practical reasons. They are chosen because they are more convenient, even though they do not necessarily represent the parent population. They are **convenience samples** (because their main virtue is that they were convenient to obtain, such as samples of patients who are visiting a medical facility, are cooperative, and are articulate) or **grab samples** (because the investigators just grabbed patients wherever they could find them). Most patients described in the medical literature, and found in most clinicians' experience, are based on biased samples of their parent population. Typically, patients are included in studies because they are under care in an academic institution; are available; are willing to be studied; are not afflicted with diseases other than the one under study; and perhaps also are particularly interesting, severely affected, or both. There is nothing wrong with this practice as long as it is understood to whom the results do (or do not) apply. However, because of this, the results of clinical research often leave the thoughtful clinician with a very large generalizability problem, from the research setting to his or her practice.

DISTRIBUTION OF DISEASE BY TIME, PLACE, AND PERSON

Epidemiology has been described as the study of the determinants of the distribution of disease in populations. Major determinants are time, place, and person. Distribution according to these factors can provide strong clues to the causes and control of disease, as well as to the need for health services.

Time

An **epidemic** is a concentration of new cases in time. The term **pandemic** is used when a disease is especially widespread, such as a global epidemic of particularly severe influenza (for example, the one in 1918–1919) and the more slowly developing but worldwide rise in HIV infection/AIDS. The existence of an epidemic is recognized by an **epidemic curve** that shows the rise (and sometimes fall) of cases of a disease over time in a population.

EXAMPLE

Figure 4.6 shows the epidemic curve for a newly recognized disease, called Severe Acute Respiratory Syndrome (SARS), in Beijing, People's Republic of China, during the spring of 2003. (10) In all, 2,521 probable cases were reported during the epidemic. Cases were called "probable" because at the time there were no hard and fast criteria for diagnosis. The working definition of a case included combinations of the following epidemiologic and clinical phenomena: contact with a patient with SARS or living or visiting an area where SARS was active, symptoms and signs of a febrile respiratory illness, chest radiograph changes, lack of response to antibiotics, and normal or decreased white blood cell count. Later, as more became known about this new disease, laboratory testing for the responsible coronavirus could be used to define a case. Cases were called "reported" to make clear that there was no assurance that all cases in the Beijing community were detected.

Figure 4.6 also indicates when major control measures were instituted. The epidemic declined in relation to aggressive quarantine measures involving the closing of public gathering places, identifying new cases early in their course, removing cases from the community, and isolating cases in facilities specifically for SARS. It is possible that the epidemic abated on its own accord, and not because of these control measures, but that is unlikely given that similar control measures in other places were also followed by a resolution of the epidemic. Whatever the cause, the decline in new cases allowed the World Health Organization to lift its advisory against travel to Beijing so that the city could resume normal international business and reopen public places.

At the simplest level, knowledge of a local epidemic helps clinicians get the right diagnosis.

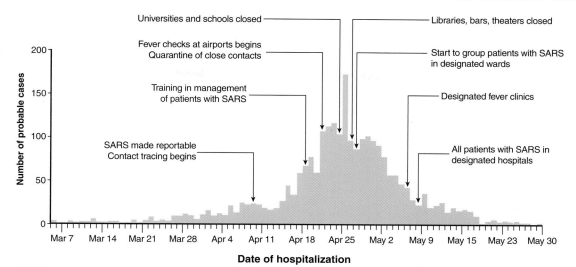

FIGURE 4.6 ■ An epidemic curve. Probable cases of severe acute respiratory syndrome in Beijing, March–May 2003, in relation to control measures. (Redrawn from Pang X, Zhu Z, Xu F, Guo J, Gong X, Liu D, et al. Evaluation of control measures implemented in the Severe Acute Respiratory Syndrome outbreak in Beijing, 2003. JAMA 2003;290:3215–3221.)

EXAMPLE

We first experienced this while serving as primary-care physicians on a military base in Germany. When one of us saw a child with a fever and rash on the hands and feet, we had only a hospital-based clerkship in pediatrics to rely on, and we were perplexed. But when we and our colleagues began seeing many such children in a short span of time, we recognized (with the help of a pediatrician friend) that we were in the midst of an outbreak of enterovirus infection ("hand, foot, and mouth disease"), which is a distinctive but mild infectious disease of children.

Place

The geographic distribution of cases indicates where a disease is more and less important and provides clues to its causes.

EXAMPLE

The incidence of colorectal cancer is very different in different parts of the world. Rates, even when adjusted for differences in age, are high in North America, Europe, and Australia and low in Africa and Asia (Figure 4.7). (11) This observation has led to the hypothesis that environmental factors may play a large part in the development of this disease. This possibility has been supported by other studies showing that people moving from countries of low incidence to those of high incidence acquire higher rates of colorectal cancer during their lifetime.

Person

When disease affects certain kinds of persons in the same time frame and in the same places as other people who are not affected, this provides clues to causes and guidance on how health-care efforts should be deployed. At the beginning of the AIDS pandemic, most cases were seen among male homosexuals who had many sexual partners and among drug addicts on the street who shared needles. This led to the early hypothesis that the disease was caused by an infectious agent transmitted in semen and blood. Laboratory studies confirmed this hypothesis and identified the human immunodeficiency virus. Identification of the kinds of people most affected also led to special efforts to prevent spread of the disease in them—for example, by targeting education about safe sex to those communities, closing public bath houses, and instituting safe-needle programs.

VALUE AND LIMITATIONS OF PREVALENCE STUDIES

Properly done prevalence studies are the very best ways to answer some important questions and are a weak way of answering others.

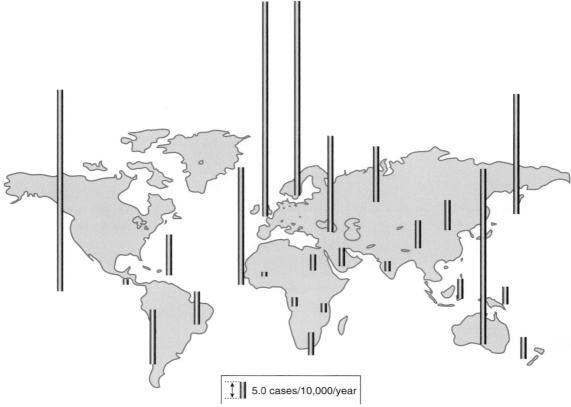

FIGURE 4.7 ▦ Estimates of colorectal cancer incidence for men and area of the globe. (From the World Cancer Research Fund/American Institute for Cancer Research. Food, Nutrition, and the Prevalence of Cancer: a Global Perspective. Washington, DC: American Institute for Cancer Research, 1997.)

What Are Prevalence Studies Good For?

Prevalence studies provide valuable information about what to expect in different clinical situations.

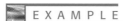 E X A M P L E

The approach to cervical lymphadenopathy depends on where and in whom it is seen. Children with persistent cervical adenopathy seen in primary-care practice have only a 0.4 percent chance that the node represents cancer, mainly lymphoma, and biopsy is not a pressing consideration. On the other hand, adults seen in primary-care practice have a 4% chance of having an underlying cancer of the head and neck. For them, clinicians should have a low threshold for lymph node biopsy, the definitive way of determining whether or not cancer is present. Rates of malignancy in referral centers are much higher, about 60% in adults with cervical adenopathy, and biopsies are usually done. The situation changes in different parts of the world. In developing countries,

mycobacterial infections are a more common cause of lymphadenopathy than cancer. Thus, knowledge of prevalence helps clinicians prioritize the diagnostic possibilities in their particular setting and for the particular patient at hand.

Cross-sectional studies are the basis for diagnostic testing. Test properties (sensitivity/specificity or likelihood ratio) are obtained in this way, as are pretest probabilities as the basis for choosing and interpreting the results of diagnostic tests (see Chapter 3).

E X A M P L E

Under what conditions is it reasonable to screen for ovarian cancer? The prevalence of treatable ovarian cancer dominates the answer to this question. The incidence in women age 50–75 years is about 0.5/1,000/year, meaning there would be 0.5 prevalent, undetected cases per 1,000 women if screening were done yearly and all cases that had arisen up until then had been detected. This prevalence is low relative to other cancers such as colorectal (about 2/1,000) and breast (about 4/1,000). It is generally accepted that the predictive value for ovarian cancer should be at least 10% because of the demands of subsequent diagnostic evaluation, which in most cases involve surgery. Positive tests lead to surgery, and nine surgeries in healthy women for every one with cancer seems to be an acceptable trade-off. Given the low prevalence, test specificity would have to be at least 99.6% (at a sensitivity of 80%) to achieve this predictive value. Current tests, such as the serum concentration of CA125 tumor marker, perform well below this level; sensitivity appears to be in the 70–80% range, but specificity is limited by false-positive results related to a wide variety of common conditions. For this reason, and in the absence of completed studies of effectiveness, no expert group in North America recommends screening for ovarian cancer in average-risk women. The low prevalence of curable disease requires that sensitivity and specificity of a screening test be extraordinarily high, higher than currently available tests. (12)

Finally, prevalence is an important guide to planning health services. In primary-care practice, being prepared for diabetes, obesity, hypertension and lipid disorders should demand more attention than planning for Hodgkin's disease, aplastic anemia, or systemic lupus erythematosis. On the other hand, some referral hospitals, such as the one in which we did our residencies, are well prepared for these diseases, and appropriately so.

When Are Prevalence Studies Not Particularly Good?

Prevalence studies provide only weak evidence of cause and effect. Causal questions are inherently about new events arising over time; that is, they are about incidence. Does disease arise more often in people exposed to a possible risk or less often after preventive care? Does treatment result in fewer bad outcomes?

One of the limitations of prevalence studies, for this purpose, is that it may be difficult to know whether the purported cause actually preceded the effect because the two are measured at the same point in time.

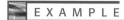

E X A M P L E

Inactivity may be a cause of cardiovascular disease. Numerous studies have found that inactive people have higher rates of cardiac events, such as sudden death and myocardial infarction, than those who exercise. The usual interpretation is that exercise protects against cardiac events. But it is at least possible that people who have early symptoms of cardiovascular disease, ones not yet recognized by patients or doctors reduce their exercise patterns, producing the observed association between exercise and cardiac events. That is, heart disease causes inactivity rather than inactivity causes heart disease. This possibility has been countered by studies in which exercise patterns were measured well before the onset of heart disease, with special efforts to rule out heart disease at that time.

If a risk or prognostic factor is certain to have preceded the onset of disease or outcome (family history or a genetic marker, for example), interpretation of the cause-and-effect sequence is less worrisome.

Another limitation is that prevalence may be the result of incidence of disease, the main consideration in causal questions; or it may be related to duration of disease, an altogether different issue. With only information about prevalence, one cannot determine how much each of the two, incidence and duration, contributes.

For these reasons, while prevalence studies may raise promising hypotheses about risk, prognosis, treatment, and prevention, these hypotheses need to be tested by strong studies that include incident cases.

POSTSCRIPT

Counting clinical events as described in this chapter may seem to be the most mundane of tasks, but it is one of the foundations of clinical science. In the nineteenth century, Pierre Louis introduced the "numerical method" of evaluating therapy. Louis had the imagination to count deaths and recoveries from febrile illness in the presence and absence of bloodletting. At the time, he was vilified for allowing lifeless numbers to cast doubt on the healing powers of the leech. Now, he is considered one of the heroes in the development of clinical research.

REVIEW QUESTIONS

The incidence of rheumatoid arthritis is 30/100,000/ year, and the prevalence is about 1/100. Choose the response that best answers the questions.

_____ **4.1.** On average, how many years does this disease last?

    A. 3
    B. 10
    C. 33
    D. 40
    E. 50

Questions 2–7 are about rates describing low back pain. For each statement, choose the rate that best describes it.

A. Cumulative incidence
B. Incidence density (person-years)
C. Point prevalence
D. Period prevalence
E. Not a rate

_____ **4.2.** 80% of people will experience back pain sometime in their lifetime.

_____ **4.3.** 31 million Americans have low back pain at any given time.

_____ **4.4.** 15%–45% of adults have back pain at some time in any year.

_____ **4.5.** 30% of adults have low back pain at any given time.

_____ **4.6.** About 2% of the U.S. workforce is compensated for back injuries each year.

_____ **4.7.** In a study of 100 patients with low back pain, 60 recovered by 6 weeks.

You are reading a report of a study of the prevalence of anemia in women and want to decide whether or not the study is scientifically sound. Choose the response that best answers the question.

_____ **4.8.** All of the following are characteristics of a good prevalence study except:

    A. Characteristics of a "case" are clearly defined.
    B. The study is done on a defined population.

    C. All members of the population should be able to experience the clinical condition of interest.
    D. Patients are followed for a sufficient period of time for outcome events to occur.
    E. The study is done on a representative sample of the population.

You have come across a study of a cohort of patients with heart failure.

_____ **4.9.** A cohort is a group of people who:

    A. have something in common at the beginning of follow-up
    B. are a random sample of a defined population
    C. experience the outcome of interest
    D. are examined at a point in time
    E. have the outcome of interest and are available for study

The following are statements about what prevalence studies are useful for. Mark each one as True or False.

_____ **4.10.** Studies of chronic diseases

_____ **4.11.** Estimating the pretest probability of disease before diagnostic testing

_____ **4.12.** Studies of cause and effect

_____ **4.13.** Studies of diseases that arise and resolve rapidly

Answers are in Appendix A.

REFERENCES

1. Bryant GD, Norman GR. Expressions of probability: words and numbers. N Engl J Med 1980;302:411.
2. Toogood JH. What do we mean by "usually"? Lancet 1980;1:1094.
3. Sedlack RE, Whisnant J, Elveback LR, Kurland LT. Incidence of Crohn's disease in Olmsted County, Minnesota, 1935–1975. Am J Epidemiol 1980;112:759–763.
4. Sands K, Vineyard G, Platt R. Surgical site infections occurring after hospital discharge. J Infect Dis 1996;173:963–970.

5. Kessler RC, Berglund P, Demler O, Jin R, Koretz D, Merikangas KR, et al. The epidemiology of major depressive disorder: Results from the National Comorbidity Survey Replication (NCS-R). JAMA 2003; 289:3095–3105.

6. Paykel ES, Brayne C, Huppert FA, Gill C, Barkley C, Gehlhaar E, et al. Incidence of dementia in a population older that 75 years in the United Kingdom. Arch Gen Psychiatry 1994;51:325–332.

7. Schwartz LM, Woloshin S. Changing disease definitions: Implications for disease prevalence. Analysis of the Third National Health and Nutrition Examination Survey, 1988–1994. Effective Clinical Practice 1999;2:76–85.

8. Jenkins C, Costello J, Hodge L. Systematic review of prevalence of aspirin induced asthma and its implications for clinical practice. BMJ 2004;328: 434–437.

9. Quinn MJ. Cancer trends in the United States— A view from Europe. J Nat Cancer Inst 2003; 95:1258–1261.

10. Pang X, Zhu Z, Xu F, Guo J, Gong X, Liu D, et al. Evaluation of control measures implemented in the Severe Acute Respiratory Syndrome outbreak in Beijing, 2003. JAMA 2003; 290:3215–3221.

11. World Cancer Research Fund/American Institute for Cancer Research. Food, Nutrition, and the Prevalence of Cancer: a Global Perspective. Washington, DC: American Institute for Cancer Research, 1997.

12. Carlson KJ. Screening for ovarian cancer. In Rose BD UpToDate 11(3). Wellesley, MA 2004.

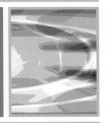

Risk: Looking Forward

The revolutionary idea that defines the boundary between modern time and the past is the mastery of risk: the notion that the future is more than a whim of the gods and that men and women are not passive before nature.

—Peter L. Bernstein, 1996

Risk generally refers to the probability of some untoward event. In this chapter, the term *risk* is used in a more restricted sense to indicate the probability that people who are exposed to certain "risk factors" will subsequently develop a particular disease more often than similar people who are not exposed.

People have a strong interest in their risk of disease. This concern is reflected in newspaper headlines and in many popular books about risk reduction. Postmenopausal hormone therapy and its relation to the risk of breast cancer and cardiovascular disease, the effect of certain genes on cancer risk, and the risk of neurological deficits after different levels of lead exposure are all examples of topics in which the public has developed a strong interest, as well as concerns about determining and managing their risk.

This chapter describes how investigators obtain estimates of risk by observing the relationship between exposure to possible risk factors and the subsequent incidence of disease. We describe methods that determine risk by following groups into the future. In

Chapter 6, we will describe methods of studying risk by looking backward in time. We also discuss several ways of comparing risks as they affect individuals and populations.

RISK FACTORS

Characteristics associated with an increased risk of becoming diseased are called **risk factors**. Some risk factors are inherited. For example, having the haplotype HLA-B27 greatly increases one's risk of acquiring the spondylarthropathies. Work on the Human Genome Project has identified many other diseases for which specific genes are risk factors, including colon and breast cancer, osteoporosis, and amyotropic lateral sclerosis. Other risk factors, such as infectious agents, drugs, and toxins, are found in the physical environment. Still others are part of the social environment. For example, bereavement after the loss of a spouse, change in daily routines, and crowding all have been shown to increase rates of disease—not only emotional illness but physical illness as well. Some of the most powerful risk factors are behavioral; examples are smoking, drinking alcohol to excess, driving without seat belts, engaging in unsafe sex, eating too much, and exercising too little.

Exposure to a risk factor means that a person, before becoming ill, has come in contact with or has manifested the factor in question. Exposure can take place at a single point in time, as when a community is exposed to radiation during a nuclear accident. More often, however, contact with risk factors for chronic disease takes place over a period of time. Cigarette smoking, hypertension, sexual promiscuity, and sun exposure are examples of risk factors, with the risk of disease being more likely to occur with prolonged exposure.

There are several different ways of characterizing the amount of exposure or contact with a putative risk factor: ever been exposed, current dose, largest dose taken, total cumulative dose, years of exposure, years since first exposure, and so on. (1) Although the various measures of dose tend to be related to one another, some may show an exposure-disease relationship, whereas others may not. For example, cumulative doses of sun exposure constitute a risk factor for non-melanoma skin cancer, whereas episodes of severe sunburn are a better predictor of melanoma. If the correct measure is not chosen, an association between a risk factor and disease may not be evident. Choice of an appropriate measure of exposure to a risk factor is usually based on all that is known about the clinical and biologic effects of the exposure, the pathophysiology of the disease and any previous epidemiological studies.

RECOGNIZING RISK

Large risks associated with effects that occur rapidly after exposure are easy for anyone to recognize. It is not difficult to appreciate the relationship between exposure and medical conditions such as chickenpox, sunburn, and aspirin overdose because these conditions follow exposure relatively rapidly and with obvious effects. But most morbidity or mortality is caused by chronic diseases for which the relationships between exposure and disease are far less obvious. It is usually impossible for individual clinicians, however astute, to recognize risk factors for chronic disease based on their own experiences with patients. This is true for several reasons, which are discussed below.

Long Latency

Many chronic diseases have long **latency periods** between exposure to a risk factor and the first manifestations of disease. Radiation exposure in childhood, for example, increases the risk for thyroid cancer in adults decades later. Similarly, hypertension precedes heart disease by decades, and calcium intake in young and middle-aged women affects osteoporosis and fracture rates in old age. When patients experience the consequence of exposure to a risk factor years later, the original exposure may be all but forgotten and the link between exposure and disease obscured.

Common Exposure to Risk Factors

Many risk factors, such as cigarette smoking or eating a diet high in cholesterol and saturated fats, have become so common in western societies that for many years it was difficult to discern their dangers. Only by comparing patterns of disease among people with and without these risk factors, using cross-national studies or investigating special subgroups—Mormons, for example, who do not smoke or vegetarians who eat diets low in cholesterol—were risks recognized that were, in fact, large.

It is now clear that about half of lifetime users of tobacco will die because of their habit; if current smoking patterns persist, it is predicted that in the 21st century, more than 1 billion deaths globally will be attributed to smoking. (2)

A relationship between the sleeping position of babies and the occurrence of Sudden Infant Death Syndrome (SIDS) is another example of a common exposure to a risk factor and the dramatic effect associated with its frequency, an association that went unrecognized until recently.

E X A M P L E

Sudden Infant Death Syndrome, the sudden, unexplained death of an infant under 1 year of age, is the leading cause of infant mortality in the first 12 months of life in the United States. Studies suggest that there are many contributing factors. In the late 1980s and 1990s, several investigations found that babies who were placed face down in their cribs were 3 to 9 times more likely to die of SIDS than those placed on their backs. (3) In 1992, the American Academy of Pediatrics issued a recommendation to place infants on their backs to sleep. Between 1992 and 1996, the percentage of babies placed in the prone position for sleep fell from 70% in 1992 to 24% in 1996, with a concomitant 40% drop in the number of SIDS cases. (4)

Low Incidence of Disease

The onset of most diseases, even ones thought to be "common," is actually uncommon. Thus, although lung cancer is the most common cause of cancer deaths in Americans, the yearly incidence of lung cancer, even in people who have smoked heavily for 25 years, is 2 to 3 in 1000. In the average physician's practice, years may pass between new cases of lung cancer. It is difficult for the clinician to draw conclusions about risks from such infrequent events.

Small Risk

Most chronic diseases are caused by several risk factors acting together. The risk associated with any one of them, taken alone, is small. To detect this risk, a large number of people must be studied to observe a difference in disease rates between exposed and unexposed persons. This is true even when both the risk factor and the disease occur relatively frequently. For example, studies of the role dietary fat plays

in the risk of breast cancer have given contradictory results. A summary of all studies found that the risk was small, with an increase of 11% to 17%, depending on the type of risk measurement used. (5) Such a small risk could be discounted as resulting from bias or chance. In contrast, it is not controversial that hepatitis B infection is a risk factor for hepatoma, because people with hepatitis B infection are hundreds of times more likely to develop liver cancer than those without it.

Common Risk

When a disease is common such as heart disease, cancer, or stroke and some of the risk factors for it are already known, it becomes difficult to distinguish a new risk factor from the others. Also, there may be less incentive to look for new risk factors, even though it is entirely conceivable that there are other important causes not yet recognized.

E X A M P L E

Cardiovascular disease is the most common cause of death in the United States (and the second most common cause worldwide). Over the past 50 years, several risk factors, including hypertension, hypercholesterolemia, cigarette smoking, diabetes mellitus, marked obesity, and physical inactivity, have been identified. However, fully half of all patients with cardiovascular disease have none of these established risk factors. Several new possible risk factors are under investigation, including a plasma marker for inflammation—C-reactive protein. In a study of more than 28,000 healthy, post-menopausal women, the baseline level of C-reactive protein was a stronger predictor of subsequent cardiovascular events than total cholesterol, HDL cholesterol or LDL cholesterol. This was true even after taking into account all classic risk factors. High C-reactive protein levels also identified women who were at risk despite their having low cholesterol levels (Figure 5.1). The authors of the study found that adding C-reactive protein levels improved the ability to predict future cardiovascular events among the women in the study. (6)

In contrast to common diseases, rare diseases and unusual or dramatic clinical presentations invite efforts to find a cause. AIDS was such an unusual syndrome that the appearance of just a few cases raised suspicion that some new agent (as it turned out, a retrovirus) might be responsible, a suspicion confirmed relatively quickly after the appearance of the disease. A previously unidentified coronavirus was confirmed as the cause of Severe Adult Respiratory

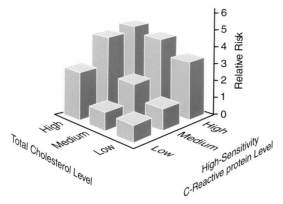

FIGURE 5.1 ▦ Levels of C-reactive protein and total cholesterol as risk factors for cardiovascular disease in women, after adjusting for other common risk factors. Using both cholesterol and C-reactive protein levels was superior to using either alone in identifying women at risk of cardiovascular disease. (Adapted from Ridker PM, Hennekens CH, Buring JE, Rifal N. C-reactive protein and other markers of inflammation in the prediction of cardiovascular disease in women. N Engl J Med 2000;342:836–843.)

Syndrome (SARS) in a matter of weeks after the first reported cases. Similarly, physicians were quick to notice when several cases of carcinoma of the vagina, a very rare condition, began appearing. A careful search for an explanation was undertaken, and maternal exposure to diethylstilbestrol (a hormone used to stabilize pregnancies in women with a history of miscarriage) was found.

Multiple Causes and Effects

There is usually not a close, one-to-one relationship between a risk factor and a particular disease. The relationship between hypertension and congestive failure is an example (Figure 5.2). Some people with hypertension develop congestive heart failure, and many do not. Also, many people who do not have hypertension develop congestive heart failure, because there are several other causes. The relationship is also difficult to recognize because hypertension causes several diseases other than congestive heart failure. Thus, al-

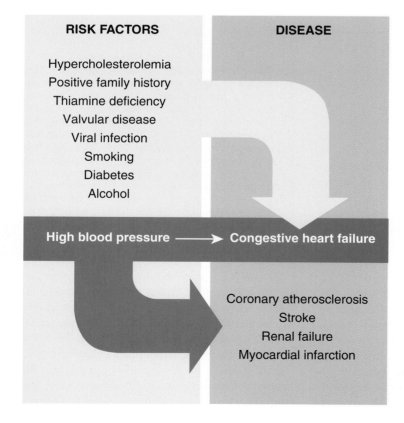

FIGURE 5.2 ▦ Relationship between risk factors and disease: hypertension and congestive heart failure. Hypertension causes many diseases, including congestive heart failure, and congestive heart failure has many causes, including hypertension.

though people with hypertension are about 3 times more likely than those without hypertension to develop congestive heart failure, and hypertension is the leading cause of the condition, physicians were not particularly aware of this relationship until the 1970s, when adequate evidence became available after careful study of large numbers of people over many years.

For all these reasons, individual clinicians are rarely in a position to recognize, let alone confirm, associations between exposure and chronic diseases. They may notice an association when a dramatic disease occurs quickly after an unusual exposure. But most diseases and most exposures do not conform to such a pattern. For accurate information about risk, clinicians must turn to the medical literature, particularly to carefully constructed studies that involve a large number of patients.

USES OF RISK

In clinical medicine, knowledge of risk factors can be used in several different ways.

Risk Factors Predict Future Disease

Risk factors are used, first and foremost, to predict the occurrence of disease. The best available information for predicting disease in an individual person is past experience with a large number of people who have a similar risk factor. How well the prediction applies to the individual depends on the similarity of the individual person to the group and is, in any case, never perfect.

The presence of even a strong risk factor does not necessarily mean that an individual is very likely to get the disease. For example, a heavy smoker (with an 80-pack-per-year history) has at least a hundred-fold greater risk of lung cancer compared to non-smokers, but he or she has about a 1 in 10 chance of getting lung cancer in the next 10 years.

Because predictions are expressed as probabilities of future events, there is a basic incompatibility between the incidence of a disease in groups of people and the chance that an individual will contract that disease. Any one person will either develop the disease or not. So, in a sense, the average is always wrong for an individual because the two are expressed in different terms, a probability versus the presence or absence of disease. Nevertheless, there is no better way than to

use probabilities to guide clinical decision making with individual patients. The goal is to continually improve predictions to make them more and more accurate for the individual at hand. For some diseases, this is increasingly possible as more and more risk factors are identified that improve the precision of predicting disease occurrence.

Risk Factors May or May Not Be Causal

The search for risk factors usually is a search for causes of disease. In clinical medicine, physicians are more comfortable with **immediate causes** of disease—infectious, physiologic, or anatomic changes leading to sickness such as a coronavirus causing SARS or hypocalcemia leading to seizures. But **distant causes**, more remote from a condition, may be important in the causal pathway. For example, lack of maternal education is a risk factor for low birth-weight infants. Yet, other factors related to education, such as poor nutrition, less prenatal care, cigarette smoking, and the like are more direct causes of low birth weight. Nevertheless, studies in India have shown that improving maternal education lowers infant mortality.

It is important to remember that just because risk factors predict disease, it does not necessarily follow that they cause disease. A risk factor may predict a disease outcome indirectly, by virtue of an association with some determinant of disease. In such a case, the risk factor is confounded with a truly causal factor.

A risk factor that is not a cause of disease is called a **marker** of disease, because it "marks" the increased probability of disease. Not being a cause does not diminish the value of a risk factor as a way of predicting the probability of disease, but it does imply that removing the risk factor might not remove the excess risk associated with it.

> ### E X A M P L E
>
> As pointed out in Chapter 1, there is strong evidence that the human papillomavirus (HPV) is a risk factor for cervical cancer, but the role of other sexually transmitted diseases, particularly *Chlamydia trachomatous,* is not as clear. Antibodies to these agents are more common among patients with cervical cancer than in women without cancer, but it is possible that *Chlamydia* is only a marker for risk of cervical cancer because promiscuity is involved in the transmission of both HPV and *Chlamydia.* If *Chlamydia* is a cause of cervical cancer, curing even asymptomatic infections might help prevent cervical cancer, but if *Chlamydia* were only a marker, treating it

would not help prevent cancer. To find out whether chlamydial infection is a marker or a cause, a study was carried out in Sweden among women in a screening program for whom Pap smears were available over many years. (7) Past *Chlamydia* infections were more common in women who subsequently developed cervical cancer even when taking into account HPV infections. Therefore, in this study, *Chlamydia trachomatous* appeared to be an independent risk factor, and not just a marker, for cervical cancer.

There are several ways of deciding whether a risk factor is a cause or merely a marker for disease. These are covered in Chapter 11.

Risk Factors Help Establish Pretest Disease Probability for Diagnostic Testing

Knowledge of risk can be used in the diagnostic process, since the presence of a risk factor increases the pretest probability of disease among patients, which is one way of improving the positive predictive value of a diagnostic test. However, in individual patients, risk factors usually are not as strong a predictor of disease as are clinical findings of early disease. As Geoffrey Rose (8) put it:

> Often the best predictor of future major diseases is the presence of existing minor disease. A low ventilatory function today is the best predictor of its future rate of decline. A high blood pressure today is the best predictor of its future rate of rise. Early coronary heart disease is better than all of the conventional risk factors as a predictor of future fatal disease.

As an example of Rose's dictum, age and sex are relatively strong risk factors for coronary artery disease, yet the prevalence of disease in the group at highest risk, older men, is only 12%. When specifics of the clinical situation, such as presence and type of chest pain and results of an electrocardiographic stress test, are considered as well, the prevalence of coronary disease can be as high as 99%. (9)

The absence of a very strong risk factor may help to rule out disease. Thus, it is reasonable to consider mesothelioma in the differential diagnosis of a pleural mass in a patient who is an asbestos worker. But mesothelioma is a much less likely diagnosis for the patient who has never been exposed to asbestos.

Risk Stratification for Screening Programs

Knowledge of risk factors can be used to improve the efficiency of screening programs by selecting subgroups of patients at substantially increased risk. Although the risk for breast cancer due to deleterious genetic mutations is very low in the general population, it is much higher in women with close relatives who developed the disease at a relatively early age; blood tests screening for gene mutations are usually reserved for women whose family history indicates they are at increased risk. Similarly, screening for colorectal cancer is recommended for the general population starting at age 50. However, people with a first-degree relative with a history of colorectal cancer are at increased risk for the disease, and several expert groups suggest that screening these people should begin at age 40.

Removing Risk Factors May Prevent Disease

If a risk factor is also a cause of disease, removing it can prevent disease whether or not the mechanism by which the disease develops is known. Some of the classic successes in the history of epidemiology illustrate this point. Before bacteria were identified, Snow noted that an increased rate of cholera occurred among people drinking water supplied by a particular company, and the epidemic subsided after he cut off that supply. In the process, he established that cholera was spread by contaminated water supplies. More recently, even before HIV had been identified, studies showed that having multiple sexual partners among homosexual men was a risk factor for acquiring AIDS. The concept of cause and its relationship to prevention is discussed in Chapter 11.

STUDIES OF RISK

The most powerful way to determine whether exposure to a potential risk factor results in an increased risk of disease is to conduct an **experiment** in which the researcher determines who is exposed. People currently without disease are divided into groups of equal susceptibility to the disease in question. One group is exposed to the purported risk factor and the other is not, but the groups otherwise are treated the same. Later, any difference in observed rates of disease in the groups could be attributed to the risk factor. Experiments are discussed in Chapter 8.

When Experiments Are Not Possible

The effects of most risk factors in humans cannot be studied with experimental studies. Consider some of the risk questions that concern us today: Are inactive people at increased risk for cardiovascular disease, everything else being equal? Do cellular phones cause brain cancer? Does a high-fat diet increase the risk of breast cancer? For such questions, it is usually not possible to conduct an experiment. First, it would be unethical to impose possible risk factors on a group of healthy people for the purposes of scientific research. Second, most people would balk at having their diets and behaviors determined by others for long periods of time. Finally, the experiment would have to go on for many years, which is difficult and expensive. As a result, it is usually necessary to study risk in less obtrusive ways.

Clinical studies in which the researcher gathers data by simply observing events as they happen, without playing an active part in what takes place, are called **observational studies**. Most studies of risk are observational studies and are either **cohort studies**, described in the rest of this chapter, or **case-control studies**, described in Chapter 6.

Cohorts

As defined in Chapter 4, the term **cohort** is used to describe a group of people who have something in common when they are first assembled and who are then observed for a period of time to see what happens to them. Table 5.1 lists some of the ways in which cohorts are used in clinical research. Whatever members of a cohort have in common, observations of them should fulfill three criteria if the obser-

vations are to provide sound information about risk of disease.

1. They do not have the disease in question at the time they are assembled.
2. They should be observed over a meaningful period of time in the natural history of the disease in question. This is so that there will be sufficient time for the risk to be expressed. If one wanted to learn whether neck irradiation during childhood results in thyroid neoplasms, a 5-year follow-up would not be a fair test of this hypothesis, because the usual time period between radiation exposure and the onset of disease is considerably longer.
3. Members of the cohort should be observed over the full period of follow-up. To the extent that people drop out of the study and their reasons for dropping out are related in some way to the outcome, the information provided by an incomplete cohort can misrepresent the true state of affairs.

Cohort Studies

In a cohort study (Figure 5.3), a group of people (a cohort) is assembled, none of whom has experienced the outcome of interest, but all of whom could experience it. (For example, in a study of risk factors for endometrial cancer, each member of the cohort should have an intact uterus.) Upon entry into the study, people in the cohort are classified according to those characteristics (possible risk factors) that might be related to outcome. For each possible risk factor, members of the cohort are classified either as *exposed* (i.e., possessing the factor in question, such as hypertension) or not ex-

TABLE 5.1 ■ Cohorts and Their Purposes

Characteristic in Common	To Assess Effect of	Example
Age	Age	Life expectancy for people age 70 (regardless of birth date)
Date of birth	Calendar time	Tuberculosis rates for people born in 1930
Exposure	Risk factor	Lung cancer in people who smoke
Disease	Prognosis	Survival rate for patients with breast cancer
Preventive intervention	Prevention	Reduction in incidence of pneumonia after pneumococcal vaccination
Therapeutic intervention	Treatment	Improvement in survival for patients with Hodgkin's disease given combination chemotherapy

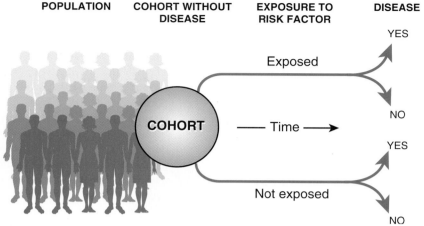

| POPULATION | COHORT WITHOUT DISEASE | EXPOSURE TO RISK FACTOR | DISEASE |

FIGURE 5.3 ▪ Design of a cohort study of risk. Persons without disease are divided into two groups—those exposed to a risk factor and those not exposed. Both groups are followed over time to determine what proportion of each group develops disease.

posed. All the members of the cohort are then observed over time to see which of them experiences the outcome, say, cardiovascular disease, and the rates of the outcome events are compared in the exposed and unexposed groups. It is then possible to see how potential risk factors relate to subsequent outcome events. Other names for cohort studies are **longitudinal studies**, which emphasize that patients are followed over time, **prospective studies**, which imply the forward direction in which the patients are pursued, and **incidence studies**, which call attention to the basic measure of new disease events over time.

The following is a description of a classic cohort study, which has made important contributions to our understanding of cardiovascular disease.

EXAMPLE

The Framingham Study (10) was begun in 1949 to identify factors associated with an increased risk of coronary heart disease (CHD). A representative sample of 5,209 men and women, aged 30–59, was selected from approximately 10,000 persons of that age living in Framingham, a small town near Boston. Of these, 5,127 were free of CHD when first examined and, therefore, were at risk of developing CHD. These people were reexamined biennially for evidence of coronary disease. The study ran for 30 years and now continues with the Framingham Offspring Study. (11) It demonstrated that the risk of developing CHD is associated with elevated blood pressure, high serum cholesterol, cigarette smoking, glucose intolerance, and left ventricular hypertrophy. There was a large difference in risk of CHD between those with none and those with all of these risk factors.

Prospective and Historical Cohort Studies

Cohort studies can be conducted in two ways (Figure 5.4). The cohort can be assembled in the present and followed into the future (a **prospective cohort study**), or it can be identified from past records and followed forward from that time up to the present (a **historical cohort study** or **retrospective cohort study**). The Framingham Study described is an example of a prospective cohort study. The decision to conduct the study was made before the cohort was assembled. Useful retrospective cohort studies are sometimes possible with large databases.

EXAMPLE

The incidence of autism increased sharply in the 1990s, coinciding with an increasing use of vaccination of young children for measles, mumps, and rubella (MMR). A report linking MMR vaccination and autism. In several children caused widespread alarm that vaccination (or the vaccine preservative, thimerosal) was responsible for the increasing incidence of autism. In some countries, MMR vaccination among young children dropped, resulting in new outbreaks and even deaths due to measles. Because of the seriousness of the situation, several studies were done to evaluate MMR vaccine as a possible risk factor. In Denmark, a retrospective cohort study included all children (537,303) born from January 1991 through December 1998. The investigators reviewed the children's country-wide health records and determined that 82% received the MMR vaccine (physicians must report vaccinations to the government in order to receive payment); 316 children were diagnosed with autism, and another 422

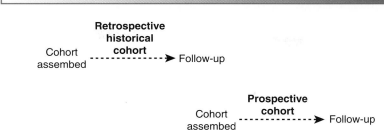

FIGURE 5.4 ▦ Retrospective and prospective cohort studies. Prospective cohorts are assembled in the present and followed forward into the future. In contrast, retrospective cohorts are made by going back into the past and assembling the cohort, such as from medical records, then following the group forward to the present.

with autistic-spectrum disorders. The frequency of autism among children who had been vaccinated was similar (in fact, slightly less) to that among children not receiving MMR vaccine. (12) This, along with other studies, provided strong evidence against the suggestion that MMR vaccine causes autism.

Case-Cohort Studies

With the increasing availability of computerized medical databases, another approach, the **case-cohort design**, takes advantage of the ability to determine the frequency of a given medical condition in a large group of people. In a case-cohort study, all exposed people are included in the study and followed for some outcome of interest. However, only a small random sample of unexposed people is studied. For efficiency, the group of unexposed people is "enriched" with those who subsequently suffer the outcome of interest. The results are then adjusted to reflect the sampling fractions used to obtain the sample. This efficient approach to a cohort study requires that frequencies of outcomes be determined in the entire group of unexposed people; thus, the need for a large, computerized, medical database.

▰ E X A M P L E

Does prophylactic mastectomy protect women who are at increased risk for breast cancer? A case-cohort study was done to examine this question in six health maintenance organizations, all of which had computerized databases of diagnoses and surgical procedures on their members. Investigators identified all women who underwent bilateral

prophylactic mastectomy over a number of years (276 women) and followed them forward over time to determine whether or not they developed breast cancer. For the comparison group, the investigators randomly sampled a similar group of women not undergoing the procedure and enriched the sample with women who subsequently developed breast cancer. "Enrichment" was accomplished by knowing who among 666,800 eligible women developed breast cancer—through examination of the computerized database. For example, the investigators randomly sampled about 1% of comparison women of a certain age who developed breast cancer, but only about .01% of women who did not. Adjustments for the sampling fractions were then made during the analysis. The results showed that bilateral prophylactic mastectomy was associated with a 99% reduction in breast cancer among women at higher risk. (13)

Advantages and Disadvantages of Cohort Studies

Most of the advantages and disadvantages of cohort studies discussed on the next page apply whether the study is prospective or historical. However, the potential for difficulties with the quality of data is different for the two. In prospective studies, data can be collected specifically for the purposes of the study and with full anticipation of what is needed. It is thereby possible to avoid biases that might undermine the accuracy of the data. On the other hand, data for historical cohorts are often gathered for other purposes—usually as part of medical records for patient care. Except for carefully selected questions, such as the relationship between vaccination and autism, the data in historical cohort studies may not be of sufficient quality for rigorous research.

Some of the advantages and disadvantages of cohort studies, for the purpose of describing risk factors, are summarized in Table 5.2. Cohort studies of risk are the best available substitutes for a true experiment when experimentation is not possible. They follow the same logic as a clinical trial and they allow measurement of exposure to a possible risk factor while avoiding any possibility of bias that might occur if exposure were determined after the outcome was already known.

The principal disadvantage is that when the outcome is infrequent, which is usually the case in studies of risk, a large number of people must be entered in a study and remain under observation for a long time before results are available. Having to measure exposure in many people, even though few get the disease, is inefficient. For example, the Framingham Study of cardiovascular disease (the most common cause of death in America) was the largest study of its kind when it began. Nevertheless, more than 5,000 people had to be followed for several years before the first, preliminary conclusions could be published. Only 5% of the people had experienced a coronary event during the first 8 years.

Another problem with prospective cohort studies results from the people under study usually being "free living" and not under the control of researchers. A great deal of effort and money must be expended to keep track of them. Cohort studies of risk, therefore, are expensive, usually costing many millions of dollars.

Because of the time and money required for cohort studies, this approach cannot be used for all clinical questions about risk. For practical reasons,

the cohort approach has been reserved for only the most important questions. This has led to efforts to find more efficient, yet dependable, ways of assessing risk. The most common of these, case-control studies, is discussed in Chapter 6.

The most important scientific disadvantage of observational studies, including cohort studies, is that they are subject to a great many more potential biases than are experiments. People who are exposed to a certain risk factor in the natural course of events are likely to differ in a great many ways from a comparison group of people not exposed to the factor. If some of these other differences are also related to the disease in question, they could account for any association observed between the putative risk factor and the disease.

This leads to the main challenge of observational studies: to deal with extraneous differences between exposed and nonexposed groups so as to mimic as closely as possible an experiment. The differences are considered "extraneous" from the point of view of someone trying to determine cause-and-effect relationships. The following example illustrates one approach to handling such differences.

EXAMPLE

Although aspirin use has been found to be protective against cardiovascular disease and against death in the setting of acute myocardial infarction, the effect of long-term aspirin use on all-cause mortality is less clear. Investigators therefore undertook a study among patients referred for stress echocardiography, to determine whether those who regularly used aspirin were at differ-

---

TABLE 5.2 ■ Advantages and Disadvantages of Cohort Studies

Advantages	Disadvantages
The only way of establishing incidence (i.e., absolute risk) directly	Inefficient because many more subjects must be enrolled than experience the event of interest; therefore, cannot be used for rare diseases
Follows the same logic as the clinical question: If persons are exposed, do they get the disease?	Expensive because of resources necessary to study many people over time
Exposure can be elicited without the bias that might occur if outcome were already known	Results not available for a long time
Can assess the relationship between exposure and many diseases	Assesses the relationship between disease and exposure to only relatively few factors (i.e., those recorded at the outset of the study)

ent risk of subsequent death than those not using aspirin. During 3 years of follow-up, aspirin users died as often as nonusers. However, aspirin users were sicker and at higher risk for death. By examining the demographic and clinical characteristics of patients, the investigators developed scores that predicted whether a patient would be using aspirin ("propensity scores"). The investigators then matched each aspirin user to a non-aspirin user with the same propensity score. Aspirin use was associated with 50% fewer deaths. (14) The use of propensity scores and matching produced two groups of similar patients except for the exposure of interest (aspirin use) and dealt with extraneous differences that were confounding the results.

Major biases in observational studies and ways of dealing them are described in Chapter 7.

WAYS TO EXPRESS AND COMPARE RISK

The basic expression of risk is **incidence**, defined in Chapter 4 as the number of new cases of disease arising during a given period of time in a defined population that is initially free of the condition. In cohort studies, the incidence of disease is compared in two or more groups that differ in exposure to a possible risk factor. To compare risks, several measures of the association between exposure and disease, called **measures of effect**, are commonly used. These measures represent different concepts of risk and are used for different purposes. Four measures of effect are discussed below. Table 5.3 summarizes the four, along with absolute risk, and Table 5.4 demonstrates their use with the example of lung cancer.

Absolute Risk

Absolute risk is the probability of an event in a population under study. Its value is the same as that for incidence, and the terms are often used interchangeably. Absolute risk is the best way for individual patients and clinicians to understand how risk factors may affect their lives. Thus, as Table 5.4 shows, although smoking greatly increases the chances of dying from lung cancer, among smokers the absolute risk of dying from lung cancer each year is about 1 in 1,000.

Attributable Risk

One might ask, "What is the additional risk (incidence) of disease following exposure, over and above that experienced by people who are not exposed?" The answer is expressed as **attributable risk**, the ab-

---

TABLE 5.3 ▦ Measures of Effect

Expression	Question	Definition[a]
Absolute risk	What is the incidence of disease in a group initially free of the condition?	$I = \dfrac{\text{\# new cases over a given period of time}}{\text{\# people in the group}}$
Attributable risk (risk difference)	What is the incidence of disease attributable to exposure?	$AR = I_E - I_{\bar{E}}$
Relative risk (risk ratio)	How many times more likely are exposed persons to become diseased, relative to nonexposed persons?	$RR = \dfrac{I_E}{I_{\bar{E}}}$
Population-attributable risk	What is the incidence of disease in a population, associated with the prevalence of a risk factor?	$AR_P = AR \times P$
Population-attributable fraction	What fraction of disease in a population is attributable to exposure to a risk factor?	$AF_P = \dfrac{AR_P}{I_T}$

[a] Where I_E = incidence in exposed persons; $I_{\bar{E}}$ = incidence in nonexposed persons; P = prevalence of exposure to a risk factor; and I_T = total incidence of disease in a population

TABLE 5.4 ■ **Calculating Measures of Effect: Cigarette Smoking and Death from Lung Cancer** [a]

Simple risks

Death rate (absolute risk) from lung cancer in nonsmokers	0.96/1000/year
Death rate (absolute risk) cancer in cigarette smokers	0.07/1000/year
Prevalence of cigarette smoking	56%
Total death rate from lung cancer	0.56/1000/year

Compared risks

Attributable risk = 0.96/1000/year − 0.07/1000/year
　　　　　　　= 0.89/1000/year

Relative risk = 0.96/1000/year ÷ 0.07/1000/year
　　　　　　= 13.7

Population − attributable risk = 0.89/1000/year × 0.56
　　　　　　　　　　　　　= 0.50/1000/year

Population − attributable fraction = 0.50/1000/year ÷ 0.56/1000/year
　　　　　　　　　　　　　　= 0.89

[a] Estimated data from Doll R, Hill AB. Mortality in relation to smoking: ten year's observation of British doctors. Br Med J 1964;1:1399–1410 and 1460–1467.

solute risk (or incidence) of disease in exposed persons minus the absolute risk in nonexposed persons. In Table 5.4 the attributable risk of lung cancer death in smokers is 0.89 per 1000. Attributable risk is the additional incidence of disease related to exposure, taking into account the background incidence of disease from other causes. Note that this way of comparing rates implies that the risk factor is a cause and not just a marker. Because of the way it is calculated, attributable risk is also called **risk difference**, the differences between two absolute risks.

Relative Risk

On the other hand, one might ask, "How many times are exposed persons more likely to get the disease relative to nonexposed persons?" To answer this question, **relative risk** or **risk ratio**, is the ratio of incidence in exposed persons to incidence in nonexposed persons. Relative risk (or an estimate of relative risk, odds ratios, taken up in Chapter 6) is the most commonly reported result in studies of risk, partly because of its computational convenience but also because it is a common metric in studies of similar risk factors but with different baseline incidence rates. Because relative risk indicates the strength of the association between exposure and disease, it is a

useful measure of effect for studies of disease etiology.

Relative risk says nothing about the magnitude of the attributable risk, which depends on absolute as well as relative risk. For example, although a large European study found that use of oral contraceptives increased the risk of acute myocardial infarction among nonsmoking women, about fourfold regardless of age, the estimated attributable risk rose from about 4 per 100,000 woman years in those younger than 35 years to more than 40 per 100,000 woman years in those 35 years and older. (15) This finding corroborates the reality that myocardial infarctions in young women are rare and the incidence rises with age, regardless of the use of oral contraceptives. Even with a large relative risk, the attributable risk might be quite small if the disease is uncommon (as demonstrated with smoking and lung cancer in Table 5.4).

Interpreting Estimates of Individual Risk

The clinical meaning attached to absolute and attributable risk, on the one hand, and relative risk, on the other, is often quite different, because these expressions of risk stand for entirely different concepts. The appropriate expression of risk depends on what question is being asked.

Risk factors for cardiovascular disease are generally thought to be weaker among the elderly than the middle-aged. This belief was examined by comparing the absolute, relative, and attributable risks of common risk factors for cardiovascular disease among different age groups. (16) An example is the risk of stroke from smoking (Table 5.5). The relative risk decreases with age, from 4.0 in persons aged 45 to 49 to 1.4 in persons aged 65 to 69. However, absolute and attributable risks increase slightly with age, mainly because stroke is more common in the elderly regardless of smoking status. Thus, the causal link between smoking and stroke decreases with age, but an elderly individual who smokes increases his or her actual risk of stroke even more than a younger person.

In most clinical situations, it is clearest simply to state the absolute risk—typically, for exposed and not exposed people. Because attributable risk represents the additional probability of disease in those exposed, it is a more meaningful expression of risk for individuals than is relative risk. On the other hand, relative risk is more useful for expressing the strength of a causal relationship.

Population Risk

Another way of looking at risk is to ask, "How much does a risk factor contribute to the overall rates of disease in groups of people, rather than individuals?"

This information is useful for deciding which risk factors are particularly important and which are trivial to the overall health of a community. This can inform those in policy positions about how to choose priorities for the deployment of health-care resources. If a relatively weak risk factor is very prevalent in a community, it could account for more disease than a very strong, but rare, risk factor.

To estimate population risk, it is necessary to take into account the frequency with which members of a community are exposed to a risk factor. **Population-attributable risk** is the product of the attributable risk and the prevalence of exposure to the risk factor in a population. It measures the excess incidence of disease in a community that is associated with a risk factor. One can also describe the fraction of disease occurrence in a population associated with a particular risk factor, the **population-attributable fraction.** It is obtained by dividing the population-attributable risk by the total incidence of disease in the population.

Figure 5.5 illustrates how the prevalence of a risk factor determines the relationship between individual and population risk. In the figure (A), the attributable risk of death according to diastolic blood pressure can be seen. Risk increases with increasing blood pressure. However, few people have extremely high blood pressure (B). When hypertension is defined as having a diastolic blood pressure >90 mm Hg, most hypertensive people are just over 90 mm Hg, and very few are in the highest category (≥115 mm Hg). As a result, the greatest percentage of excess deaths in the population (58.4%) is attributable to lower levels of hypertension, 90–105 mm Hg (see C). Paradoxically, then, physicians could save more lives with effective treatment of lower, rather than higher, levels of hypertension. This fact, so counterintuitive to clinical thinking, has been termed "the prevention paradox." (17)

Measures of population risk are less frequently encountered in the clinical literature than are measures of absolute, attributable, and relative risks. But a particular clinical practice is as much a population for the doctor as is a community for health policymakers. Also, how the prevalence of exposure affects community risk can be important in the care of individual patients. For instance, when patients cannot give a history or when exposure is difficult for them to recognize, physicians depend on the usual prevalence of exposure to estimate the likelihood of various

TABLE 5.5 ■ Comparing Relative Risk and Attributable Risk in the Relationship of Smoking, Stroke, and Age[a]				
	Incidence (Absolute risk per 1000)			
Age	Non-smokers	Smokers	Relative Risk	Attributable Risk
45–49	7.4	29.7	4.0	22.3
50–54	17.2	37.0	2.2	19.8
55–59	27.9	64.7	2.3	36.7
60–64	47.4	76.9	1.6	29.5
65–69	80.2	110.4	1.4	30.2

[a] Adapted from Psaty BM, Koepsell TD, Manolio TA, Longstreth WT, Wagner EH, Wahl PW, et al. Risk ratios and risk differences in estimating the effect of risk factors for cardiovascular disease in the elderly. J Clin Epidemiol 1990;43:961–970.

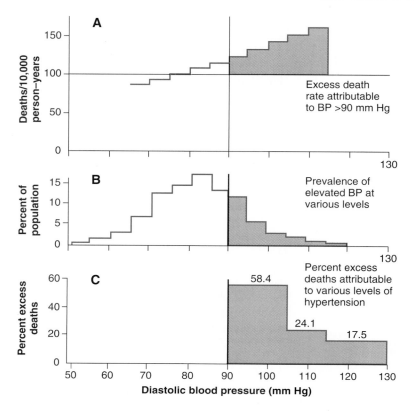

FIGURE   5.5 ■ Relationships among attributable risk, prevalence of risk factor, and population risk for hypertension. Although the attributable risk for death (excess death) increases as blood pressure levels increase, most excess deaths caused by hypertension are due to modest blood pressure elevation because mild hypertension is much more prevalent than severe hypertension. (Adapted from The Hypertension Detection and Follow-Up Cooperative Group. Mild hypertensives in the hypertension detection and follow-up program. Ann N Y Acad Sci 1978; 304:254–266.)

diseases. When considering treatable causes of cirrhosis in a North American patient, for example, it would be more useful to consider alcohol than schistosomes, inasmuch as few North Americans are exposed to *Schistosoma mansoni*. Of course, one might take a very different stance in the Nile delta, where schistosomiasis are prevalent, and the people, who are mostly Muslims, rarely drink alcohol.

REVIEW QUESTIONS

Questions 5.1 to 5.9 are based on the following example:

Deep venous thrombosis (DVT) is a serious condition that occasionally can lead to pulmonary embolism and death. (18) The incidence of DVT is increased with the use of oral contraceptives (OC). In 1993, a genetic mutation, Factor V Leiden, was identified as causing a hereditary prothrombin condition associated with DVT. Heterozygotes have 4 to 10 times— and homozygotes have 50 to 100 times—the risk of

DVT of the general population. These two risk factors, OC and Factor V Leiden, interact. In women without the genetic mutation, incidence of DVT rises from about 0.8/10,000 women/year among those not on OC to 3.0/10,000 women/year for those taking the pill. The baseline incidence of DVT in heterozygotes for Factor V Leiden is 5.7/10,000 women/year, rising to 28.5/10,000 women/year among those taking OC. Mutations for Factor V Leiden occur in about 5% of whites but are absent in Africans and Asians.

For questions 5.1 to 5.6, select the one best answer for each group of women described.

A. 7.1/10,000/year
B. 5.7/10,000/year
C. 28.5/10,000/year
D. 35.6/10,000/year
E. 0.8/10,000/year
F. 3.8/10,000/year
G. 3.0/10,000/year
H. 9.5/10,000/year
I. 4.7/10,000/year
J. 4.4/10,000/year

____ **5.1.** Absolute risk of DVT in women who neither have the mutation nor take OC.

____ **5.2.** Absolute risk of DVT in women who do not have the mutation but take OC.

____ **5.3.** Absolute risk of DVT in women who are heterozygous for the mutation but do not take OC.

____ **5.4.** Risk of DVT in women who are heterozygous for the mutation and take OC, relative to women without the mutation who take OC.

____ **5.5.** Risk of DVT in women who take OC but do not have the mutation, relative to those without the mutation who do not take OC.

____ **5.6.** Risk of DVT in women who are heterozygous for the mutation but do not take OC, relative to those without the mutation who do not take OC.

In a population with 100,000 white women, all of whom take OC, calculate:

5.7. The difference in risk for women who are heterozygous for Factor V Leiden and those without the mutation.

5.8. The population-attributable risk for DVT in women who are heterozygous for Factor Leiden V.

Answer the following question and give your reasoning:

5.9. Would you prescribe an oral contraceptive to a woman who was known to be heterozygous for a Factor V Leiden mutation? Why or why not?

Circle the best response.

5.10. All of the following statements are true about both prospective and retrospective cohort studies except:

A. They measure incidence of disease directly.

B. They allow assessment of possible associations between exposure and many diseases.

C. They allow investigators to decide beforehand what data to collect.

D. They avoid bias that might occur if measurement of exposure is made after the outcome of interest is known.

Answers are in Appendix A.

REFERENCES

1. Weiss NS, Liff JM. Accounting for the multicausal nature of disease in the design and analysis of epidemiologic studies. Am J Epidemiol 1983;117:14–18.
2. Vineis P, Alavanja M, Buffler P, Fontham E, Franceschi S, Gao YT, et al. Tobacco and cancer: recent epidemiological evidence. J Natl Cancer Inst 2004;96:99–106.
3. Guntheroth WG, Spiers PS. Sleeping prone and the risk of sudden infant death syndrome. JAMA 1992; 267:2359–2362.
4. Willinger M, Hoffman HJ, Wu KT, Hou JR, Kessler RC, Ward SL, et al. Factors associated with the transition to nonprone sleep positions of infants in the United States: The National Infant Sleep Position Study. JAMA 1998;280:329–335.
5. Boyd NF, Stone J, Vogt KN, Connelly BS, Martin LJ, Minkin S. Dietary fat and breast cancer risk revisited: A meta-analysis of the published literature. Br J Cancer 2003;89:1672–1685.
6. Ridker PM, Hennekens CH, Buring JE, Rifal N. C-reactive protein and other markers of inflammation in the prediction of cardiovascular disease in women. N Engl J Med 2000;342:836–843.
7. Wallin KL, Wiklund F, Luostarinen T, Angstrom T, Anttila T, Bergman F, et al. A population-based prospective study of *Chlamydia trachomatis* infection and cervical carcinoma. Int J Cancer 2002;101: 371–374.
8. Rose G. Sick individuals and sick populations. Int J Epidemiol 1985;14:32–38.
9. Diamond GA, Forrester JS. Analysis of probability as an aid in the clinical diagnosis of coronary-artery disease. N Engl J Med 1979;300:1350–1358.
10. Dawber TR. The Framingham Study: The Epidemiology of Atherosclerotic Disease. Cambridge, MA: Harvard University Press, 1980.
11. Kannel WB, Feinleib M, McNamara PM, Garrison RJ, Castelli WP. An investigation of coronary heart disease in families. The Framingham Offspring Study. Am J Epidemiol 1979;110:281–290.
12. Madsen KM, Hviid A, Vestergaard M, Schendel D, Wohlfahrt J, Thorsen P, et al. A population-based study of measles, mumps, and rubella vaccination and autism. N Engl J Med 2002;347:1477–1482.
13. Geiger AM, Yu O, Herrinton LJ, Barlow WE (on behalf of the CRN PROTECTS Group). A case-cohort

study of bilateral prophylactic mastectomy efficacy in community practices. Am J Epidemiol 2004;159: S99.

14. Gum P, Thamilarasan M, Watanabe J, Blackstone EH, Lauer MS. Aspirin use and all-cause mortality among patients being evaluated for known or suspected coronary artery disease: A propensity analysis. JAMA 2001;286:1187–1194.

15. WHO Collaborative Study of Cardiovascular Disease and Steroid Hormone Contraception. Acute myocardial infarction and combined oral contraceptives: results of an international multicentre case-control study. Lancet 1997;349:1202–1209.

16. Psaty BM, Koepsell TD, Manolio TA, Longstreth WT, Wagner EH, Wahl PW, et al. Risk ratios and risk differences in estimating the effect of risk factors for cardiovascular disease in the elderly. J Clin Epidemiol 1990;43:961–970.

17. Hofman A, Vandenbroucke JP. Geoffrey Rose's big idea. Br Med J 1992;305:1519–1520.

18. Vandenbroucke JP, Rosing J, Bloemenkemp KW, Middleidorp S, Helmerhorst FM, Bouma BN, et al. Rosendaal FR. Oral contraceptives and the risk of venous thombosis. N Engl J Med 2001;20:1527–1535.

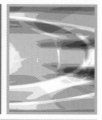

Risk: Looking Backward

KEY WORDS

Latency period
Case-control study
Retrospective studies
Control

Population-based case-
  control studies
Nested case-control study
Matching
Overmatching

Recall bias
Odds ratio
Estimated relative risk
Framing

I shall propose nothing dictated merely from theory; but shall confirm all by experience and facts, the surest and most unerring guides.

—James Lind, 1753

Cohort studies are a wonderfully logical and direct way of studying risk, but they have practical limitations. Most chronic diseases take a long time to develop. The **latency period**, or the period of time between exposure to a risk factor and the expression of its pathologic effects, is measured in decades for most chronic diseases. For example, smoking precedes coronary disease, lung cancer, and chronic bronchitis by 20 or more years, and osteoporosis with fractures occurs in the elderly because of diet and exercise patterns throughout life. Also, relatively few people in a cohort develop the outcome of interest, even though it is necessary to measure exposure in, and to follow-up, all members of the cohort. The result is that cohort studies of risk require a lot of time and effort, not to mention money, to get an answer. The situation is even worse when the disease is uncommon.

Some of these limitations can be overcome by making modifications to cohort methods, such as retrospective cohort or case-cohort designs, described in the preceding chapter. In this chapter, we describe another way of studying the relationship between a potential risk (or protective) factor and disease more efficiently: case-control studies. This approach has two main advantages over cohort studies. First, it is more efficient because it bypasses the need to collect data on a large number of people, most of whom do not get the disease. Second, it is faster. It is not necessary to wait from measurement of exposure until effects occur.

But efficiency and timeliness come at a cost: Managing bias is a more difficult and sometimes uncertain task in case-control studies. Also, these studies produce only an estimate of relative risk and no direct information on the other measures of effect such as absolute risk, attributable risk, and population risks that were described in the preceding chapter.

The respective advantages and disadvantages of cohort, case-control, and prevalence studies are summarized in Table 6.1.

Despite the drawbacks, the trade-off between scientific strength and feasibility is often worthwhile. Indeed, case-control studies are indispensable for studying risk for very uncommon diseases.

E X A M P L E

It has long been suspected that phenylpropanolamine, a constituent of appetite suppressants and cough and cold remedies, might cause hemorrhagic stroke, especially in young women. However, hemorrhagic stroke is quite uncommon; the rate is 0.6 per million women age 35 to 54 years per day. If the risk of phenylpropanolamine were studied in a cohort, hundreds of millions of women-days would have to be accumulated to observe just a few hundred cases, which would be barely enough to detect even a large relative risk with statistical confidence. A case-control study overcame this problem. The investigators identified 702 patients with hemorrhagic stroke in 43 U.S. hospitals and twice as many controls in the same areas as cases. The study was able to estimate the relative risk of stroke in women taking appetite suppressants containing phenylpropanolomaine, which was about 16. (1)

The case-control method was first made explicit around 1960. By the 1990s, this method comprised several percent of clinical research articles in major medical journals. (2)

This chapter is titled "Risk: Looking Backward" because case-control studies involve looking backward from disease to exposure, in contrast to cohort studies, which look forward from exposure to disease.

CASE-CONTROL STUDIES

The basic design of a **case-control study** is diagrammed in Figure 6.1. Two samples are selected: patients who have developed the disease in question and otherwise similar people who have not developed the disease. The researchers then look backward in time to measure the frequency of exposure to a possible risk factor in the two groups. For this reason, case-control studies are sometimes called **retrospective studies**, which should not be confused with retrospective cohort studies (described in the preceding chapter). The resulting data can be used to estimate the relative risk of disease related to the possible risk factor.

TABLE 6.1 ■ Summary of Characteristics of Cohort, Case-Control, and Prevalence Designs

Cohort	Case-Control	Prevalence
Begins with a defined population at risk	Population at risk may be undefined	Begins with a defined population
Cases not selected but ascertained by surveillance	Cases selected by investigator from an available pool of patients	Cases not selected but ascertained by a single examination of the population
Controls, the comparison group (i.e., noncases), not selected—they evolve naturally	Controls selected by investigator to resemble cases	Noncases include those free of disease at the single examination
Exposure measured before the development of disease	Exposure measured, reconstructed, or recollected after development of disease	Exposure measured, at the same time as disease
Risk or incidence of disease and relative risk measured directly	Risk or incidence of disease cannot be measured directly: Relative risk of exposure can be estimated by the odds ratio	Risk or incidence of disease cannot be measured directly: Relative risk of exposure can be estimated by the odds ratio

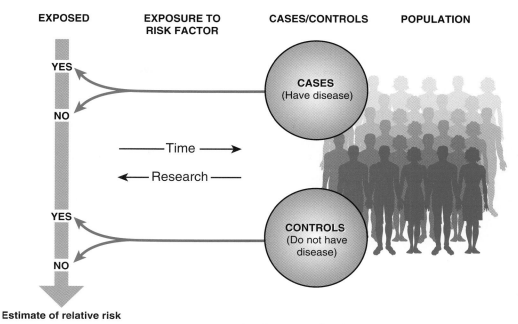

EXPOSED   EXPOSURE TO   CASES/CONTROLS   POPULATION
                 RISK FACTOR

YES

        CASES
        (Have disease)

NO

          → Time →

          ← Research ←

YES

        CONTROLS
        (Do not have
        disease)

NO

Estimate of relative risk

FIGURE 6.1 ▪ Design of case-control studies.

EXAMPLE

Does habitual, vigorous physical activity protect against primary cardiac arrest in people without apparent heart disease? Investigators in Seattle conducted a case-control study to answer this question. (3) How was it done? (See Figure 6.2.)

First, the investigators obtained a sample of cases of primary cardiac arrest, which is cardiac arrest without an apparent antecedent cause such as sepsis or trauma, arising in a defined population. The existence of an emergency medical information system in Seattle made this possible. Cases were selected from 1,250 people living in Seattle and suburban King County, Washington, who had suffered out-of-hospital primary cardiac arrest during a defined period of time. Paramedics attended nearly all instances of primary cardiac arrest in the area at the time, so their records included most cases in the population.

Second, the investigators needed controls that were otherwise similar but had not had primary cardiac arrest. Controls were selected by dialing randomly selected telephone numbers in the same area; most people in the area had telephones in their homes. Cases and controls had to meet the same criteria for entry: be 25 to 75 years of age, have no clinically recognizable heart disease, have had no prior disease that limited activity; and have a spouse who could provide information about habitual exercise (the exposure of interest). In summary, entry criteria sought to ensure that cases and controls were members of the same base population and had similar opportunities to engage in physical activity. In addition, controls were matched to cases on age, sex, and urban or suburban residence.

Third, the investigators needed a reliable measure of exposure—in this case, habitual exercise. Spouses of both cases and controls were asked about leisure-time activity. In the subset of patients with primary cardiac arrest who survived, it was possible to ask cases themselves about their own exercise patterns to check the validity of spouses' reports.

In this study, based on 163 eligible cases and controls, the estimated relative risk of primary cardiac arrest was 62% lower in persons at the highest level of high-intensity, leisure-time activity compared with sedentary people.

The word **control** comes up in other situations, too. It is used in experimental studies to refer to people, as well as animals, cell lines, and genetic material, that have not gotten the study intervention. In diagnostic laboratories, controls refer to specimens that have a known amount of the mate-

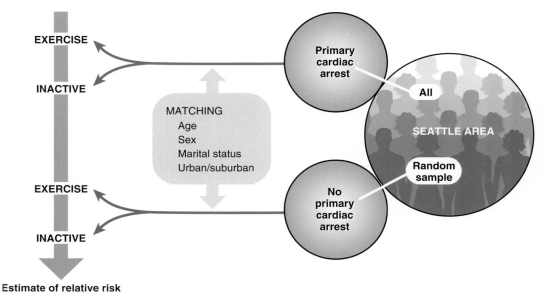

FIGURE 6.2 ■ A case-control study of exercise and risk of sudden death. (From Siscovick DS, Weiss NS, Hall-strom AP, Inui TS, Peterson DR. Physical activity and primary cardiac arrest. JAMA 1982;248:3113–3117.)

rial being tested. As a verb, *control* is used to describe the process of taking into account, neutralizing, or subtracting the effects of variables that are extraneous to the main question. Here, the term is used in the context of case-control studies.

DESIGN OF CASE-CONTROL STUDIES

The validity of case-control studies depends on the care with which cases and controls are selected, how exposure is measured, and how extraneous variables are controlled for.

Selecting Cases

The cases in case-control research should be new (incident) cases, not existing (prevalent) ones. The reasons are based on the concepts discussed in Chapter 4. The prevalence of a disease at a point in time is a function of both the incidence and duration of that disease. Duration is in turn determined by the rate at which patients leave the disease state (because of recovery or death) or persist in it (because of a slow course or successful palliation). It follows from these relationships that risk factors for prevalent disease may be risk factors for incidence, duration, or both; the relative contributions of the two cannot be determined. As an

illustration, if prevalent cases were studied, an exposure that causes a rapidly lethal form of the disease would lower the proportion of prevalent cases that are exposed, reducing in relative risk and thereby suggesting that exposure is less harmful than it really is or even that it is protective.

At best, the study should include all the cases or a representative sample of all cases that arise in a defined population. For example, the study of exercise and primary cardiac arrest included all cases arising in the Seattle area who met entry criteria. In this way, one can be assured that the cases are not atypical examples of either disease or exposure because of where and how they happened to be found. Referral centers, because of the reputation of their staff and facilities, may attract particularly severe or atypical cases or those with unusual exposures—the wrong sample if the underlying research question in case-control studies is about ordinary occurrences of disease and exposures. The following is an example of a case-control study based on a national sample.

EXAMPLE

Is vasectomy a risk factor for prostate cancer? Several studies have suggested that it might be, although none was especially strong, and the hypothesis is biologically implausible. Investigators in New Zealand addressed this question in a national sample. Cases were all of the 3,186 men developing prostate cancer during a 34-month period, and all were identified from a national cancer registry. Controls were identified from the general electoral roll and matched to cases by age. Cases and controls were interviewed by telephone to establish whether they had had a vasectomy. There was no association between vasectomy and prostate cancer; the estimated relative risk was 0.92. (4)

Some case-control studies, especially older ones, have identified cases in hospitals and referral centers where uncommon diseases are most likely to be found. This way of choosing cases is convenient, but it raises validity problems. Not only might the cases be unusual, but also it is difficult in this situation to be confident that controls, however they are chosen, are truly similar to cases in all ways other than exposure, which is critical to the validity of this kind of study (see Selecting Controls section below). Fortunately, it is rarely necessary to take this scientific risk these days because there are many databases that make true population sampling possible.

However the cases may be identified, it should be possible for them to be exposed to the risk factor and to experience the outcome. For example, in the study of exercise and sudden death, cases and controls had to be able to exercise to a similar degree to be eligible.

It goes without saying that diagnosis should be rigorously confirmed for cases (and excluded for controls), and the criteria made explicit. In the exercise study, cases of sudden and unexpected death from causes other than suspected heart disease, such as trauma, drug overdose, or respiratory arrest, were excluded based on information in the paramedics' reports. Other causes of sudden death, for example, subarachnoid hemorrhage and ruptured abdominal aortic aneurysm, were also excluded after examination of death certificates.

Selecting Controls

The validity of a case-control study depends above all on the comparability of cases and controls. They are comparable if the controls would have been cases who had developed the condition under study. In other words, to be comparable, cases and controls should be members of the same base population and have an equal opportunity of being exposed.

The Population Approach

The best approach to meeting these requirements is to ensure that controls are a random sample of all noncases in the same population that produced the cases, such as the approach used in the study of exercise and primary cardiac arrest (Figure 6.2). Studies in which cases and controls are a complete or probability sample of a defined population are called **population-based case-control studies**. In the primary cardiac arrest study, controls were selected by dialing random telephone numbers in the same area as the cases were identified. This sample approximated a random sample of the same population because nearly everyone in the area had a telephone.

Another way to ensure that cases and controls are comparable is to draw them from the same cohort. In this situation, the study is said to be a **nested case-control study** (it is "nested" in the cohort). An advantage of this approach, relative to simply analyzing the data as a cohort study, is that analyses are more efficient. In the cohort analysis, all people in the cohort (exposed and nonexposed) would be included in a follow-up study, although relatively few of them will get the disease. Nested case-control studies are similar to population-based cohort studies except that, in the latter, cases and controls are entering and leaving the population continually.

Cases and controls should meet the same criteria for inclusion in the study. In the primary cardiac arrest example,

1. Both were in the same age range, because the very young are more likely to have atypical causes and the very old have age itself as a dominant risk factor.
2. Neither had a history of heart disease; the study was of "primary" cardiac arrest, which is the first manifestation of heart disease.
3. Neither had other diseases that prevented them from exercising, so that they could be exposed.
4. Both had a spouse, so that a comparable history of exposure could be obtained.
5. Both lived in the same study area.

If different criteria for cases and controls were allowed, systematic differences between them, other than for exposure, might have accounted for any differences found. That is, the exposure-disease relationship might have been confounded.

Hospital and Community Controls

If population- or cohort-based sampling is not possible, a fallback position would be to select controls in such a way that the selection *seems* to produce controls that are comparable to cases. For example, if cases are selected from a hospital ward, the controls would be selected from patients with different diseases, apparently unrelated to the exposure and disease of interest, in the same hospital. Studying people in health-care settings is more fallible than population- or cohort-based sampling because hospitalized patients are usually a biased sample of all people in the community, the people to whom the results should apply.

Another approach is to obtain controls from the community served by the hospital. However, many hospitals do not draw patients exclusively from the surrounding community—some people in the community go to other hospitals, and some people in other communities pass up their own neighborhood hospital to go to the study hospital. As a result, cases and controls may be substantially different in ways that distort the exposure-disease relationship.

Multiple Control Groups

If none of the available control groups seems ideal, one can see how choice of controls affects results by selecting several control groups with apparently complementary scientific strengths and weaknesses. Typically, one group of controls is selected from the same institution and another from the community. If similar estimates of relative risk are obtained using different control groups, this is evidence against bias because it is unlikely that the same biases would affect otherwise dissimilar groups in the same direction and to the same extent. If the estimates of relative risks are different, it is a signal that one or both are biased, and an opportunity exists to investigate where the bias lies.

EXAMPLE

In a case-control study of estrogen and endometrial cancer, cases were identified from a single teaching hospital. Two control groups were selected: one from among gynecologic admissions to the same hospital and the second from a random sample of women living in the area served by the hospital. Other diseases such as hypertension, diabetes, and gallbladder disease, were much more common among the cases and in the hospital control group, which presumably reflected the various forces that led to hospitalization. Despite these differences, the two control groups reported much less long-term estrogen use than did the cases and yielded very similar estimates of relative risk (4.1 and 3.6). The authors concluded that "this consistency of results with two very different comparison groups suggests that neither is significantly biased and that the results . . . are reasonably accurate." (5)

Multiple Controls per Case

Having several control groups per case group should not be confused with having several controls per case. If the number of cases is limited, as is often true with rare diseases, the study can provide more information when there is more than one control per case. More controls produce a gain in the ability to detect an increase or decrease in risk if it exists, a property of a study called "statistical power" (see Chapter 10). As a practical matter, the gain is worthwhile up to about three or four controls per case, after which little is gained by including more controls.

Matching

If some characteristics seem especially strongly related to either exposure or disease, such that one would want to be sure that they are comparable in cases and controls, they can be matched. With **matching**, for each case with a set of characteristics, one or more controls that possess the same characteristics are selected. Researchers commonly match for age, sex, and residence because these are frequently related to both exposure and disease. But matching often extends beyond these demographic characteristics when other factors are known to be strongly associated with disease risk.

Matching increases the useful information obtainable from a set of cases and controls because it reduces differences between groups in determinants of disease other than the one being considered, and thereby supports a more powerful (sensitive) test of association. But matching carries a risk. If the investigator happens to match on a factor that is itself related to the exposure under study, there is an increased chance that the matched case and control will have the same history of exposure. For example, in a study of non-steroidal, anti-inflammatory drugs (NSAIDs) and renal failure, if cases and controls were matched for the presence of arthritic symptoms, which are commonly treated with NSAIDs, more matched pairs would have the same history of NSAID use. This process, called **overmatching**, can bias the study toward finding no effect and so diminish the ability of a study to detect an increased or decreased estimated relative risk.

Measuring Exposure

The validity of case-control studies also depends on avoiding bias in measurement of exposure. The safest approach to measuring exposure is to depend on complete, accurate records that were collected before disease developed. With such records, knowledge of disease status cannot bias reporting of exposure. Examples include pharmacy records for studies of prescription drug risks; surgical records for studies of surgical complications; and stored blood specimens for studies of risk related to biochemical abnormalities.

However, many important exposures can only be measured by asking cases and controls or their proxies. Among these are exercise, diet, and over-the-counter and recreational drug use. The following example illustrates this.

EXAMPLE

What are the risk factors for suicide in China? Investigators studied 519 people who had committed suicide and 536 people who had died from other injuries. Both groups came from 23 geographically representative sites in China. (6) Exposure was measured through interviews with family members and close associates. The author noted that as with other studies that depended on a "psychological autopsy" for measurement of exposure, "interviewers were aware of the cause of death of the deceased (suicide or other injury) so we could not completely eliminate potential interviewer bias." They went on to explain that "we tried to keep this bias to a minimum by using the same interview schedule for cases and controls, employing objective measures of potential risk factors, independently obtaining evidence from two sources (family members and close associates), and giving extensive training to interviewers."

They also chose controls who had died from injuries to match for one important characteristic that might affect responses in the interview. This was the recent death of a family member or associate.

The study identified eight predictors of suicide: high depression symptom score, previous suicide attempt, acute stress just prior to death, low quality of life, high chronic stress, severe interpersonal conflict in the two days before death, a blood relative with previous suicide behavior, and a friend or associate with previous suicide behavior.

When cases and controls are asked to recall their previous exposures, measurement is prone to error. Having the disease under study may affect their responses—so might their existing beliefs about whether exposure and disease are related.

Bias can occur in three general ways. First, exposure itself can be affected by the presence of disease. This can be a particular problem when the exposure under study is a medical treatment. Early manifestations of the disease may lead to treatment, while the study question is just the other way around: whether treatment affects disease. If this problem is anticipated, it can be dealt with, as the following example illustrates.

EXAMPLE

Do beta-blocker drugs prevent first myocardial infarctions in patients being treated for hypertension? A case-control study addressed this question. (7) Because angina is a major indication for use of beta-blockers, the investigators carefully excluded any subjects with a history suggesting angina or other manifestation of coronary heart disease. They found that patients with hypertension treated with beta-blockers had a reduced risk of nonfatal myocardial infarctions, even after those with angina or other evidence of coronary disease were carefully excluded.

Second, having the disease in question can affect patients' recollection of exposure. This is called **recall bias**. A relatively young woman with myocardial infarction might be more likely to report use of birth control pills than a similarly young woman without a myocardial infarction. A man with prostate cancer might be more likely to report a prior vasectomy. With all the publicity surrounding the possible risks of various environmental and drug exposures, it is entirely possible that victims of disease would remember their exposures more often than people without the disease.

There are two ways of protecting against recall bias. First, alternative sources of the same information, whether written documents such as medical (or other) records or interviews with relatives, allow investigators to check for inconsistency. Second, the specific purpose of the study should be concealed from the people being studied. It would be unethical not to inform participants in research about the general nature of the study question, but to provide detailed information about specific questions and hypotheses could so bias the resulting information as to commit another breach of ethics—involving subjects in a worthless research project.

Third, the presence of disease can also affect the measurement or recording of exposure. This bias should be understandable to all students of physical diagnosis. If a resident admitting a relatively young woman with acute myocardial infarction is aware of the reported association with use of birth control pills, he or she might be likely to question the patient more intensely about birth control pill use and to record this information more carefully. Interviewers who are aware of a possible relationship between exposure and disease would be remarkable indeed if they conducted identical interviews, and recorded with identical thoroughness, for cases and controls. Protections against this kind of bias are the same as those mentioned above: multiple sources of information and blinding the data gatherers by keeping them in the dark about the hypothesis under study.

THE ODDS RATIO: AN ESTIMATE OF RELATIVE RISK

How do we calculate risk in a case-control study? Figure 6.3 shows how risk is calculated for cohort and case-control studies. In the following, the study of exercise and primary cardiac arrest is used as an example.

In a cohort study, the susceptible cohort is divided into two groups at the outset—exposed (A + B) to exercise and not exposed (C + D) to exercise. Cases of primary cardiac arrest emerge naturally over time in the exposed group (A) and the unexposed group (C). This provides appropriate numerators and denominators to calculate the incidences of primary cardiac arrest in the exposed [A/(A + B)] and unexposed [C/(C + D)] cohorts. It is also possible to calculate the relative risk:

$$\text{Relative risk} = \frac{\text{Incidence of disease in the exposed}}{\text{Incidence of disease in the unexposed}}$$
$$= \frac{A/(A + B)}{C/(C + D)}$$

Case-control studies, on the other hand, begin with the selection of a group of cases of primary cardiac arrest (A + C) and another group of controls without primary cardiac arrest (B + D). There is no way of knowing disease rates because these groups are determined not by nature but by the investigators' selection criteria. Therefore, an incidence rate of disease among those exposed to exercise and those not exposed cannot be computed. Consequently, it

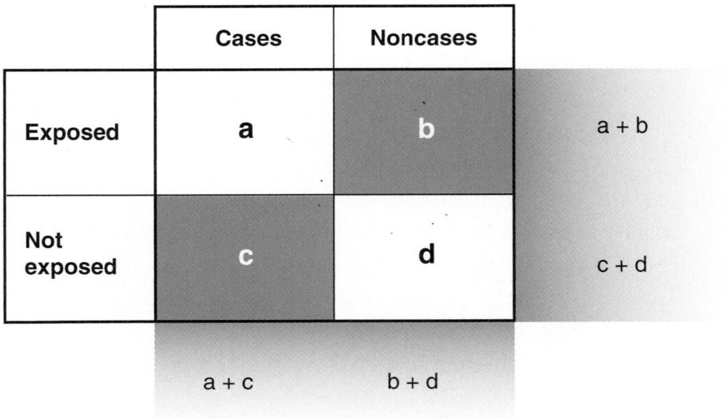

	Cases	Noncases	
Exposed	a	b	a + b
Not exposed	c	d	c + d
	a + c	b + d	

COHORT STUDY

Relative risk =
$$\frac{a/(a + b)}{c/(c + d)}$$

CASE-CONTROL STUDY

Odds ratio =
$$\frac{\dfrac{a/(a + c)}{c/(a + c)}}{\dfrac{b/(b + d)}{d/(b + d)}} = \frac{a/c}{b/d} = \frac{ad}{bc}$$

FIGURE 6.3 ■ Calculation of relative risk from a cohort study and odds ratio (estimated relative risk) from a case-control study.

is not possible to obtain a relative risk by dividing incidence among exercisers by incidence among nonexercisers. What does have meaning, however, is the relative frequency of exposure to exercise among the cases and controls.

One approach to comparing the frequency of exposure among cases and controls provides a measure of risk that is conceptually and mathematically similar to the relative risk. This is the **odds ratio**, defined as the odds† that a case is exposed divided by the odds that a control is exposed:

$$\frac{[A/(A + C) \div C/(A + C)]}{[B/(B + D) \div D/(B + D)]}$$

The odds ratio simplifies to

$$\frac{A/C}{B/D} \quad \text{or} \quad \frac{AD}{BC}$$

As is seen in Figure 6.3, the odds ratio can be obtained by multiplying diagonally across the table and dividing these cross-products.

If the frequency of exposure is higher among cases, the odds ratio will exceed 1, indicating increased risk. Thus, the stronger the association between the exposure and disease, the higher the odds ratio. Conversely, if the frequency of exposure is lower among cases, the odds ratio will be less than 1, indicating protection. The meaning of the odds ratio, therefore, is analogous to that of relative risk obtained from cohort studies. Because of the similarity of the information conveyed by the odds ratio and the relative risk, some investigators report odds ratios as **estimated relative risks**.

The odds ratio is approximately equal to the relative risk only when the incidence of disease is low because of assumptions that must be made in the calculations. How low must the rates be for the odds ratio to be an accurate estimate of relative risk? The answer depends in part on the size of the relative risk. (8) In general, however, bias in the estimate of relative risk becomes large enough to matter as disease rates in unexposed people become greater than about 1/100. Fortunately, most diseases, particularly those examined by means of case-control studies, have considerably lower rates. In general, as outcomes become more frequent the odds ratio tends to overestimate the relative risk when it is greater than 1 and underestimate the relative risk when it is less than 1.

CONTROLLING FOR EXTRANEOUS VARIABLES

Once the data are collected, other options remain for dealing with extraneous variables. These were mentioned in Chapter 5 and will be described in more detail in Chapter 7. Briefly, one can examine strata of patients who have comparable characteristics, or one can mathematically adjust for differences between cases and controls. Of course, these can only be done for characteristics that were already suspected to affect the exposure-disease relationship and were measured in the study.

INVESTIGATION OF A DISEASE OUTBREAK

Up to this point, we have described use of the case-control method to identify risk factors for chronic diseases. The same method is used to identify risk factors for outbreaks (small epidemics) of acute diseases, typically infectious diseases. Often, the microbiologic cause of the disease is obvious early in the epidemic, after diagnostic evaluation of cases. But the mode of transmission may not be as obvious, and information on how the disease was spread is needed to stop the epidemic. This information also increases understanding of possible modes of transmission, which might be useful in the control of future epidemics.

EXAMPLE

During a four-week period, 555 persons who lived in or had visited a town in Pennsylvania developed hepatitis A, and three of them died. All had eaten at a restaurant in the town, and most had eaten there within a four-day period, which was about 4 weeks before the epidemic (the typical incubation period for hepatitis A is 2 to 6 weeks). Figure 6.4 shows the distribution of dates for dining at the restaurant and onset of disease. A case-control study was done to identify menu items or ingredients associated with illness. Cases were 181 patients who had onset of illness during the epidemic period, had acute hepatitis A virus infection confirmed by laboratory tests, had eaten at the restaurant during the four-day period, and had eaten there only once during the 2- to 6-week period before the onset of their illness. Controls were people who had eaten at the same restaurant during the same four-day period but did not have hepatitis. Cases and controls were asked what foods they had eaten at the restaurant.

Cases were more likely than controls to have eaten mild salsa (odds ratio = 24.2) and chili con questa

---

† For a reminder of what *odds* means, see page **49**.

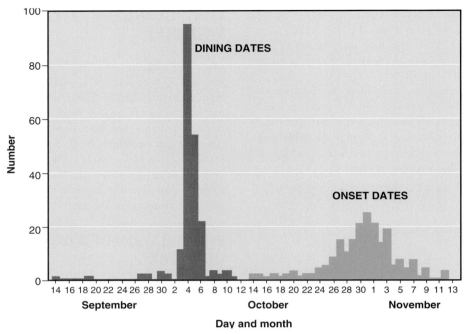

FIGURE 6.4 ■ Number of hepatitis A cases by date after eating at a restaurant and illness onset. (From Dato V, Weltman A, Waller K, Ruta M, Hembree C, Evanson S, et al. Hepatitis A outbreak associated with green onions at a restaurant—Monaca, Pennsylvania 2003. MMWR 2003;52:1155–1157.)

(odds ratio = 5.2), both of which contained uncooked or mildly heated, fresh green onions. Other menu items also contained green onions, and the odds ratio for eating any menu item containing green onions was 20.2. Consumption of white onions was also associated with hepatitis A but not after taking into account green onion consumption; that is, the two were confounded. The green onions used in the restaurant were traced back to one or more farms in Mexico where similar epidemics related to green onions had arisen. (9)

This example also illustrates how epidemiologic and laboratory methods can complement each other. Cases were confirmed by laboratory testing. Also, the genetic sequence of the outbreak strain was very similar to the sequences of the hepatitis A virus identified in other outbreaks linked to green onions.

SCIENTIFIC STANDARDS FOR CASE-CONTROL RESEARCH

It has been suggested that one should judge the validity of a case-control study by considering how a randomized, controlled trial of the same question would have been conducted. (10) Of course, one could not actually do the study that way. But a randomized, controlled trial (described in more detail in Chapter 8) would be the scientific standard against which to consider the effects of the various compromises that are inherent in a case-control study.

Just as one would enter into a trial only those patients who could take the experimental intervention if it were offered, so would one in a case-control study select cases and controls who could have been exposed. For example, the study of whether exercise protects against primary cardiac arrest included men and women who had no impediments to exercise, such as chronic disease. Similarly, cases and controls were subjected to similar efforts to discover primary cardiac arrest if it occurred. These and other parallels between clinical trials and case-control studies can be exploited when trying to think through just what could go wrong, how serious a problem might be, and what could be done about it.

RISK COMMUNICATION

As summarized in this and the preceding chapter, risk can be described in quantitative terms. Although we have used as the main examples studies of risk factors for developing disease, the same kinds of studies, and the same kinds of metrics, can be used to describe other clinically-important phenomena such as factors related to the outcome of disease, the effectiveness of preventive or therapeutic interventions, and the rate of complications following a test or procedure.

How effectively do clinicians communicate risk to patients? This is an important question because risk communication is the common ground for discussions with patients about their options and choices for care. Also, risk communication honors the ethical responsibility to give patients information in a way they can understand, so that they can participate knowledgeably in health-care decisions.

However, communicating risk is a thorny issue for several reasons. For one thing, most people are not very numerate. One study reported that a third of respondents thought that 1,000 flips of a fair coin would result in fewer than 300 heads. (11) Also, different ways of presenting the same risk information, called **framing**, produce different perceptions. (12) Table 6.2 summarizes some of these framing effects. Personal experience also affects perceptions. People weigh risks more heavily whenever they or someone close to them has actually experienced the outcome. The risk seems even larger when experience with it is recent or especially memorable.

For all these reasons, clinicians are in the uncomfortable position of knowing that they can manipulate perceptions of risk and that risk perception is very patient-specific, and to some extent, unpredictable. Unfortunately, clinicians know far less about how to produce an accurate perception.

Given the difficulties of risk communication, it seems best to describe risk in several different ways, with the hope that these ways will complement one another and, taken together, produce a fair perception of risk. Actual frequencies, expressing the base rates, should certainly be one of the ways. Thus, explaining that "the risk of thromboembolism is 1 per 14,000 women and is increased to 2 per 14,000 after taking the contraceptive pill" would certainly create a different impression of risk than "the contraceptive pill leads to a twofold increase in the risk of thromboembolism." (13) Large denominators can be made more familiar by anchoring them in common experiences. For example, 14,000 might be described to someone in our town as "about the number of people who would fit into a college basketball arena."

Pictures may communicate more effectively than numbers. Figure 6.5 is an example, showing outcome (pain at 2–7 days after treatment) for 100 children with otitis media treated with antibiotics. Most of the children (79) would have a good outcome even without antibiotics, 7 would have a good outcome because of antibiotics, and 14 would have a bad outcome regardless of antibiotic treatment. Except for the most numerate among us, such as mathematics majors, this kind of visual presentation seems to summarize rates in a much more digestible way than do tables with numbers.

TABLE 6.2 ■ The Effects of Presentation of Risk Information on Perceptions of Risk

Information on relative risk is more persuasive than the same information presented as absolute risk.

"Loss" framing (e.g., the potential for losses from not being screened for cancer) influences decisions more than "gain" framing.

Positive framing (e.g., chance of survival) is more effective than negative framing (e.g., chance of death) in persuading people to take risky options with treatments.

More information and information that is more understandable to the patient are associated with a greater wariness to take treatment or tests.

The risk following inaction is perceived as greater than the same risk following action.

(Adapted from Edwards A, Elwyn G, Mulley A. Explaining risks: Turning numerical data into meaningful pictures. BMJ 2002;324:827–830.)

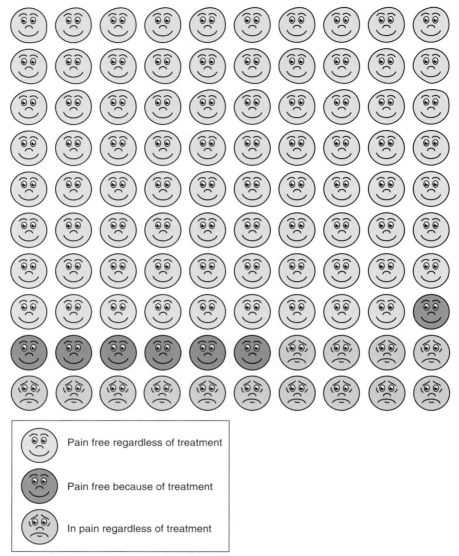

Pain free regardless of treatment

Pain free because of treatment

In pain regardless of treatment

FIGURE 6.5 ■ Communicating quantitative risk information by a picture. Ear pain 2–7 days after onset of otitis media in 100 children treated with antibiotics. Most children would have a good outcome even without antibiotics, 7 would have a good outcome because of antibiotics, and 14 would have a bad outcome regardless of antibiotic treatment. (From http://nntonline.net/ebm/newsletter/200210/200210.asp [accessed November 18, 2004], October 2002 Newsletter)

REVIEW QUESTIONS

For questions 6.1 to 6.6, select the most appropriate option for each attribute.

A. Cohort study
B. Case-control study
C. Both A and B
D. Neither A nor B

_____ **6.1.** Incidence in exposed and unexposed people can be obtained directly from the study.

_____ **6.2.** It is not necessary to measure exposure in everyone in the study who might get the disease.

_____ **6.3.** The study can be done on a sample of the population.

_____ **6.4.** The study cannot be done until enough time has passed after exposure for disease to develop.

_____ **6.5.** The only measure of risk is the odds ratio.

_____ **6.6.** Prevalence of disease is measured in a sample of a population.

Circle the best response.

6.7. Case-control studies would be useful for answering all of the following questions except:

A. Do cholesterol-lowering drugs prevent coronary heart disease?
B. What is the incidence of complications from fiberoptic cholecystectomy?
C. Is drinking alcohol a risk factor for breast cancer?
D. How effective are antibiotics for otitis media?
E. Are complications more common with fiberoptic cholecystectomy than with conventional (open) surgery?

6.8. All of the following are true for odds ratio except:

A. It is an estimate of relative risk.
B. It is the only measure of risk that can be obtained directly from a case-control study.
C. It tends to be biased toward 1 (neither risk or protection) at high rates of disease.
D. It is the ratio of incidence in exposed divided by incidence in nonexposed.
E. It can be calculated without data on incidence.

6.9. For case-control studies, sampling cases and controls from a defined population or cohort accomplishes which of the following?

A. Ensures that unusually severe or difficult cases are included.
B. Tends to include cases and controls that are similar to each other except for exposure.
C. Ensures that unusual exposures are included.
D. Is the only way of including incident (new) cases of disease.
E. Matches cases and controls on important variables.

Answers are in Appendix A.

REFERENCES

1. Kernan WN, Viscoli CM, Brass LM, Broderick JP, Brott T, Feldmann E, et al. Phenylpropanolamine and the risk of hemorrhagic stroke. N Engl J Med 2000;343:1826–1832.
2. McDermott MM, Lefevre F, Feinglass J, Reifler D, Dolan N, Potts S, et al. Changes in study design, gender issues, and other characteristics of clinical research published in three major medical journals from 1971 to 1991. J Gen Intern Med 1995;10:13–18.
3. Siscovick DS, Weiss NS, Hallstrom AP, Inui TS, Peterson DR. Physical activity and primary cardiac arrest. JAMA 1982;248:3113–3117.
4. Cox B, Sneyd MJ, Paul C, Delahunt B, Skegg DCG. Vasectomy and risk of prostate cancer. JAMA 2002; 287:3110–3115.
5. Hulka BS, Fowler WC Jr, Kaufman DG, Grimson RC, Greenberg BG, Hogue CJ, et al. Estrogen and endometrial cancer: Cases and two control groups from North Carolina. Am J Obstet Gynecol 1980; 137:92–101.
6. Phillips MR, Yang G, Zhang Y, Wang L, Ji H, Zhou M. Risk factors for suicide in China: A national case-control psychological autopsy study. Lancet 2002; 360:1728–1736.

7. Psaty BM, Koepsell TD, LoGerfo JP, Wagner EH, Inui TS. Beta-blockers and primary prevention of coronary heart disease in patients with high blood pressure. JAMA 1989;261:2087–2094.

8. Feinstein AR. The bias caused by high value of incidence for p1 in the odds ratio assumption that 1-p1 is approximately equal to 1. J Chron Dis 1986;39:485–487.

9. Dato V, Weltman A, Waller K, Ruta MA, Hembree C, Highbaugh-Battle A et al. Hepatitis A outbreak associated with green onions at a restaurant—Monaca, Pennsylvania 2003. MMWR 2003;52: 1155–1157.

10. Feinstein AR, Horwitz RI. Double standards, scientific methods, and epidemiologic research. N Engl J Med 1982;307:1611–1617.

11. Schwartz LM, Woloshin S, Black WC, Welch HG. The role of numeracy in understanding the benefit of screening mammography. Ann Intern Med 1997;127: 966–72.

12. Edwards A, Elwyn G, Mulley A. Explaining risks: turning numerical data into meaningful pictures. BMJ 2002;324:827–830.

13. Gigerenzer G. Why does framing influence judgment? J Gen Intern Med 2003;18:960–961.

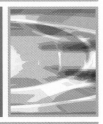

Prognosis

> *The physician who cannot inform his patient what would be the probable issue of his complaint, if allowed to follow its natural course, is not qualified to prescribe any rational treatment for its cure.*
>
> *—Hippocrates 460–375 B.C.*

When people become sick, they have a great many questions about how their illness will affect them. Is it dangerous? Could I die of it? Will there be pain? How long will I be able to continue my present activities? Will it ever go away altogether? Most patients and their families want to know what to expect, even in situations where little can be done about their illness.

Prognosis is a prediction of the course of disease following its onset. In this chapter, we review the ways in which the course of disease can be described. Also, we consider the biases that can affect these descriptions and how these biases can be controlled. The intention is to give readers a better understanding of a difficult but indispensable task—predicting patients' futures as closely as possible. The objective is to avoid expressing prognoses with vagueness when unnecessary and with certainty when misleading.

Doctors and patients want to know the general course of the illness. But they want to go further and tailor this information to their particular situation as much as possible. For example, even though HIV infection is almost certainly fatal in the long run, individuals with the infection may live from a few months to a decade or more, and patients want to know where on this continuum their particular case likely falls.

Studies of prognosis are similar to cohort studies of risk. Patients are assembled who have something in common, such as a particular disease or illness in the case of prognostic studies, the group is followed forward in time, and clinical outcomes are measured. Conditions that are associated with an outcome of the disease, called **prognostic factors**, are identified. Prognostic factors are analogous to risk factors, except they represent a different part of the disease spectrum; from disease to outcomes. Case-control studies of people with the disease who do and do not have a bad outcome can also estimate the relative risk associated with various prognostic factors, but they are unable to provide information on outcome rates (see Chapter 6).

DIFFERENCES IN RISK AND PROGNOSTIC FACTORS

Risk and prognostic factors differ from each other in several ways.

Patients Are Different

Studies of risk factors usually deal with healthy people, whereas studies of prognostic factors are of outcomes in sick people.

Outcomes Are Different

Risk and prognosis describe different phenomena. For risk, the event being counted is the onset of disease. For prognosis, a range of disease consequences is counted, including death, complications, disability, and suffering.

Rates Are Different

Risk factors are usually for low-probability events. Yearly rates for the onset of various diseases are on the order of 1/1,000 to 1/100,000 or less. As a result, relationships between exposure and disease are difficult to confirm in the course of day-to-day activities, even for astute clinicians. Prognosis, on the other hand, describes relatively frequent events. Several percent of patients with acute myocardial infarction die during the several-day period following onset. Often, clinicians can form good estimates of short-term prognosis from their own personal experience. They may be less able to sort out, without the assistance of research, the various factors that are related to long-term prognosis or the complex ways in which prognostic factors are related to one another.

Risk and Prognostic Factors Are Different

Variables associated with an increased risk are not necessarily the same as those marking a worse prognosis. Often, they are considerably different for a given disease. For example, low blood pressure decreases one's chances of having an acute myocardial infarction, but it is a bad prognostic sign when present during the acute event (Figure 7.1). On the other hand, some patient characteristics do have a similar effect on both risk and prognosis. For example, both the risk of experiencing an acute myocardial infarction and the risk of dying of it increase with age.

CLINICAL COURSE AND NATURAL HISTORY OF DISEASE

Prognosis can be described as either a clinical course or the natural history of disease. The term **clinical course** describes the evolution (prognosis) of a disease that has come under medical care and has been treated in a variety of ways that affect the subsequent course of events. Patients usually receive medical care at some time in the course of their illness when they have diseases that cause symptoms such as pain, failure to thrive, disfigurement, or unusual behavior. Examples include type 1 diabetes mellitus, carcinoma of the lung, and rabies. Once disease is recognized, it is likely to be treated.

The prognosis of disease without medical intervention is termed the **natural history** of disease. Natural history describes how patients will fare if nothing is done about their disease. A great many

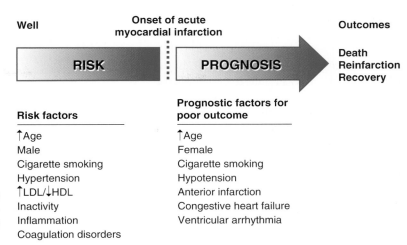

FIGURE 7.1 ■ Risk and prognostic factors for acute myocardial infarction. The prognostic factors listed are for worse outcomes.

medical conditions, even in countries with advanced health-care systems, do not come under medical care. They remain unrecognized because they are asymptomatic or because people consider them one of the ordinary discomforts of daily living. Examples include mild depression, low-grade anemia, and cancers that are occult and slow growing, such as some cancers of the thyroid and prostate. For some conditions, only a minority of afflicted patients seeks medical care.

EXAMPLE

Irritable bowel syndrome is a common condition involving abdominal pain and disturbed defecation not caused by other diseases. How often do patients with this condition visit doctors? Investigators surveyed a random sample of 1,021 middle-aged adults living in a county in Minnesota, 835 of whom responded. (1) Of these, 26% reported abdominal pain more than six times in the prior year, 17.9% reported chronic diarrhea, and 17.4% reported chronic constipation; 17% met accepted criteria for irritable bowel syndrome. Only 9% of this sample (about a third of those with bowel symptoms) had seen a doctor for abdominal pain or for disturbed defecation in the prior year. For the most part, characteristics of the abdominal complaints did not account for whether or not these people sought health care for their symptoms.

ELEMENTS OF PROGNOSTIC STUDIES

At best, studies of prognosis are population-based or include a complete description of patients and the setting in which they were identified. They begin

observation at a specified point in time in the course of disease, they include follow-up on patients for an adequate period of time, and they measure all relevant outcomes.

The Patient Sample

Studies of prognosis, like those of risk, are best done on a population of all people with the disease in question in a defined geographic region. In this way, one can be confident that the patients being described are an unbiased sample of all such patients. The existence of national medical records makes population-based studies possible in some countries.

EXAMPLE

Dutch investigators studied the risk of complications of pregnancy in women with type 1 diabetes mellitus. (2) The sample included all of the 323 women in the Netherlands with type 1 diabetes who had become pregnant during a year (1999–2000) and had been under care in one of the nation's 118 hospitals. Most pregnancies were planned, and during pregnancy, most women took folic acid supplements and had good glycemic control. Nevertheless, complication rates were much higher than in the general population. Neonatal morbidity (one or more complications) occurred in 80%, and rates of congenital malformations and macrosomia were threefold to twelvefold higher than in the general population. This study suggests that optimal glycemic control alone was not good enough to prevent complications of pregnancy in women with type 1 diabetes.

Most studies of prognosis, however, are based on clinical samples not directly related to geographic populations. For them, it is especially important to describe patients' characteristics (such as age, severity of disease, and comorbidity), the setting where they were found, and how they were sampled. This allows those who rely on the study's results to decide whether it is appropriate to generalize from experience with these patients to other situations.

Zero Time

Cohorts in prognostic studies should begin from a point in time in the course of disease, called **zero time**. This time should be specified clearly and be the same well-defined point, such as at the time of the onset of symptoms, time of diagnosis, or beginning of treatment for all patients in the cohort. If observation is begun at different points in the course of disease for the various patients in a cohort, description of their prognosis will lack precision. The timing of recovery, recurrence, death, and other such events would be difficult to interpret or be misleading. The term **inception cohort** is used to describe a group of people that is assembled at the onset, or inception, of their disease.

Changes in zero time can result in a different prognosis, even if each patient had the same course of disease.

EXAMPLE

Patients with lung cancer are assigned a stage, which depends in part on the sensitivity of diagnostic tests used to detect extent of disease and how aggressively they are used. Feinstein and colleagues found that a recent cohort of patients with lung cancer had a better six-month survival, stage for stage, than a cohort from an earlier era. (3) Did this represent progress in the treatment of this disease? Actually, new ways of staging patients seemed to have accounted for the difference. Recent patients had undergone many new diagnostic imaging procedures. When "old" diagnostic data were applied to old and new cohorts, members of the recent cohort tended to be classified at a more advanced stage. Metastases that had been found with the newer imaging techniques had gone undetected with the old staging evaluation. This resulted in a "zero-time shift" with newer staging techniques, in which patients migrated to a worse prognostic stage than they would have during the earlier era. Survival in the recent cohort was higher for each stage, even though individual patients' actual prognosis was apparently the same. The investigators called this the "Will Rogers phenomenon" after the humorist who said of the geographic migration in the United States during the economic depression of the 1930s, "When the Okies left Oklahoma

and moved to California, they raised the average intelligence in both states." This is an example of how a change in zero time, in this case related to advances in technology, changed apparent (but not actual) prognosis.

Follow-Up

Patients must be followed for a long enough period of time for most of the clinically important outcome events to have occurred. Otherwise, the observed rate will understate the true one. The appropriate length of follow-up depends on the disease. It is a few weeks for studies of surgical site infections and several years for studies of the onset of AIDS and its complications in patients with HIV infection.

Outcomes of Disease

Descriptions of prognosis should include the full range of manifestations of disease that would be considered important to patients. This means not only death and disease but also pain, anguish, and inability to care for one's self or pursue usual activities. The five Ds—Death, Disease, Discomfort, Disability, and Dissatisfaction—are a simple way to summarize important clinical outcomes (see Table 1.3 in Chapter 1).

In their efforts to be "scientific," physicians tend to value precise or technologically measured outcomes over others, sometimes at the expense of clinical relevance. As discussed in Chapter 1, clinical effects that cannot be directly perceived by patients, such as radiologic reduction in tumor size, normalization of blood chemistries, improvement in ejection fraction, or change in serology, are not clinically useful ends in themselves. It is appropriate to substitute these biologic phenomena for clinical outcomes only when the two are known to be related to each other. Thus, hypercalcemia is an important clinical outcome of hyperparathyroidism only at levels at which it causes symptoms such as drowsiness and thirst or when there is research evidence that it will eventually lead to symptoms or complications such as bone demineralization or kidney stones. If an outcome cannot be linked to something patients can recognize, the information should not be used to guide patient care, even though it may be of considerable value in understanding the origins and mechanisms of disease.

Composite outcomes are a set of separate outcomes that are combined into a single outcome variable. In a study of cardiovascular disease, for example, the primary outcomes might be the occurrence of either fatal coronary heart disease or non-fatal myocardial infarction. Composite outcomes are often used when the individual elements share a common cause and treatment. Because they comprise more outcome events than the component outcomes alone, they are more likely to show a statistical effect.

Health-related quality of life is measured by broad, composite measures of **health status.** A simple quality of life measure, used by a collaborative group of cancer researchers, is shown in Table 7.1. This "performance scale" combines symptoms and function, such as the ability to walk. Others are much more extensive; the Sickness Impact Profile contains more than 100 items and a dozen categories. Still others are specifically developed for individual diseases. The main issue is that the value of a prognosis study is strengthened to the extent that such measures are reported along with obvious measures such as death and recurrence of disease.

DESCRIBING PROGNOSIS

It is convenient to summarize the course of disease as a single rate—the proportion of people experiencing an event in a fixed time period. Some rates used for this purpose are shown in Table 7.2. These rates have in common the same basic components of incidence: events arising in a cohort of patients over time.

TABLE 7.1 ■ A Simple Measure of Quality of Life. The Eastern Collaborative Oncology Group's Performance Scale

Performance Status	Definition
0	Asymptomatic
1	Symptomatic, fully ambulatory
2	Symptomatic, in bed <50% of the day
3	Symptomatic, in bed >50% of the day
4	Bedridden
5	Dead

TABLE 7.2 ■ Rates Commonly Used to Describe Prognosis

Rate	Definition[a]
5-year survival	Percent of patients surviving 5 years from some point in the course of their disease
Case fatality	Percent of patients with a disease who die of it
Disease-specific mortality	Number of people per 10,000 (or 100,000) population dying of a specific disease
Response	Percent of patients showing some evidence of improvement following an intervention
Remission	Percent of patients entering a phase in which disease is no longer detectable
Recurrence	Percent of patients who have return of disease after a disease-free interval

[a] Time under observation is either stated or assumed to be sufficiently long so that all events that will occur have been observed.

A Trade-Off: Simplicity Versus More Information

Summarizing prognosis by a single rate has the virtue of simplicity. Rates can be committed to memory and communicated succinctly. Their drawback is that relatively little information is conveyed. Large differences in prognosis can be hidden within similar summary rates.

Figure 7.2 shows 5-year survival for patients with four conditions. For each condition, about 10% of the patients are alive at 5 years. However, the clinical courses are otherwise quite different in ways that might be very important to patients. Early survival in patients with dissecting aneurysms is very poor, but if they survive the first few months, their risk of dying is little affected by having had the aneurysm (Figure 7.2A). Patients with locally-invasive, non-small cell lung cancer experience a relatively constant mortality rate throughout the 5 years following diagnosis (Figure 7.2B). Most patients with HIV infection and the beginning of AIDS-defining illnesses survive at first but over the years develop complications and die, at least until recently for patients with expert care and meticulous attention to

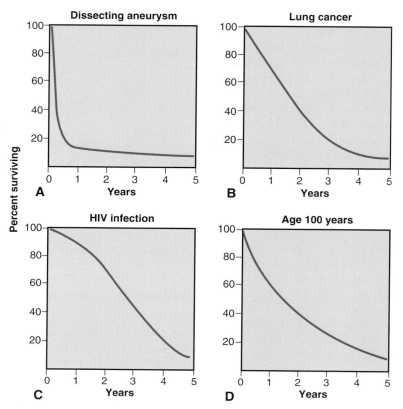

FIGURE 7.2 ▦ A limitation of 5-year survival rates: Four conditions with the same 5-year survival rate of 10%.

medications (Figure 7.2C). Figure 7.2D is presented as a benchmark. Only at age 100 do people in the general population have a 5-year survival rate comparable to that of patients with the three diseases.

Survival Analysis

When interpreting prognosis, it is preferable to know the likelihood, on average, that patients with a given condition will experience an outcome at any point in time. Prognosis expressed as a summary rate does not contain this information. However, figures can summarize information about average time to event for any point in the course of disease. In the following discussion, we take the usual approach of describing outcomes in terms of "survival," but the same methods apply to the reverse (time to death) and to any other outcome event such as cancer recurrence, cure of infection, freedom from symptoms, or inactive arthritis.

Survival of a Cohort

The most straightforward way to learn about survival is to assemble a cohort of patients who have the condition of interest, are at the same point in the course of their illness (such as onset of symptoms, diagnosis, or beginning of treatment), and are kept under observation until all can experience the outcome of interest. For a small cohort, one might then represent these patients' clinical course as shown in Figure 7.3A. The plot of survival against time displays steps corresponding to the death of each of the 10 patients in the cohort. If the number of patients were increased, the size of the steps would diminish. If a very large number of patients were studied, the figure would approximate a smooth curve (Figure 7.3B). This information could then be used to predict the year-by-year, or even week-by-week, prognosis of similar patients.

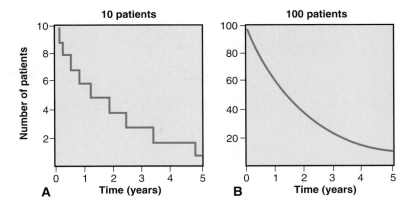

FIGURE 7.3 ▪ Survival of two cohorts, small and large, when all members are observed for the full period of follow-up.

Unfortunately, obtaining the information in this way is impractical for several reasons. Some of the patients would undoubtedly drop out of the study before the end of the follow-up period, perhaps because of another illness, a move from the study area, or dissatisfaction with the study. These patients would have to be excluded from the cohort even though considerable effort may have been exerted to gather data on them up to the point at which they dropped out. Also, it would be necessary to wait until all of the cohort's members had reached each point in follow-up before the probability of surviving to that point could be calculated. Because patients ordinarily become available for a study over a period of time, at any point in calendar time there would be a relatively long follow-up for patients who had entered the study first, but only brief experience with those who had entered recently. The last patient who entered the study would have to reach each year of follow-up before any information on survival to that year would be available.

Survival Curves

To make efficient use of all available data from each patient in the cohort, **survival analysis** has been developed to estimate the survival of a cohort over time. The usual method is called **Kaplan-Meir analysis** after its originators. Survival analysis can be applied to any outcomes that are dichotomous and occur only once during follow-up (e.g., time to coronary event or to recurrence of cancer). When an event other than survival is described, the general term **time-to-event analysis** is used.

Figure 7.4 shows a simplified survival curve. On the vertical axis is the estimated probability of surviving, and on the horizontal axis is the period of time following the beginning of observation.

The probability of surviving to any point in time is estimated from the cumulative probability of surviving each of the time intervals that preceded it. Time intervals can be made as small as necessary; in Kaplan-Meir analyses, the intervals are between each new event, such as death, and the preceding one, however short or long that is. Most of the time, no one dies and the probability of surviving is 1. When a patient dies, the probability of surviving at that moment is calculated as the ratio of the number of patients surviving to the number at risk of dying at that time. Patients who have already died, dropped out, or have not yet been followed up to that point are not at risk of dying, and so are not used to estimate survival for that time. The probability of surviving does not change during intervals in which no one dies, so, in practice, the probability of surviving is recalculated only for times when there is a death. Although the probability assigned at any given interval is not very accurate, because either nothing has happened or there has been only one event in a large cohort, the overall probability of surviving up to each point in time (the product of all preceding probabilities) is remarkably accurate.

When patients are lost from the study at any point in time, for any reason other than the outcome event, they are referred to as **censored**, and they are no longer counted in the denominator. In survival analysis, it is assumed that being censored is not related to prognosis. To the extent that this is not true, a survival analysis may yield biased estimates of survival in cohorts.

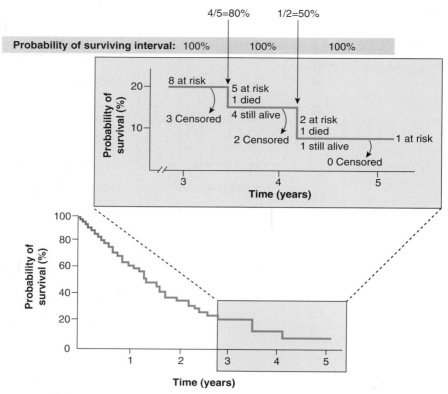

FIGURE 7.4 ▦ Example of a survival curve, with detail for one part of the curve.

A part of the survival curve in Figure 7.4 (from 3 to 5 years after zero time) is presented in detail to illustrate the data used to estimate survival: patients at risk, patients no longer at risk (censored), and patients experiencing outcome events at each point in time.

Survival Curves That Include Other Information

Variations on the basic survival curve increase the amount of information they contain. The numbers of patients at risk at various points in time may be shown to give some idea of the contribution of chance to the observed rates. Figure 7.5 illustrates this for a study of the conversion of lone atrial flutter to atrial fibrillation. The proportion with, rather than without, the outcome event may be indicated on the vertical axis; the resulting curve will sweep upward and to the right. The precision of survival

estimates, which declines with time because fewer and fewer patients are still under observation, can be demostrated by confidence intervals at various points in time (see Chapter 10). Sometimes tics (not shown in Figure 7.5) are added to the survival curves to indicate each time a patient is censored.

Interpreting Survival Curves

Several points must be kept in mind when interpreting survival curves. First, the vertical axis represents the *estimated* probability of surviving for members of a hypothetical cohort, not the percent surviving for an actual cohort.

Second, points on a survival curve are the best estimate, for a given set of data, of the probability of survival for members of a cohort. However, the precision of these estimates depends, as do all observations of samples, on the number of patients on

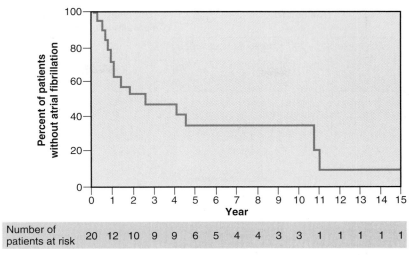

Number of patients at risk	20	12	10	9	9	6	5	4	4	3	3	1	1	1	1	1

FIGURE 7.5 ▦ A survival curve showing number of patients observed for each of the 15 years of follow-up. Time without conversion to atrial fibrillation for patients with atrial flutter and hypertension. (From Halligan SC, Gersh BJ, Brown RD Jr, Rosales G, Munger TM, Shen WK et al. The natural history of lone atrial flutter. Ann Intern Med 2004;140:265–268.)

whom the estimate is based. One can be more confident that the estimates on the left-hand side of the curve are sound, because more patients are at risk during this time. But at the tail of the curve, on the right, the number of patients on whom estimates of survival are based may become relatively small because deaths, dropouts, and late entrants to the study result in fewer and fewer patients being followed for that length of time. As a result, estimates of survival toward the end of the follow-up period are imprecise and can be strongly affected by what happens to relatively few patients. For example, in Figure 7.5 only one patient was under observation at year 15. If that one remaining patient happened to die, the probability of surviving would fall from 8% to zero. Clearly, this would be a too literal reading of the data. Therefore, estimates of survival at the tails of survival curves must be interpreted with caution.

Finally, the shape of some survival curves, particularly those in which most patients experience the event of interest, gives the impression that an outcome event occurs more frequently early in follow-up than later on, when the slope reaches a plateau. But this impression is deceptive. As time passes, rates of survival are being applied to a diminishing number of patients, causing the slope of the curve to flatten even if the rate of outcome events did not change. For example, Figure 7.2D shows the survival curve

for a relatively constant outcome rate over time, and it flattens out on the right.

FALSE COHORTS

True cohort studies should be distinguished from those masquerading as cohort studies (Figure 7.6). In the latter, patients are included because they have the disease in question and are currently available—perhaps because they are being seen in a specialty clinic. Their clinical course is then described by going back in time and seeing how they have fared from the time they were first seen up to the present. Such groups of patients are sometimes called **false cohorts, survival cohorts,** or **available patient cohorts,** although they are not really cohorts at all.

Reports of survival cohorts are misleading when they are presented as true cohorts describing the course of disease from its inception. They represent a biased view of the course of disease because they include only those patients who are available for study some time after their disease began. All of the patients must have remained under care to be included. For lethal conditions, the patients in a survival cohort are the ones who are fortunate enough to have survived and so are available for observation years later. For diseases that remit, the patients are the ones who are unfortunate enough to have

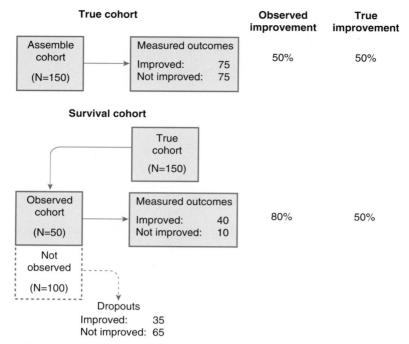

FIGURE 7.6 ■ Comparison of a true and false cohort. In the false cohort, some of the patients present at the beginning are not included in the follow-up.

persistent disease. Also, patients are assembled at various times throughout the course of their disease rather than at the beginning (as in a true inception cohort study). In effect, survival cohorts describe the past history of prevalent cases and not what one would expect over the time after the onset of disease.

Reports of survival cohorts are relatively common in the medical literature, particularly in the form of **case series**—descriptions of groups of patients with a disease. Such reports can make an important contribution, primarily by describing early experiences with newly defined syndromes and providing hypotheses about prognosis, but they represent tentative, not conclusive, observations.

EXAMPLE

Silicone breast implants have been suspected of causing connective tissue diseases such as scleroderma and rheumatoid arthritis. An early case series described 156 women with silicone breast implants and rheumatic disease complaints referred to three rheumatologists who were known for their interest in silicone implants and rheumatic disease. (4) Serologic tests in these women were compared to those of women without implants (but who did have fibromyalgia) and to tests in women with im-

plants but no rheumatic symptoms. The clinical findings in most of the women with implants and complaints did not fulfill criteria for rheumatoid arthritis and most of these women had normal immunologic tests. However, 14 patients had scleroderma-like illness and abnormal serology that was not found in the comparison groups. Because this case series was a biased sample of patients with implants, the authors were cautious about their findings, concluding that "the hypotheses raised in this study and others should be tested in large, population-based studies." A summary of 20 studies (some of which were population-based) published several years later found no evidence that breast implants were associated with an increased risk of any of the connective tissue diseases. (5)

IDENTIFYING PROGNOSTIC FACTORS

Often, we want to go beyond a simple description of prognosis in a homogeneous group of patients to compare prognosis in patients with different characteristics—that is, potential prognostic factors. Multiple survival curves, one for patients with each of the characteristics, are represented on the same figure where they can be visually (and statistically) compared.

EXAMPLE

Abdominal aortic aneurysms tend to increase in size over time. The risk of rupture, which is rapidly fatal, increases with aneurysm size. Rupture can be prevented with elective surgery, in which the aneurysm is replaced by a graft, but the surgery itself is somewhat risky. This situation presents a difficult question: When in the course of the aneurysm should one intervene with surgery? The answer depends in part on the risk of rupture associated with various aneurysm sizes. Investigators took advantage of a natural experiment to provide an answer. They observed 198 patients with abdominal aortic aneurysms, which were at least 5cm in diameter, and for whom surgery was not planned because the patients either had medical contraindications to surgery or refused it. (6) During up to 5 years of follow-up (average 1.5 years), 45 of these patients (23%) had probable rupture as determined by medical records, eyewitness accounts, and autopsy reports. The investigators compared the probability of rupture according to the last recorded size of the aneurysm, using a time-to-event analysis (Figure 7.7).

Rupture was common in all patients, it increased with size, and it was highest in patients with aneurysms of >7.0cm. in diameter.

The effects of possible prognostic factors, relative to one another, can be summarized by a **hazard ratio**, which is analogous to a risk ratio (relative risk). Hazard ratios are derived from time-to-event analyses. Also, survival curves can be compared after taking into account other factors related to prognosis, so that the independent effect of just one variable is examined (see mathematical modeling below).

PREDICTION RULES

A combination of variables often provides a more precise prognosis than any of these variables taken one at a time. **Clinical prediction rules** estimate the

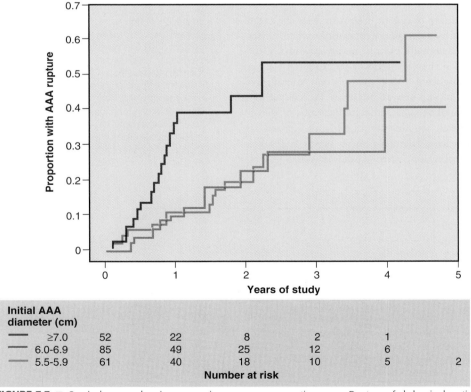

Initial AAA diameter (cm)					
≥7.0	52	22	8	2	1
6.0-6.9	85	49	25	12	6
5.5-5.9	61	40	18	10	5	2

Number at risk

FIGURE 7.7 ■ Survival curves showing comparison among prognostic groups. Rupture of abdominal aortic aneurysm (AAA) according to the most recent diameter. (From Lederle FA, Johnson GR, Wilson SE et al. Rupture of large abdominal aortic aneurysms in patients refusing or unfit for elective surgery. JAMA 2002; 287:2968–2972.)

probability of outcomes according to a set of patient characteristics (see Chapter 3).

> ### E X A M P L E
>
> How well can we predict the chances of death among patients hospitalized for heart failure? A set of predictive variables was identified in a cohort of 2,624 patients admitted to multiple hospitals in Canada. (7) The predictive variables included older age, lower systolic blood pressure, higher respiratory rate, and higher urea nitrogen level (a measure of renal function), as well as several coexistent diseases. These variables were combined into a risk index, which weighted the relative importance of each. One-year mortality rate was 2.7% for patients with very low-risk scores and 74.7% in patients with very high-risk scores (Figure 7.8). The results were reproduced in a separate cohort of 1,407 patients, suggesting that the predictive ability of the model was not confined to the particular patients used to derive it.

BIAS IN COHORT STUDIES

In cohort studies of risk or prognosis, bias can create apparent differences between groups when differences do not actually exist in nature or obscure differences when they really do exist. Potential for bias can be recognized more easily when one knows where it is most likely to occur in the course of a study. Some of the characteristic locations of bias in cohort research are illustrated in Figure 7.9 and are described below. Many of these biases have their counterparts in case-control studies as well.

Susceptibility Bias

A form of selection bias called **susceptibility bias** occurs when groups of patients assembled for study differ in ways other than the variables under study. These extraneous variables, not the particular variables being studied, may determine the outcome. A comparable term is **assembly bias**. Groups being compared are not equally susceptible to the outcome of interest for reasons other than the factor under study.

Susceptibility bias in prognostic studies may be due to one or more differences among cohorts, including the extent of disease, the presence of other diseases, the point of time in the course of disease, and prior treatment. The following illustrates how susceptibility bias was recognized and dealt with.

> ### E X A M P L E
>
> The clinical course of diffuse, large-B-cell lymphoma is currently predicted by the International Prognostic Index (IPI). The prediction is based on five clinical characteristics: age, tumor stage, serum lactic dehydrogenase concentration, performance status, and number of extranodal disease sites. However, even within IPI risk categories, prognosis is quite variable. If it were possible to improve prediction, aggressiveness of treatment could be matched to prognosis.
>
> Investigators used gene-expression signatures to predict prognosis. (8) They studied 36 genes whose expression had been found in other studies to be related to survival for this lymphoma. Six were strong predictors in the data. They developed a prediction rule based on these six and found that it also predicted clinical course in two

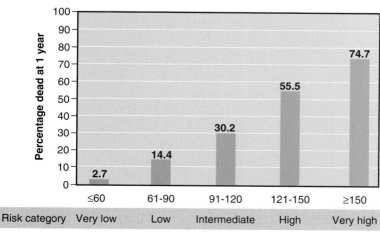

FIGURE 7.8 ▪ Example of a clinical prediction rule. One-year mortality rate for patients hospitalized for heart failure according to risk scores based on 10 variables. (From Lee DS, Austin PC, Rouleau JL, Liu PP, Naimark D, Tu JV, et al. Predicting mortality among patients hospitalized for heart failure: derivation and validation of a clinical model. JAMA 2003;290: 2581–2587.)

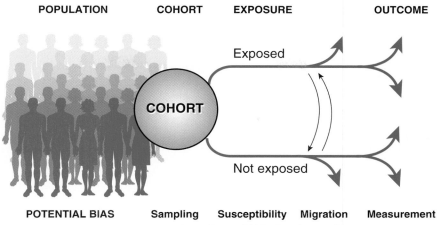

POPULATION   COHORT   EXPOSURE   OUTCOME

Exposed

COHORT

Not exposed

POTENTIAL BIAS   Sampling   Susceptibility   Migration   Measurement

FIGURE 7.9 ■ Locations of potential bias in cohort studies.

separate groups of patients. But was the prognostic information contributed by these six genes independent of information already available in the IPI? Simpler predictors such as age might have accounted for the differences in clinical course attributed to the six-gene model but this possibility was ruled out. Low-, medium-, and high-risk patients (according to the six-gene model) had a very different clinical course when applied separately to patients classified as low-, medium-, and high-risk according to the IPI. Therefore, prediction by the six-gene model could not be attributed to systematic differences in the age, tumor stage, and the like in the prognostic groups (susceptibility bias). The new model added information after the best previously available prediction was taken into account.

Migration Bias

Migration bias, another form of selection bias, can occur when patients in one subgroup of a cohort leave their original group, dropping out of the study altogether or moving to one of the other groups under study. If these changes take place on a sufficiently large scale, they can affect the validity of conclusions.

In nearly all studies, some members of an original group drop out over time. If these **dropouts** occur randomly, such that the characteristics of lost subjects in one group are on the average similar to those lost from the other, then no bias would be introduced. This is so whether or not the number of dropouts is large or the number of dropouts is similar in the groups. But ordinarily the characteristics of

lost subjects are not the same in various groups. The reasons for dropping out include death, recovery, and side effects of treatment and are often related to prognosis and so may also affect one group more than another. As a result, groups in a cohort that were comparable at the outset may become less so as time passes. As the proportion of people in the cohort who are not followed up increases, the potential for bias increases.

Patients may also move from one group to another in the cohort during their follow-up, a phenomenon called **crossover**. Whenever this occurs, the original reasons for patients being in one group or the other no longer apply. If exchange of patients between groups takes place on a large scale, it can diminish the observed difference in risk compared to what might have been observed if the original groups had remained intact.

Migration bias from crossover is more often a problem in risk than in prognosis studies, because risk studies go on for many years.

EXAMPLE

What proportion of patients having poliomyelitis develop the post-polio syndrome, involving muscle weakness, pain, and fatigue, years later? To answer this question, investigators identified a cohort of 939 patients who had poliomyelitis and were admitted to the two hospitals serving their region from 1950 to 1955. (9) The cohort included 95% of the polio cases on record at the local health department during those years, suggesting that the investigators had identified a relatively complete sample of cases in their region. In the late 1980s (32–39 years after the acute illness), investigators were able to trace 667 of these patients; 41 had died of other causes, leaving 626 members of the cohort who could have experienced the outcome (post-polio syndrome). Of these, 551 (88%) provided data on their current symptoms. In all, 137 of the 551 (25%) met criteria for post-polio syndrome.

How much could the missing cases, if they were different from those who provided data, have biased the estimate of the rate of post-polio syndrome? To find out, a **best-case/worst-case analysis** could have been done, looking at the effects of making assumptions about potential bias. (This approach will be explained in detail later in this chapter.) In the worst case, if all of the 75 patients who did not provide outcome data had the syndrome, the rate would have been 137 + 75/551 + 75 = 34%. If, on the other hand, none of these 75 patients had the syndrome, the rate would have been 137/551 + 75 = 22%. Therefore, even if the worst possible bias had been present, inability to get data from 75 members of the cohort would not have changed the rate estimate greatly.

If more plausible bias were assumed—that patients with missing data were twice as likely (or half as likely) to develop the syndrome—the actual rate might have been as high as 28% or as low as 23%, which would be very close to the estimate from available data. Therefore, migration bias related to incomplete follow-up was unlikely to have had important effects on the study's conclusions.

This example illustrates the potentially biasing effects of dropouts during a long period of follow-up and how they can be estimated. The analysis did not take into account possible differences in the 272 patients who could not be traced, the effects of which could be estimated in a similar way.

Measurement Bias

Measurement bias is possible when patients in one subgroup of a cohort stand a better chance of having their outcomes detected than those in another subgroup. Obviously, some outcomes, such as death, cardiovascular catastrophes, and major cancers, are so obtrusive that they are unlikely to be missed. But for less clear-cut outcomes, including specific cause of death, sub-clinical disease, side effects, or disability, measurement bias can occur because of differences in the methods with which the outcome is sought or classified.

Measurement bias can be minimized in three general ways: Ensure that those who record outcome events are unaware of the group to which each patient belongs, set up careful rules for deciding

whether or not an outcome event has occurred (and follow the rules), and apply efforts to discover outcome events equally for all patients in the study.

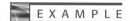 EXAMPLE

Clinical trials of anticoagulants depend on accurate measurement of pulmonary embolus, the main outcome event. Ventilation-perfusion lung scans are the standard for diagnosis, but their interpretation is subjective. In one study, agreement among radiologists was 65 to 79% (depending on the criteria) after taking into account chance agreement. (10) Possibilities for increasing agreement for key study variables include use of explicit standards for interpretation of scans (three sets of criteria are in general use) and "blinding" radiologists to treatment group so that knowledge of how patients were treated cannot affect the radiologists' interpretations of scans.

DEALING WITH SELECTION BIAS AND CONFOUNDING

To determine whether a factor is independently related to risk or prognosis, it is ideal to compare cohorts with and without the factor, everything else being equal. But in real life, "everything else" usually is not equal in observational studies.

What can be done about this problem? There are several possible ways of **controlling**† for differences between groups. Controlling is a general term for any process aimed at removing the effects of extraneous variables while examining the independent effects of one variable. These methods can be applied during the design or analysis of research (Table 7.3). Strategies for these are described below. One or more of these strategies should be applied in any observational study that attempts to describe the effect of one variable independent of other variables that might affect the outcome. The basic question is, "Are the differences between groups in risk or prognosis related to the particular factor under study or to some other factor(s)?"

---

†Unfortunately, control also has several other meanings: the non-exposed people in a cohort study (a confusing use of the term); the patients in a clinical trial who do not receive the experimental treatment; and non-diseased people (noncases) in a case control study.

TABLE 7.3 ■ **Methods for Controlling Selection Bias**

		Phase of Study	
Method	*Description*	*Design*	*Analysis*
Randomization	Assign patients to groups in a way that gives each patient an equal chance of falling into one or the other group	+	
Restriction	Limit the range of characteristics of patients in the study	+	
Matching	For each patient in one group, select one or more patients with the same characteristics (except for the one under study) for a comparison group	+	+
Stratification	Compare rates within subgroups (strata) with otherwise similar probability of the outcome		+
Simple adjustment	Mathematically adjust crude rates for one or a few characteristics so that equal weight is given to strata of similar risk		+
Multivariable	Adjust for differences in a large number of factors related to outcome, using mathematical modeling techniques		+
Best case/worst case	Describe how different the results could be under the most extreme (or simply very unlikely) assumption about selection bias		+

Randomization

The best way to balance all extraneous variables between groups is to assign patients to groups randomly so that each patient has an equal chance of falling into the exposed or unexposed group. A special feature of **randomization** is that it not only balances variables known to affect prognosis, but it also balances those that are unknown. Thus, randomization goes a long way toward protecting against incorrect conclusions about risk or prognostic factors.

Unfortunately, it is usually not possible to randomize risk or prognostic factors. The special situations in which it is possible to allocate exposure randomly, in studies of the effects of treatment on prognosis, will be discussed in Chapter 8.

Restriction

Patients who are enrolled in a study can be confined to only those possessing a narrow range of characteristics, a strategy called **restriction**. When this is done, characteristics cannot be very different in the groups being compared. For example, the effect of age on prognosis after acute myocardial infarction could be studied in white males who have uncomplicated anterior myocardial infarctions. However, this approach is limiting. Although restriction on entry to a study can certainly produce homogeneous subgroups of patients, it does so at the expense of generalizability. In the course of excluding potential subjects, cohorts may be selected that are not representative of most patients with the condition. Also, after restriction it is no longer possible, in that study, to learn anything more about the effects of excluded variables.

Matching

Matching is another way to make patients in two groups similar. In its simplest form, for each patient in one group one or more patients with the same characteristics (except for the factor of interest) is selected for a comparison group. Often, patients are matched for age and sex because these variables are strongly related to risk or prognosis for many diseases. But matching for other variables such as stage or severity of disease, rate of progression, and prior treatments, may be useful as well. An example of matching in a case-control study of exercise and sudden death was described in Chapter 6.

Although matching is commonly done and can be very useful, it has limitations. Matching controls bias only for those variables involved in the match. Also, it is usually not possible to match for more than a few variables because of practical difficulties in finding patients who meet all of the matching criteria. Moreover, if categories for matching are relatively crude, there may be room for substantial differences between matched groups. For example, if women in a study of risk for birth of a child with Down syndrome were matched for maternal age within 10 years, there could be a nearly tenfold difference in frequency related to age if most of the women in one group were 30 and most in the other 39 years old. Finally, as with restriction, once one matches on a variable, its effects on outcomes can no longer be evaluated in the study. For example, the study of exercise and primary cardiac arrest (in Chapter 6) matched on age and sex, so it was not possible to learn from that study whether the effect of exercise was different at different ages or in men versus women. For these reasons, while matching may be done for a few characteristics that are especially strongly related to outcome, investigators rely on other ways of controlling for bias as well.

Stratification

With **stratification**, data are analyzed and results presented according to subgroups of patients, or **strata**, of similar characteristics. We shall describe this approach using as an example difference in hospital mortality for a common surgical procedure. This is especially relevant these days because of several high-profile examples of "report cards" for doctors and hospitals, and the concern that the reported differences may be related to patient rather than provider or hospital characteristics.

EXAMPLE

Suppose we want to compare the operative mortality rates for coronary bypass surgery at hospitals A and B. Overall, hospital A noted 48 deaths in 1,200 bypass operations (4%), and hospital B experienced 64 deaths in 2,400 operations (2.6%).

The crude rates suggest that hospital B is superior. Or do they? Perhaps patients in the two hospitals were not otherwise of comparable prognosis. On the basis of age, myocardial function, extent of occlusive disease, and other characteristics, the patients can be divided into subgroups based on preoperative risk; then the operative mortality rates within each category (stratum) of risk can be compared.

Table 7.4 shows that when patients are divided by preoperative risk, the operative mortality rates in each risk stratum are identical in two hospitals: 6% in high-risk patients, 4% in medium-risk patients, and 0.67% in low-risk patients. The crude rates were misleading because of important differences in the risk characteristics of the patients treated at the two hospitals: 42% of hospital A's patients and only 17% of hospital B's patients were high risk.

An advantage of stratification is that it is a relatively transparent way of recognizing and controlling for bias.

Standardization

If an extraneous factor is especially strongly related to outcomes, two rates can be compared without bias related to this factor if they are adjusted to equalize the weight given to the factor. This process, called **standardization** (or **adjustment**), shows what the overall rate would be if strata-specific rates were applied to a population made up of similar proportions of people in each stratum.

EXAMPLE

In this example, we standardize hospitals A and B to the same distribution of risk groups. The crude rates do not take into account dissimilar risks in the two hospitals. The mortality rate of 6% for high-risk patients receives a weight of 500/1,200 in hospital A and a much lower weight of 400/2,400 in hospital B. The other risk strata were also weighted differently in the two hospitals. The result is a crude rate for hospital A, which is the sum of the rate in each stratum times its weight: (500/1,200 × 0.06) + (400/1,200 × 0.04) + (300/1,200 - 0.0067) = 0.04. Similarly, the crude rate for hospital B is (400/2,400 × 0.06) + (800/2,400 × 0.04) + (1,200/2,400 × 0. 0067) = 0.026.

If equal weights were used when comparing the two hospitals, the comparison would be fair (free of the effect of different proportions in the various risk groups). The choice of weights does not matter, as long as it is the same in the two hospitals. Weights could be based on those existing in either of the hospitals or any reference population. If each stratum were weighted 1/3, then the standardized rate for hospital A = (1/3 × 0.06) + (1/3

TABLE 7.4 ■ Example of Stratification: Hypothetical Death Rates After Coronary Bypass Surgery in Two Hospitals, Stratified by Preoperative Risk

	Hospital A			Hospital B		
Preoperative Risk	Patients	Deaths	Rate (%)	Patients	Deaths	Rate (%)
High	500	30	6	400	24	6
Medium	400	16	4	800	32	4
Low	300	2	0.67	1,200	8	0.67
Total	1,200	48	4	2,400	64	2.6

$\times$ 0.04) + (1/3 $\times$ 0.0067) = 0.036, which is exactly the same as the standardized rate for hospital B. The consequence of giving equal weight to strata in each hospital is to totally remove the apparent excess risk of hospital A.

The difference between the crude operative mortality rates in the two hospitals results from the bias introduced by the differences in patients' preoperative risk. Of primary interest are the differences attributable to the hospitals and their surgeons, not to the patients per se. The difference in the crude mortality rates is confounded by the differences in patients, and standardization removed this unwanted (extraneous) effect, allowing comparisons of hospital survival that are unbiased by preoperative mortality.

Multivariable Adjustment

In most clinical situations, many variables act together to produce effects. The relationships among these variables are complex. They may be related to one anther as well as to the outcome of interest. The effect of one might be modified by the presence of others, and the joint effects of two or more might be greater than the sum of their individual effects.

Mathematical modeling is a way of combining data on all the variables, based on certain assumptions about their distributions and relationships. Modeling makes it possible to consider the effects of many variables simultaneously. Another term for this approach is **multivariable analysis.** Modeling is used to adjust (control) for the effects of many variables to determine the independent effects of one. This method also can select, from a large set of variables, those that contribute independently to the overall variation in outcome. Modeling can also arrange variables in order of the strength of their contribution. **Cox proportional**

hazard model is a type of multivariable technique used when the outcome is the time to an event (as in survival analyses). Case-control studies typically rely on **logistic regression**, which is specifically for dichotomous outcomes.

Multivariable analysis is the only feasible way of dealing with many variables at one time. Randomization also controls for multiple variables, but during the design and conduct phases of a study. Matching can account for only a few variables at a time, and stratified analyses of many variables run the risk of having too few patients in some strata. The disadvantage of modeling is that for most of us it is a "black box," making it difficult to recognize where the method might be misleading. Typically, modeling is used in addition to, not in place of, matching and stratified analysis.

Sensitivity Analysis

When important data are not available, it is possible to estimate their potential effects on the study by assuming various degrees of maldistribution of the variable between the groups being compared and seeing how it would affect the results. The general term for this process is **sensitivity analysis**. Another term, with the same meaning, is **"what if" analysis**. A special case is the best-case/worst-case analysis, in which one assumes the best and worst possible distribution; an example of this approach has already been presented in the example of migration bias (page 118).

E X A M P L E

A randomized study of treatment for mild diabetes found that patients who were given tolbutamide, a first-generation oral agent for type II diabetes, experienced a greater risk of dying from cardiovascular disease than those given insulin or diet alone. The results were criticized because data on smoking, which is known to be associated with cardiovascular death, were not collected and could not be taken into account in the analysis. It was suggested that if cigarette smokers were unequally distributed among the groups, such that there were more smokers among those receiving tolbutamide than in the other groups, then the difference in death rates might be related to smoking, not tolbutamide. However, Cornfield (11) pointed out that even if cigarette smokers in the tolbutamide group exceeded those in the control group by 20%, a situation that would have been extremely unlikely by chance (1/50,000), smoking would not have accounted for the observed difference. Thus, bias in the distribution of smokers was unlikely to have accounted for the observed differences. Some, but not all, subsequent studies of this class of drugs have confirmed an increased risk of cardiovascular disease, although controversy remains.

Overall Strategy for Controlling Bias

Except for randomization, all ways of dealing with extraneous differences between groups share a limitation: They are effective against only those variables that are singled out for consideration. They do not deal with risk or prognostic factors that are not known at the time of the study, or they are known but not taken into account.

For this reason, and the complementary strengths and weakness of the various methods, one does not rely on only one or another method of controlling for bias but rather uses several methods together, layered one on another.

E X A M P L E

In a study of whether the presence of ventricular premature contractions decreases survival in the years following acute myocardial infarction, one might:

1. Restrict the study to patients who are not very old or young and who do not have unusual causes, such as mycotic aneurysm, for their infarction
2. Match for age, a factor strongly related to prognosis but extraneous to the main question
3. Examine the results separately for strata of differing clinical severity. This includes the presence or absence of congestive heart failure or other diseases, such as chronic obstructive pulmonary disease
4. Using multivariable analysis, adjust the crude results for the effects of all the variables other than the arrhythmia, taken together, that might be related to prognosis.

GENERALIZABILITY AND SAMPLING BIAS

Published accounts of disease prognosis based on experience in special centers can paint a misleading picture of prognosis in less selected patients. This is true even when a study is well done, biases are carefully controlled for, and the reported prognosis is correct for the particular sample of patients. Because of the sample of patients used, it may be that the study findings are not generalizable to most other patients with the condition or to your patient. **Sampling bias** occurs when patients selected for study are systematically different from those the results are generalized to.

E X A M P L E

Febrile seizures are common, occurring in 2–4% of children. It is important to know how likely such seizures are to recur. If they recur often, treatment with anticonvulsant drugs might be worthwhile. If febrile seizures are usually one-time phenomena, explanation and reassurance is in order. Figure 7.10 summarizes recurrence rates for febrile seizures reported in 21 studies, grouped according to whether the children were identified in a community sample or a referral center.(12) Recurrence rates in population-based studies (on the left) were low, about 3%. On the other hand, rates in hospital clinics and specialty referral units (on the right) varied but in general were much higher, with a range of 5 to 75%.

Applying results from referral centers to community practice would result in falsely high estimates of the likelihood of recurrent seizures. On the other hand, using the results of population-based studies for children seen in referral centers would also be inaccurate, underestimating rates for those children. Therefore, the children studied should match the setting in which the information is used.

BIAS, PERHAPS, BUT DOES IT MATTER?

Clinical epidemiology is not an error-finding game. Rather, it is meant to characterize the credibility of a study so that clinicians can decide how much to rely on its results when making high-stakes decisions about patients. It would be irresponsible to ignore results of studies that meet high standards, just as

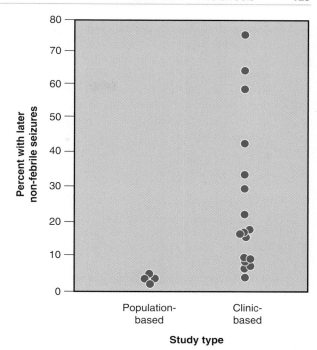

FIGURE 7.10 ▦ Example of sampling bias. Recurrent seizures in infants with febrile seizures in population-based and clinic-based studies. (Redrawn from Ellenberg JH, Nelson KB. Sample selection and the natural history of disease: Studies of febrile seizure. JAMA 1980;243: 1337–1340.)

clinical decisions need not be bound by the results of weak studies.

With this in mind, it is not enough to recognize that bias might be present in a study. One must go on to determine whether or not bias is actually present in the particular study. Beyond that, one must decide whether the consequences of bias are sufficiently large that they actually change the conclusions in a clinically important way. A sensitivity analysis, even if just a rough-and-ready one, can be helpful for this purpose. If damage to the study's conclusions is not very great, then the presence of bias is of little practical consequence and the study is still useful.

REVIEW QUESTIONS

Read the following and circle the best option.

7.1. A patient wants your advice about recovery after an attack of acute low back pain. The best available study of this question describes time-to-recovery for a large cohort of patients with low back pain. Patients were followed from onset to 1 year, when nearly all had recovered. The study found that several variables were related to prognosis: severity of pain at onset, presence of lumbar disk disease, neurologic deficits such as weakness and numbness, activity following the attack, and spinal manipulation. Which approach would provide the most information in tailoring prognosis to your particular patient?

A. Stratified analysis
B. Matching
C. Multivariable analysis
D. Restriction
E. Sensitivity analysis

7.2. Investigators wish to describe the clinical course of multiple sclerosis. They take advantage of a clinical trial, already completed, in which control patients received usual care. Patients in the trial had been identified at referral centers, had been enrolled at the time of diagnosis, and had met rigorous entry criteria. After 10 years, all patients remained under observation, and 40% were still able to walk. This study was most limited by:

A. Inconsistent zero time
B. Generalizability
C. Measurement bias
D. Migration bias
E. Failure to use time-to-event methods

7.3. A study describes the clinical course of patients who have an uncommon neurologic disease. Patients are identified at a referral center that specializes in this disease. Their medical records are reviewed for patient characteristics and treatments and are then related to their current status. This study is best described as a:

A. Cohort study
B. Case-control study
C. Case series
D. Cross-sectional study
E. A randomized controlled trial

Questions 7.4–7.8 are based on the following study:

Time to recurrence after surgery for lung cancer is described in a time-to-event analysis. Thirty patients are enrolled at the time of curative-intent surgery. Patients are entered in the study over a 2-year period and followed up with for as long as 5 years. Some die of other diseases, or drop out of the study during follow-up. By the end of follow-up, three patients were still under observation and free of disease.

Read the following statements about this study and mark each one as True or False.

_____ **7.4.** The recurrence rate at 5 years is 27/30 = 90%.

_____ **7.5.** The estimated time to recurrence at the end of follow-up is sensitive to what happens to just a few patients.

_____ **7.6** A major disadvantage of this study is that all of the patients were not enrolled at the same calendar time.

_____ **7.7.** This study depends on the assumption that censored patients are similar to those who remain in the study

_____ **7.8.** This analysis provides an estimate of what time-to-recurrence would be in a cohort of similar patients.

Answers are in Appendix A.

REFERENCES

1. Talley NJ, Zinsmeister AR, Van Dyke C, Melton LJ 3rd. Epidemiology of colonic symptoms and the irritable bowel syndrome. Gastroenterology 1991;101: 927–934.

2. Evers IM, de Valk HW, Visser GHA. Risk of complications of pregnancy in women with type 1 diabetes: Nationwide prospective study in the Netherlands. BMJ 2004;328:915–920.

3. Feinstein AR, Sosin DM, Wells CK. The Will Rogers phenomenon: Stage migration and new diagnostic techniques as a source of misleading statistics for survival in cancer. N Engl J Med 1985;312:1604–1608.

4. Bridges AJ, Conley C, Wang G, Burns DE, Vasey FB. A clinical and immunologic evaluation of women with silicone breast implants and symptoms of rheumatic disease. Ann Intern Med 1993;118: 929–936.

5. Janowsky EC, Kupper KL, Hulka BS. Meta-analysis of the relation between silicone breast implants and the risk of connective-tissue diseases. N Engl J Med 2000;342:781–790.

6. Lederle FA, Johnson GR, Wilson SE, Ballard DJ, Jordan WD Jr, Blebea J, et al. Rupture of large abdominal aortic aneurysms in patients refusing or unfit for elective surgery. JAMA 2002;287:2968–2972.

7. Lee DS, Austin PC, Rouleau JL, Liu PP, Naimark D, Tu JV. Predicting mortality among patients hospitalized for heart failure: derivation and validation of a clinical model. JAMA 2003;290:2581–2587.

8. Lossos IS, Czerwinski DK, Alizadeh AA, Wechser MA, Tibshirani R, Botstein D, et al. Prediction of survival in diffuse large-B-cell lymphoma based on the expression of six genes. N Engl J Med 2004;350: 1828–1837.

9. Ramlow J, Alexander M, LaPorte R, Kaufmann C, Kuller L. Epidemiology of post-polio syndrome. Am J Epid 1992;136:769–786.

10. Hagen PJ, Hartmann IJ, Hoekstra OS, Stokkel MP, Postmus PE, Prins MH: Antelope Study Group. Comparison of observer variability and accuracy of different criteria for lung scan interpretation. J Nucl Med 2003;44:739–744.

11. Cornfield J. The University Group Diabetes Program: A further statistical analysis of the mortality findings. JAMA 1971;217:1676–1687.

12. Ellenberg JH, Nelson KB. Sample selection and the natural history of disease. Studies of febrile seizures. JAMA 1980;243:1337–1340.

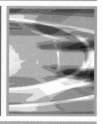

Treatment

Treatments should be given "not because they ought to work, but because they do work."
—*L.H. Opie*

Once the nature of a patient's illness has been established and its expected course predicted, the next question is, what can be done about it? Is there a treatment that improves the outcome of disease? This chapter describes the evidence used to decide whether a well-intentioned treatment is actually effective.

IDEAS AND EVIDENCE

The discovery of new treatments requires rich sources of promising possibilities and rigorous ways of establishing that the treatments are, in fact and on average, effective (Figure 8.1).

Ideas

Ideas about what might be a useful treatment arise from virtually any activity within medicine. Ideas are called **hypotheses** to the extent that they are assertions about the natural world made for the purposes of empiric testing. Some therapeutic hypotheses are suggested by the mechanisms of disease at the molecular level. Drugs against antibiotic-resistant

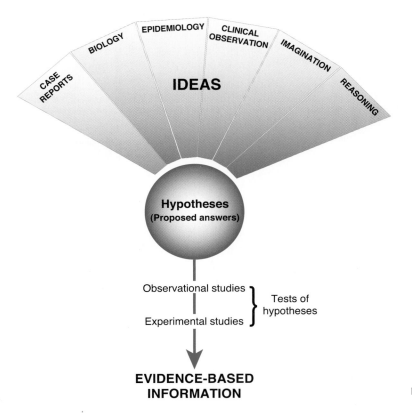

FIGURE 8.1 ▪ Ideas and evidence.

bacteria are developed through knowledge of the mechanism of resistance. Hormone analogues are based on the structure of native hormones.

Other hypotheses about treatments have come from astute observations by clinicians. These observations are shared with their colleagues in **case reports**, which are detailed descriptions of a single case or just a few cases. The following is an example of a case report that led to a new class of drugs for influenza. At the time, the drug, amantadine, was already in use for prevention of influenza, a totally unrelated disease.

EXAMPLE

". . . . A 58-year-old woman with moderately severe, bilateral Parkinson's disease recounted to us that three months before, while taking amantadine hydrochloride 100 mg twice daily, to prevent the flu, she experienced a remarkable remission in her symptoms of rigidity, tremor, and akinesia. These promptly returned on stopping the drug after six weeks. Her husband corroborated all of this." (1)

More recently, the drug minoxidil, which was developed for hypertension, was found to improve male pattern baldness. Tamoxifen, developed for contraception, was found to prevent breast cancer in high-risk women.

Other sources of ideas about effective treatments include beliefs about herbal remedies, some of which are supported by centuries of experience. Aspirin, atropine, digitalis, and taxol are examples of naturally occurring substances that have become established as orthodox medicines after rigorous testing.

Still other ideas come from trial and error. Some anticancer drugs have been found by methodically screening huge numbers of substances for activity in laboratory models.

Ideas about treatment, but more often prevention, have also come from epidemiologic studies of populations. Burkitt observed that colonic diseases, such as irritable bowel syndrome, diverticulitis, appendicitis, and colorectal cancer, are less common in African countries, where diet is high in fiber, than in developed countries, where dietary intake of fiber is low. This observation has led to efforts to prevent bowel diseases with high-fiber diets. Similarly, comparisons across regions have suggested the value of fluoride to prevent dental caries.

Testing Ideas

Some treatment effects are so prompt and powerful that their value is self-evident even without formal testing. Clinicians do not have reservations about the value of antibiotics for bacterial pneumonia, surgery for appendicitis, or colchicine for an acute attack of gout. Clinical experience was sufficient.

In contrast, many diseases, including most chronic diseases, involve treatments that are considerably less dramatic. The effects are slower and smaller. It is then necessary to put ideas about treatments to a formal test, through clinical research, because a variety of circumstances, such as coincidence, faulty comparisons, spontaneous changes in the course of disease, or wishful thinking, can obscure the true relationship between treatment and outcomes.

When knowledge of the pathogenesis of disease, based on work with laboratory models or physiologic studies in humans, has become extensive, it is tempting to predict effects in humans on this basis alone. However, relying solely on current understanding of mechanisms without testing ideas using strong clinical research on intact humans can lead to unpleasant surprises.

E X A M P L E

Some strokes are caused by cerebral infarction in the area of the brain distal to an obstructed segment of the internal carotid artery. It should be possible to prevent strokes in people with these lesions by bypassing the diseased segment so that blood can flow to the threatened area normally. It is technically feasible to connect the superficial temporal artery to the internal carotid artery distal to an obstruction. Because its value seemed self-evident on physiologic grounds and because of the documented success of an analogous procedure, coronary artery bypass surgery, this new surgery became widely used.

The EC/IC Bypass Study Group conducted a randomized controlled trial of temporal artery bypass surgery. (2) Patients with cerebral ischemia and an obstructed internal carotid artery were randomly allocated to surgical versus medical treatment. The operation was a technical success; 96% of anastomoses were patent just after surgery. Yet, the surgery did not help the patients. Mortality and stroke rates after 5 years were nearly identical in the surgically and medically treated patients, but deaths had occurred earlier in the surgically treated patients.

This study illustrates how treatments that make good sense, based on what we know about the mechanisms of disease, may be found ineffective in human terms when put to a rigorous test. Of course, it is not always the case that ideas are debunked; the value of carotid endarterectomy, suggested on similar grounds, has been confirmed.

Knowledge of pathogenesis, worked out in laboratory models, may be disappointing in human studies because the laboratory studies are in highly simplified settings. They usually exclude, or control for, many real-world influences on disease such as variation in genetic endowment, the physical and social environment, and individual behaviors and preferences.

Clinical experience and tradition also need to be put to a test.

E X A M P L E

Bed rest has been advocated for a large number of medical conditions. Usually, there is a rationale for it. For example, it has been thought that the headache following lumbar puncture might result from a leak of cerebrospinal fluid through the needle track causing stretching of the meninges. However, a review of 39 trials of bed rest for 15 different conditions found that outcome did not improve for any condition. Outcomes were worse with bed rest in 17 trials, including not only lumbar puncture, but also acute low back pain, labor, hypertension during pregnancy, acute myocardial infarction, and acute infectious hepatitis. (3)

Therefore, it is almost always necessary to test therapeutic hypotheses by means of clinical research, in which data are collected on the clinical course of treated and untreated patients. As one author put it, treatments should be given "not because they ought to work, but because they do work." (4)

STUDIES OF TREATMENT EFFECTS

Treatment is any intervention, which may include prescribing drugs, performing surgery, or counseling, that is intended to improve the course of disease once it is established. Treatment is a special case of **interventions** in general that might be applied at any point in the natural history of disease, from disease prevention to palliative care at the end of life. Interventions can take any form, including relaxation therapy, laser surgery, or changes in the organization and financing of health care. Regardless of the nature of a well-intentioned intervention, the principles by which it is judged superior to other alternatives are the same.

Observational and Experimental Studies of Treatment Effects

Two general methods are used to establish the effects of interventions: observational and experimental studies. The two differ in their scientific strength and feasibility.

In **observational studies** of interventions, investigators simply observe what happens to patients who for various reasons do or do not get exposed to an intervention. Observational studies of treatment are a special case of studies of prognosis in general, in which the prognostic factor of interest is a therapeutic intervention. What has been said about cohort studies (especially in Chapters 5 and 7) applies to observational studies of treatment as well. The main advantage of these studies is feasibility. The main drawback is the possibility that there are systematic differences in treatment groups, other than the treatment itself, that can lead to misleading conclusions about the effects of treatment.

Experimental studies are a special kind of cohort study in which the conditions of study—that is, selection of treatment groups, nature of interventions, management during follow-up, and measurement of outcomes—are specified by the investigator for the purpose of making unbiased comparisons. These studies are generally referred to as **clinical trials**. Clinical trials are more highly controlled and managed than are cohort studies. The investigators are conducting an experiment, analogous to those done in the laboratory. They have taken it upon themselves (with their patients' permission) to isolate for study the unique contribution of one factor by holding constant, as much as possible, all other determinants of the outcome.

Randomized controlled trials, in which treatment is randomly allocated, are the standard of excellence for scientific studies of the effects of treatment. They are described in detail below, along with alternative ways of studying the effectiveness of interventions.

RANDOMIZED CONTROLLED TRIALS

The structure of a randomized controlled trial is shown in Figure 8.2. All elements are the same as for a cohort study except that treatment is assigned by randomization rather than by physician or patient choice. The "exposures" are treatments, the "outcomes" are any of the 5 Ds described in Chapter 1 (see also Table 1.3), and the measure of effect is the degree of improvement.

The patients to be studied are first selected from a larger number of patients with the condition of interest. They are then divided, using randomization, into two groups (or more) of comparable prognosis. One group, called the **experimental group**, is exposed to an intervention that is believed to be better than current alternatives. The other group, called a **control group** (or **comparison group**), is treated the same in all ways except that its members are not exposed to the experimental intervention. Patients in the control group may receive a

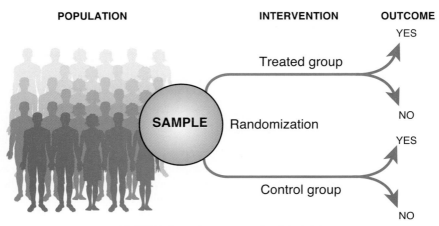

FIGURE 8.2 ■ The structure of a clinical trial.

placebo, usual care, or the current best available treatment. There may be more than one control group. The course of disease is then recorded in both groups, and differences in outcome are attributed to the intervention.

The main reason for structuring clinical trials in this way is to avoid bias (systematic error) when comparing the respective effects of two or more kinds of treatments. The validity of clinical trials depends on how well they have created equal distribution of all determinants of prognosis, other than the one being tested, in treated and control patients.

The individual elements of clinical trials are described in detail below.

Sampling

Clinical trials typically require patients to meet rigorous inclusion and exclusion criteria. These are designed to increase the homogeneity of patients in the study, to strengthen internal validity, and to make it easier to distinguish the "signal" (treatment effect) from the "noise" (bias and chance).

The usual **inclusion criterion** is that patients really do have the condition being studied. To be on the safe side, strict diagnostic criteria are applied. Patients with unusual, mild, or equivocal manifestations of disease may be left out in the process, restricting generalizability.

Of the many possible **exclusion criteria,** several account for most of the losses:

1. Patients with **comorbidity,** diseases other than the one being studied, are typically excluded because the care and outcome of these other diseases can muddy the contrast between experimental and comparison treatments and their outcomes.

2. Patients are excluded if they are not expected to live long enough to experience the outcome events of interest.

3. Patients with contraindications to one or the other treatment cannot be randomized.

4. Patients who refuse to participate in a trial are excluded. Patients may not want one of the treatments, may not want their medical care decided by a flip of a coin, or may not want treatment performed by someone other than their own physician. Unfortunately, patients who refuse to participate are usually systematically different—whether in socioeconomic

class, severity of disease, other health-related problems, or in other ways—from those who agree to participate, which can limit generalizability of the trial's results.

5. Patients who do not follow instructions during the early stages of the trial are also excluded. This avoids wasted effort and the reduction in internal validity that occurs when patients do not take their assigned intervention, move in and out of treatment groups, or leave the trial altogether.

For these reasons, patients in clinical trials are usually a highly selected, biased sample of all patients with the condition of interest. As heterogeneity is restricted, the internal validity of the study is improved; in other words, there is less opportunity for differences in outcome that are not related to treatment itself. But exclusions come at the price of diminished generalizability.

E X A M P L E

Figure 8.3 summarizes how patients were selected for a randomized controlled trial of asthma management. (5) The investigators invited 1,410 patients with asthma in 81 general practices in Scotland to participate. Only 458 of those invited, about one third, agreed to participate and could be contacted. An additional 199 were excluded, mainly because they did not meet eligibility criteria, leaving 259 patients (18% of those invited) to be randomized. While the study invited patients from community practices, those who actually participated in the trial were highly selected and quite unlike most patients in the community.

Because of the high degree of selection in trials, it may require considerable faith to generalize the results of clinical trials to ordinary practice settings.

Large, simple trials are a way of overcoming the generalizability problem. (6) Trial entry is simplified so that most patients developing the study condition are eligible. Participating patients have to accept random allocation of treatment, but their care is otherwise the same as usual, without a great deal of extra testing related to the trial. Follow-up is for a simple, clinically important outcome, such as death. This approach not only improves generalizability, it also makes it easier to recruit large numbers of participants at a reasonable cost so that moderate effect sizes (large effects are implausible for most clinical questions) can be detected.

CRITERIA FOR INCLUSION	NUMBER REMAINING

Population sampled
  Patients in 81 general practices
462,526

Invited to participate
  Patients with asthma
1,410

Agreed to participate
Able to contact
458

Met eligibility criteria
  Asthma for at least 1 year
  Age 18 or older
  Treated with inhaled corticosteroid
  No asthma visit in past 2 months
  Able to use peak flow meter
  No serious illness
  No substance abuse
  Not pregnant
  Other
318

Able and willing to cooperate
  Gave informed consent
259

Randomized
259

FIGURE 8.3 ■ Sampling of patients for a randomized controlled trial of asthma management. (Source: Hawkins G, McMahon AD, Twaddle S, Wood SF, Ford I, Thomson NC. Stepping down inhaled corticosteroids in asthma: Randomized controlled trial. BMJ 2003;326:1115–1121.)

Intervention

The intervention itself can be described in relation to three general characteristics: generalizability, complexity, and strength.

First, is the intervention one that is likely to be implemented in usual clinical practice? In an effort to standardize therapy so that it can be easily described and reproduced in other settings, investigators may cater to their scientific, not their clinical colleagues by studying treatments that are not feasible in usual practice that the results of the trial are not generally useful.

Second, does the intervention reflect a complexity that is normal for real-world treatment plans? Clinicians regularly make decisions from among alternative treatment plans, each of which has many elements. Single, highly specific interventions make for tidy science, because they can be described precisely and applied in a reproducible way, but they may have weak effects. Multifaceted interventions which are often more effective are also amenable to careful evaluation as long as their essence can be communicated and applied in other settings.

EXAMPLE

Approximately one in three persons over 65 years of age and living in the community fall each year. Some of these falls result in fractures. The falls have many causes, including physical weakness and lack of agility, drug side effects such as drowsiness or unsteadiness, and hazards in the home environment such as loose rugs or lamp cords. Therefore, prevention of falls is also likely to require attention to many aspects of daily living tailored to the individual patient's circumstances. Some randomized controlled trials of fall prevention have studied the effects of a multidisciplinary team assessing all of these factors and modifying them as necessary. One such trial has shown a 27% reduction in falls. (7) This kind of intervention may be more difficult to reproduce, but it resembles the complexity of real-life interventions in practice.

Third, is the intervention in question sufficiently different from alternative managements that it is reasonable to expect that the outcome will be affected? Some diseases can be reversed by treating a single, dominant cause. Treating hyperthyroidism with radioisotope ablation or surgery is one example. But most diseases arise from a combination of factors acting in concert. Interventions that change only one of them, and only a small amount, cannot be expected to result in strong treatment effects. If the conclusion of a trial evaluating such interventions is that a new treatment is not effective, it should come as no surprise. For this reason, the first trials of a new treatment tend to enroll those patients who are most likely to respond to treatment and to maximize dose and compliance.

Comparison Groups

The value of a treatment can only be judged by comparing its results to those of some alternative course of action. The question is not whether a point of comparison is used, but how appropriate it is. Results can be measured against one or more of several kinds of comparison groups.

- **No Intervention.** Do patients who are offered the experimental treatment end up better off than those offered nothing at all? Comparing treatment with no treatment measures the total effects of care, both specific and nonspecific.
- **Observation.** Do treated patients do better than other patients who are simply observed? A great deal of special attention is directed toward patients in clinical trials. People have a tendency to change their behavior when they are the target of special interest and attention in a study, regardless of the specific nature of the intervention they might be receiving. This phenomenon is called the **Hawthorne effect**. The reasons are not clear, but some seem likely. Patients become anxious to please their doctors and to make them feel successful. Also, patients who volunteer for trials want to do their part to see that "good" results are obtained.
- **Placebo Treatment.** Do treated patients do better than similar patients given a **placebo**—an intervention intended to be indistinguishable from the active treatment (whether in physical appearance, color, taste, or smell) but which does not have a specific, known mechanism of action? Sugar pills and saline injections are examples of placebos. It has been shown that placebos, given with conviction, relieve severe, unpleasant symptoms, such as postoperative pain, nausea, or itching, of about one-third of patients, a phenomenon called the **placebo effect**.

  Placebo effects have different meaning for researchers and clinicians. Researchers are more likely to be interested in measuring specific

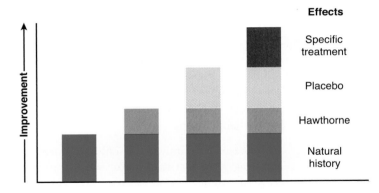

Effects

Specific
treatment

Placebo

Hawthorne

Natural
history

FIGURE 8.4 ■ Total effects of treatment are the sum of spontaneous improvement (natural history) as well as nonspecific and specific responses.

effects—ones that are consistent with current theories about the causes and treatment of disease. They consider the placebo effect the baseline against which to measure specific effects. Clinicians, on the other hand, should welcome the placebo effect and attempt to maximize it (or any other way of making patients feel better).

- **Usual Care.** Do patients given the experimental treatment do better than those receiving usual care? This is the only meaningful (and ethical) question if usual care is already known to be effective.

The cumulative effects of these various reasons for improvement in treated patients are diagrammed in Figure 8.4.

Allocating Treatment

To study the effects of a clinical intervention free of other effects, the best way to allocate patients to treatment groups is by means of **random allocation (randomization)**. Patients are assigned to either the experimental or the control treatment by one of a variety of disciplined procedures—analogous to flipping a coin—whereby each patient has an equal (or at least known) chance of being assigned to any one of the treatment groups.

Random allocation of patients is preferable to other methods of allocation because only randomization has the ability to create truly comparable groups. All factors related to prognosis, whether or not they are known before the study takes place or have been measured, tend to be equally distributed in the comparison groups. Patients in one group are, on the average, as likely to possess a given characteristic as patients in another.

In the long run, with a large number of patients in the trial, randomization usually works as described

above. However, random allocation does not guarantee that the groups will be similar. Dissimilarities between groups can arise by chance alone, particularly when the number of patients randomized is small. To assess whether this kind of "bad luck" has occurred, authors of randomized controlled trials often present a table comparing the frequency of a variety of characteristics in the treated and control groups, especially those known to be related to outcome. These are called **baseline characteristics** because they are present before randomization and so should be equally distributed in the treatment groups.

> ### E X A M P L E
>
> Table 8.1 shows some of the baseline characteristics for women in a Women's Health Initiative study, a randomized trial of 16,608 women followed for an average of 5.6 years, comparing the effects of menopausal hormone supplements (estrogen plus progestin) with placebo. This analysis was for risk of fracture. (8) The table lists several characteristics that were already believed from other studies to be associated with risk of fractures. Thus, women who were older, fair skinned, thin, prone to ingest very little calcium, smokers, and had already had falls or fractures were more likely to have a new fracture, the outcome event, whether or not they were offered hormones in the trial. Each of these characteristics was similarly distributed in the two treatment groups. Also (not shown) bone mineral density was similar in the two groups. These comparisons, at least for characteristics that are known to be risk factors and were measured, strengthen the belief that randomization actually produced groups with similar risks for fractures. This trial showed that women in the estrogen plus progestin group had 24% fewer fractures than those in the placebo group.

It is reassuring to see that important characteristics have, in fact, fallen out nearly equally in the groups being compared. In any case, this is bound to be so in such a large trial. If the groups are substan-

TABLE 8.1 ▥	Example of a Table Comparing Baseline Characteristics: A Randomized Trial of Estrogen Plus Progestin Versus Placebo on the Risk of Fractures in Women.

Characteristics	Percent with Characteristic for Each Group	
	Estrogen plus Progestin (8,506 women)	*Placebo (8,102 women)*
Age 70–79 years	21.3	21.8
White	83.9	84.0
Body mass index <25	30.5	30.8
Total calcium intake <600 mg/d	24.4	24.2
Current smoker	10.5	10.5
≥2 falls in past 12 months	12.8	12.4
History of fracture	38.8	39.1

(Source: Cauley JA, Robbins J, Chen Z, Cummings SR, Jackson RD, La Croix AZ, et al. Effects of estrogen plus progestin on risk of fracture and bone mineral density. The women's health initiative randomized trial. JAMA 2003;290:1729–1738.)

tially different, it suggests that something has gone wrong with the randomization process. Smaller differences, which are to be expected, can be controlled for during data analysis (see Chapter 7).

In some situations, especially small trials, it is best to make sure that at least some of the characteristics known to be strongly associated with outcome occur equally in treated and control patients, in order to reduce the risk of bad luck. Patients are gathered into groups (strata) having similar levels of a prognostic factor (such as age for most chronic diseases) and are randomized separately within each stratum. This is a process called **stratified randomization** (see Figure 8.5). The final groups are bound to be comparable, at least for the characteristics that were used to create the strata. Some investigators do not favor stratified randomization, arguing that whatever differences arise by bad luck are unlikely to be large and can be adjusted for mathematically after the data have been collected.

Differences Arising After Randomization

Not all patients in a clinical trial participate as originally planned. Some are found not to have the disease they were thought to have when they entered the trial. Others drop out, do not take their medications, are taken out of the study because of side effects or other illnesses, or somehow obtain the other study treatment or treatments that are not part of the study at all. This

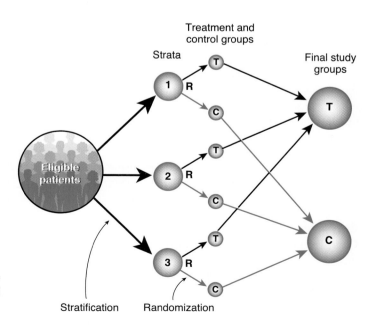

FIGURE 8.5 ▥ Diagram of stratified randomization. T = treated group, and C = control group. R = randomization.

results in treatment groups that might have been comparable just after randomization becoming less so as time passes. There are several reasons:

Patients Do Not Have the Disease Under Study

It is sometimes necessary (both in clinical trials and in practice) to begin treatment before it is certain whether the patient actually has the disease for which the treatment is designed.

E X A M P L E

The clinical diagnosis of influenza is based on typical symptoms of fever, aching, and respiratory complaints during the winter months, especially during an epidemic. Laboratory tests take time and treatment must begin before confirmation of the diagnosis. The efficacy of a new drug for influenza, a neurominidase inhibitor, was tested in a randomized controlled trial. (9) Adults with influenza-like illness for ≤ 48 hours were randomly allocated to the new drug or placebo. Of 417 people randomized, 282 (63%) were later found to have confirmed influenza. The median time for alleviation of all major symptoms in patients with influenza was one day less in those given the new drug. The effect would have been less in all patients offered the drug. Rapid diagnostic tests are being developed and will make a more accurate diagnosis available at the time treatment is started.

When patients are enrolled in a study and later turn out not to have the index disease, there is a price to pay. The main disadvantage of this approach is the inefficiency of enrolling and gathering data on patients who do not contribute to the study's results. Patients who could benefit from the experimental treatment are mixed with others who cannot, so the effect size is reduced relative to a trial that includes only patients with the disease. This decreases the chances, for a given number of patients in the trial, that an effect will be found (see Chapter 10). However, this kind of trial has the important advantage of providing information on the consequences of a decision that a clinician must make (see the Intention-to-Treat and Explanatory Trials section in this chapter).

Compliance

Compliance is the extent to which patients follow medical advice. The term **adherence** may be preferable because it connotes a less subservient relationship between patient and doctor. Compliance is another characteristic that comes into play after randomization.

Although noncompliance suggests a kind of willful neglect of good advice, other factors also contribute. Patients may misunderstand which drugs and doses are intended, may run out of prescription medications, may confuse various preparations of the same drug, or may have no money or insurance to pay for drugs. Taken together, these may limit the usefulness of treatments that have been shown to work under favorable conditions.

Compliance is particularly important in medical care outside the hospital. In hospitals, many factors act to constrain patients' personal behavior and render them compliant. Hospitalized patients are generally sicker and more frightened. They are in strange surroundings, dependent upon the skill and attention of the staff for everything, including their life. What is more, doctors, nurses, and pharmacists have developed a well-organized system for ensuring that patients receive what is ordered for them. As a result, clinical experience and medical literature developed on the wards may underestimate the importance of compliance outside the hospital, where most patients and doctors are and where following doctors' orders is less common.

In clinical trials, patients are typically selected for their compliance. During a **run-in period**, in which placebo is given and compliance monitored, noncompliant patients can be detected and excluded before randomization.

Co-interventions

After randomization, patients may receive a variety of interventions other than the ones being studied. If these occur unequally in the two groups and affect outcomes, they can introduce systematic differences (bias) between the groups that were not present when the groups were formed.

Comparisons of Responders to Nonresponders

In some clinical trials, particularly those involving cancer, the outcomes of patients who initially improve after treatment (responders) are compared with outcomes in those who do not (nonresponders). The implication is that one can learn something about the efficacy of treatment in this way.

This approach is scientifically unsound and misleading because response and nonresponse might be associated with many characteristics related to outcome, including stage of disease, rate of progression, compliance, dose and side effects of drugs, and the presence of other diseases. If no patient actually improved because of the treatment, and patients were destined to follow various clinical courses for other reasons, then some patients (the ones who happened to be doing well) would be called "responders" and others (the ones having a bad course) would be considered "nonresponders." Responders would, of course, have a better outcome whether or not they received the experimental treatment.

Blinding

Participants in a trial may change their behavior or reporting of outcomes in a systematic way (i.e., be biased) if they are aware of which patients receive which treatment. One way to minimize this effect is by **blinding**, an attempt to make the various participants in a study unaware of the treatment group patients have been randomized to so that this knowledge cannot cause them to act differently, and thereby damage the internal validity of the study. **Masking** is a more appropriate metaphor, but blinding is the time-honored term.

Blinding can take place in a clinical trial at four levels (Figure 8.6). First, those responsible for allocating patients to treatment groups should not know

which treatment will be assigned next so that the knowledge does not allow them to break the randomization plan. **Allocation concealment** is a common term for this form of blinding. Without it, some investigators might be tempted to enter patients in the trial out of order, to ensure that individuals get the treatment that seems best for them. Second, patients should be unaware of which treatment they are taking so that they cannot change their compliance or reporting of symptoms because of their knowledge of this information. Third, physicians who take care of patients in the study should not know which treatment each patient is on; then they cannot, even subconsciously, manage them differently. Finally, when the researchers who assess outcomes are unaware of which treatment individual patients have been offered, that knowledge cannot affect their measurements.

The terms **single-blind** (patients) and **double-blind** are sometimes used, but their meanings are ambiguous. In a study of physicians' interpretations and textbook definitions of blinding, physicians identified 10, 17, and 15 unique interpretations of single-, double-, and triple-blinded, randomized controlled trials, and textbooks provided 5, 9, and 7 different definitions, respectively. (10) It is better simply to describe what was done. A trial in which

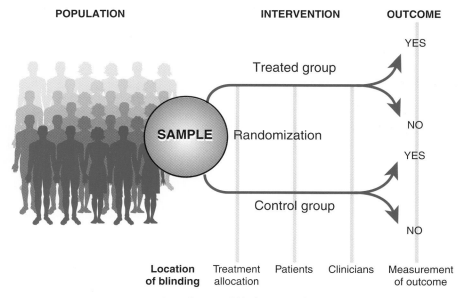

FIGURE 8.6 ▓ Locations of potential blinding in randomize controlled trials.

there is no attempt at blinding is called an *open* or in the case of drug trials, an **open label** trial.

Blinding is often made possible for studies of drug effects by using a placebo. However, for many important clinical questions, such as the effects of surgery, radiotherapy, diet, or the organization of medical care, blinding of patients and their physicians is difficult if not impossible.

Even when blinding appears to be possible, it is more often claimed than successful. Physiologic effects, such as lowered pulse rate with beta-blocking drugs or bone marrow depression with cancer chemotherapy, are regular features of some medications. Symptoms such as gastrointestinal upset or drowsiness are a characteristic of some drugs. These effects can signal to patients whether they are taking the active drug or placebo.

EXAMPLE

Zinc lozenges were compared with placebo lozenges in a randomized controlled trial of 100 people with a common cold. (11) Average time to complete resolution of symptoms was 4.4 days in the zinc group and 7.6 days in the placebo group. However, side effects were much more common in the zinc group than in the placebo group. Bad taste was reported in 80% versus 30% and nausea in 20% versus 4%, respectively. Critics of the study suggested that although the trial was called "double-blind," many patients would have known that they were taking the active drug and that this might have affected reporting of symptoms. In fact, other studies of zinc for the common cold have had mixed results, so the effectiveness of zinc for this purpose is uncertain.

In some trials, patients and doctors are asked whether they believe the patient is taking an active drug or placebo. Their answers provide objective evidence of whether efforts to mask patients were successful.

EXAMPLE

A double-blind, randomized trial was conducted to see if propranolol, a beta-blocking drug, could prevent a myocardial infarction in patients who had already had one. (12) At the conclusion of the trial but before unblinding, patients and clinic personnel were asked to guess the treatment group assignment of each patient. For patients, 79.9% guessed propranolol correctly and 57.2% placebo correctly. Physicians and clinic personnel were similarly accurate. Though clinic personnel seemed to be aided in their guessing by observation of heart rate, it was unclear how patients knew.

Assessment of Outcomes

Assessment of outcome and how it can be affected by measurement bias has been discussed (see Chapter 7), as have the dangers of substituting intermediate outcomes for clinically important ones (Chapter 1). The discussion about these issues applies also to randomized controlled trials.

Options for describing effect size for clinical trials are summarized in Table 8.2. The options are similar to summaries of risk and prognosis but related to change in outcome resulting from the intervention.

INTENTION-TO-TREAT AND EXPLANATORY TRIALS

The results of a randomized controlled trial can be analyzed and presented in two general ways: according to the treatment to which the patients were randomized or according to the one they actually received. The correct presentation of results depends on the question being asked (Figure 8.7).

One question is: Which treatment option is best at the time the decision must be made? To answer this question, analysis is according to which group the patients were assigned (randomized), regardless of whether they actually received the treatment they were supposed to receive. This method of analyzing trial results is called an **intention-to-treat analysis**. An advantage of this approach is that the question

---

TABLE 8.2 ■ Summarizing Treatment Effects[a]

Summary Measure[b]	Definition
Relative risk reduction	$\dfrac{\text{Control event rate} - \text{Treated event rate}}{\text{Control event rate}}$
Absolute risk reduction	Control event rate − Treated event rate
Number needed to treat	$\dfrac{1}{\text{Control event rate} - \text{Treated event rate}}$

[a] Laupacis A, Sackett DL, Roberts RS. An assessment of clinically useful measures of the consequences of treatment. New Engl J Med 1988;318:1728–1733.
[b] For continuous data, in which there are measurements at baseline and after treatment, analogous measures are based on the mean values for treated and control groups either after treatment or for the difference between baseline and posttreatment values.

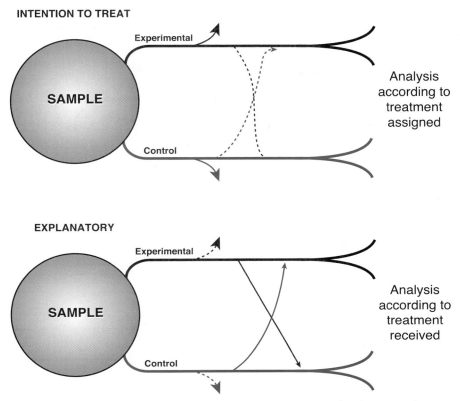

INTENTION TO TREAT

SAMPLE

Experimental

Control

Analysis
according to
treatment
assigned

EXPLANATORY

SAMPLE

Experimental

Control

Analysis
according to
treatment
received

FIGURE 8.7 ■ Diagram of group assignment in intention-to-treat and explanatory analyses.

corresponds to the one actually faced by clinicians; they either offer a treatment or not. Also, the groups compared are as originally randomized, so this comparison has the full strength of a randomized trial. The disadvantage is that when many patients do not receive the treatment to which they were randomized, differences in effectiveness between experimental and control interventions will tend to be obscured, increasing the chances of observing a misleadingly small effect or no statistical effect at all. If the study shows no difference, it will be uncertain whether the experimental treatment is truly ineffective or was just not received.

Another question is whether the experimental treatment itself is better. For this question, the proper analysis is according to the treatment each patient actually received, regardless of the treatment to which they were randomized. Trials analyzed in this way are called **explanatory trials** because they assess whether actually taking the treatments, rather than just being offered them, makes the difference. The problem with this approach is that unless most patients receive the treatment to which they are assigned, the study no longer represents a randomized trial; it is simply a cohort study. One must be concerned about dissimilarities among groups, other than the experimental treatment, and must use one or more methods such as restriction, matching, stratification, or adjustment to achieve comparability, just as one would for any nonexperimental study.

To the extent that patients in a trial follow the treatment to which they were randomized, these two analyses will give similar results.

EFFICACY AND EFFECTIVENESS

Clinical trials are also classified according to whether they describe the results of an intervention in ideal or real-world situations (Figure 8.8).

First, can treatment work under *ideal* circumstances? Trials that answer this question are called **efficacy trials**. Elements of ideal circumstances include patients who accept the interventions

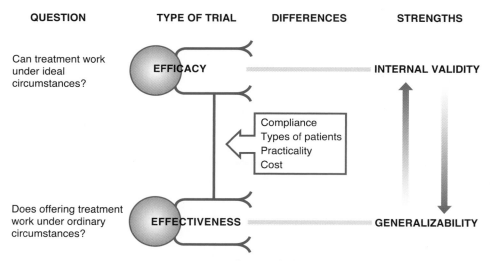

FIGURE 8.8 ▦ Efficacy and effectiveness

offered to them and follow instructions faithfully; the best possible care; and the absence of extraneous effects from other diseases.

Second, does treatment work under *ordinary* circumstances? Trials designed to answer this kind of question are called **effectiveness trials**. All the usual elements of patient care may be part of effectiveness trials. Patients may not take their assigned treatment. Some may drop out of the study, and others find ways to take the treatment they were not assigned. The doctors and facilities may not be the best. In short, effectiveness trials describe results as most patients would experience them.

Ordinarily, efficacy trials are restricted to compliant patients, so it makes relatively little difference whether analysis is by intention to treat or as an explanatory trial. Effectiveness trials are usually analyzed by intention to treat.

TAILORING THE RESULTS OF TRIALS TO INDIVIDUAL PATIENTS

Clinical trials involve pooling the experience of many patients who may be dissimilar, both to one another and to the patients to whom the trial results will be generalized. Trials describe what happens on the average. How can more precise estimates for individual patients be obtained? Two ways are to examine trial subgroups and to study individual patients using rigorous methods similar to those in randomized trials.

Subgroups

Patients in clinical trials can be sorted into subgroups, each with a specific combination of characteristics, such as age, severity of disease, and comorbidity, that might affect outcome. The number of such subgroups is limited only by the number of patients in the subgroups, and this number has to be large enough to provide reasonably stable estimates. Patients in each subgroup have been randomly allocated to treatment groups, as long as the characteristics used to define the subgroups existed before randomization. So, results in each subgroup represent, in effect, a small trial-within-a-trial. It is possible to match the characteristics of a given patient to those of one of the subgroups. (For example, the patient might be elderly and have severe disease but no comorbidity.) Treatment effectiveness in the matched subgroup will more closely approximate that of the individual patient and will be limited mainly by statistical risks of false-positive and false-negative conclusions, which are described in the Subgroup Analysis section in Chapter 10.

Trials of *N* = 1

Rigorous clinical trials, with proper attention to bias and chance, can be done with individual patients, one at a time. (13) The method—called **trials of *N* = 1**—is an improvement over the more informal process of trial and error that is time-honored in clinical practice. A patient is given one or another treatment, such as an active treatment or placebo, in random order, each for a brief period of time, such as a week or two. Patient and physician are blinded to which treatment is given. Outcomes, such as a simple preference for a treatment or a symptom score, are assessed after each period and subjected to statistical analysis.

This method is useful when activity of disease is unpredictable, response to treatment is prompt, and there is no carryover effect from period to period. Examples of diseases for which the method can be used include migraine headaches, asthma, and fibrositis.

N of 1 trials can be useful for guiding clinical decision making. However, they are possible for only a relatively small proportion of patients who have conditions that occur frequently and resolve rapidly and who are willing to go on and off "active" drug and placebo in this way. A placebo intervention must be possible if *N* of 1 trials can be used to screen interesting clinical hypotheses and select those that are promising enough to be evaluated using a full randomized controlled trial involving many patients.

Effectiveness in Individual Patients

A treatment that is effective on the average may not work on an individual patient. Therefore, results of valid clinical research provide a good reason to begin treating a patient, but experience with that patient is a better reason to continue or not. When managing an individual patient, it is useful to ask the following series of questions:

- Is the treatment known (by randomized controlled trial) to be efficacious for any patients?
- Is the treatment known to be effective, on the average, in patients like mine?
- Is the treatment working in my patient?
- Are the benefits worth the discomforts and risks (according to the patient's values and preferences)?

By asking these questions and not simply following the results of trials alone, one can guard against ill-founded choice of treatment or stubborn persistence in the face of poor results.

LIMITATIONS OF RANDOMIZED TRIALS

Randomized controlled trials are the gold standard of intervention studies. Usually, they put things on a sound footing. However, even the existence of several well-conducted randomized controlled trials of a clinical question does not necessarily settle a question. For example, controversy about the effectiveness of screening mammography remains, even though eight randomized trials involving thousands of women have been published. Critics have questioned various aspects of the individual trials such as the quality of mammography, age to which screening effects should be attributed, and the correctness of randomization procedures.

Clinical trials also suffer from practical limitations. There may not be enough patients with the disease of interest, at one time and place, to carry out a scientifically sound trial. This can be overcome by **multicenter trials.** Patients and their physicians may be reluctant to have their treatment choice decided by investigators through a random process. Clinical trials are expensive, costing hundreds of millions of dollars for some large trials. Years may pass before results are available, which may be politically unacceptable for severe, emotion-laden diseases such as AIDS and cancer.

Some practices are established without the benefit of randomized trials, and the trials are no longer feasible. A practice may have become so well established, in the absence of conclusive evidence of its benefit, that it is difficult to convince physicians and patients that a trial is needed. It could be argued that if the treatment effect is not really known, then the only ethical approach is to do the trial (it can be considered unethical to continue to use treatments of uncertain benefit). But this argument demands a level of analytic reasoning that is uncommon among patients and their physicians. Because of this problem, some physicians have advocated "randomization from the first patient," beginning trials just after a new treatment is introduced. Others argue that it is better to conduct rigorous clinical trials somewhat later, after the best way to deliver the treatment has been worked out, so that a good example of the intervention is tested. In any case, it is generally agreed that if a controlled trial is postponed too long, the opportunity to do it at all may be lost.

For these reasons, guidance from clinical trials is not available for many important treatment decisions. But clinical decisions must be made nonetheless.

ALTERNATIVES TO RANDOMIZED TRIALS

What are the alternatives to randomized controlled trials and how credible are they?

Comparisons Across Time and Place

Experimental and control patients can be assembled from different times and places. This approach is convenient. The problem is that time and place are almost always strongly related to prognosis, making bias a substantial possibility. Studies that attempt to make fair comparisons between groups of patients arising in different eras, or in different settings, have a particularly difficult task.

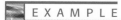

E X A M P L E

Some adenomas in the colon and rectum, usually seen as polyps, develop into cancer. This suggests that removing polyps might prevent colorectal cancer. The National Polyp Study followed a cohort of patients with colorectal polyps assembled at several U.S. referral centers. The polyps were removed, and the patients remained under surveillance for new polyps, which were also removed when found. (14) Over an average of 5.9 years of follow-up, five patients developed asymptomatic, early-stage, colorectal cancers. For comparison, the investigators calculated expected rates in three other cohorts of patients who had not had surveillance. Two of these three reference groups were of patients with polyps, and one described population-based rates for average risk people. The reference groups were assembled as much as a decade earlier than the study and were from various places in the United States and England. The results are summarized in Figure 8.9. Colon cancer rates in patients whose polyps had been removed were 76%–90% lower than in the three comparison cohorts.

Could this difference have been found because the cohorts did not really have a similar prognosis at inception (before surveillance)? Perhaps, but the differences were so large that it is difficult to believe that all of them could have resulted from bias. However, while a protective effect of removing colon polyps seems very likely, the magnitude of the effect is uncertain because of the many differences between the study and comparison cohorts.

The results of current treatment are sometimes compared to experience with similar patients in the past, called **historical controls** or **nonconcurrent controls**. This design has many pitfalls. Methods of diagnosis change with time, as does average prognosis. Supporting treatments, such as antibiotics, nutritional supplementation, and thrombosis prevention, improve with time, creating a general improvement in prognosis that might not be attributable to the specific treatment given in a later time period.

When historical controls are used, the shorter the period between selection of treated groups and control groups—and the less other aspects of medical care have changed during the interval—the safer the comparison. Thus, some oncologists study a succession of chemotherapeutic regimens by comparing results of the newest regimen with those of the immediately preceding one, often given as recently as the previous year. In general, however, choosing **concurrent controls** (for example, patients treated during the same period of time) provide a better way of avoiding bias.

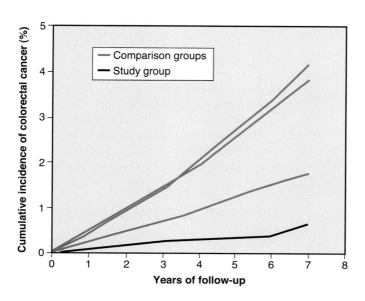

FIGURE 8.9 ▪ Example of nonconcurrent conrol groups. A cohort study of effectiveness with comparison to cohorts from other times and places. (Source: Winawer SJ, Zauber AG, Ho MN, O'Brien MJ, Gottlieb LS, Sternberg SS, et al. Prevention of colorectal cancer by colonoscopic polypectomy. N Engl J Med 1993;329:1977–1981.)

Uncontrolled Trials

Uncontrolled trials describe the course of disease in a single group of patients before and after exposure to an intervention. Another name for this design is a **before-after study**. The assumption of this approach is that any improvement observed after treatment is the result of treatment. This assumption may be unwarranted for the reasons described below.

Unpredictable Clinical Course

When the clinical course of a disease is quite predictable, a separate control group is less important. We know that subacute bacterial endocarditis without antibiotics and rabies invariably lead to death and that bowel infarction will rarely improve without surgery.

However, most diseases do not have such predictable outcomes. In situations in which the clinical course is extremely variable, for a given patient and from one patient to another, before-after studies are unreliable.

E X A M P L E

Benign prostatic hyperplasia is a common condition of middle-aged and elderly men. Symptoms caused by urinary obstruction and irritation include urinary frequency, urgency, nocturia, hesitancy, and poor stream. The condition is generally thought to be uniformly progressive. However, studies of the natural history of this condition show that change over time is unpredictable; some men get worse, while many stay the same or improve. Figure 8.10 shows change in symptoms in 97 men over 5 years and illustrates how unpredictable the natural history is. (15) Could these men have experienced fewer symptoms with time because they just got used to the symptoms? Perhaps, but physical measures of prostate disease, such as residual urine and voiding detrusor pressure, showed similar changes over time. Therefore, one cannot count on a predictable, downhill course against which to compare treated men in an uncontrolled trial.

Nonspecific Effects

In uncontrolled trials, there is no way of separating Hawthorne and placebo effects from treatment effects. On the other hand, when there are control patients who receive the same attention as the treated ones, as well as a placebo, these effects cancel out in the comparison.

Regression to the Mean

Treatments are often tried because a manifestation of disease, such as a particularly high blood pressure or fever, is extreme or unusual. In this situation, subsequent measurements are likely to show improvement for purely statistical reasons. As discussed in Chapter 2, patients selected because they represent an extremely high value in a distribution are likely, on the average, to have lower values on later measurements. If those patients are treated after first being found abnormal and the effects of treatment are assessed by subsequent measurements, improvement could be expected even if treatment were ineffective.

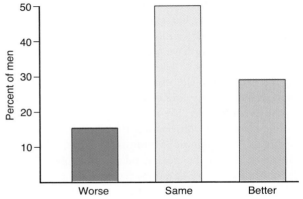

FIGURE 8.10 ■ The unpredictable course of disease. Change in symptoms over 5 years in 97 men with benign prostatic hyperplasia. (Source: Ball AJ, Feneley RCL, Abrams PH. The natural history of untreated "prostatism." British J Urology 1981;53:613–616.)

Predictable Improvement

The usual course of some diseases is to improve; if so, therapeutic efforts may coincide with improvement but not cause it. For example, patients tend to seek care for many acute, self-limited diseases, such as upper respiratory infections or gastroenteritis, when symptoms are at their worst. They may begin to recover after seeing the doctor because of the natural course of events regardless of what was done for them.

OBSERVATIONAL STUDIES OF INTERVENTIONS

Observational (cohort or case-control) studies of treatment effects take into account the fact that therapeutic decisions must be made for sick patients regardless of the quality of existing evidence on the subject. In the absence of a consensus favoring one mode of treatment over others, various treatments are given. As a result, in the course of ordinary patient care, large numbers of patients receive various treatments and go on to manifest their effects. When experience with these patients is captured and properly analyzed, it can be used to guide therapeutic decisions.

Unfortunately, it is often difficult to be sure that observational studies of treatment involve unbiased comparisons. Decisions about treatment are determined by a great many factors, including severity of illness, concurrent diseases, local preferences, and patient cooperation. Patients receiving the various treatments are likely to differ not only in their treatment but in other ways as well.

Especially troubling is **confounding by indication,** which occurs, in the case of a drug, when whatever has made the doctor prescribe a drug (the "indications") is the cause of the observed outcome, not the drug itself. For example, patients may be offered a new surgical procedure because they are a good surgical risk or have nonaggressive disease, and so seem most likely to benefit from the procedure. To the extent that the reasons for choice of treatment are known, they can be taken into account like any other confounder. But many are not known.

In practice, are observational studies a reliable substitute for randomized controlled trials? With controlled trials as the gold standard, most observational studies of most questions get the right answer. (16) However, there are dramatic exceptions.

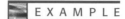

> **E X A M P L E**
>
> Observational studies, both cohort and case-control, have consistently shown that women who take menopausal hormones (estrogen and progestin) are at decreased risk of cardiovascular disease. A randomized controlled trial was undertaken to test this important observation. 16,606 postmenopausal women ages 50–79 years were randomized to estrogen plus progestin or placebo and followed up for a mean of 5.2 years. (17) Coronary heart disease (nonfatal myocardial infarction and coronary heart disease death) was 29% *higher* in the women randomized to estrogen and progestin.

Reasons for the discrepancy between observational and experimental studies of this question are uncertain. Women in the observational studies who chose to use hormone replacement therapy may have had healthier lifestyles than those who did not. Also, if patients believed that hormone therapy was effective, they may have been less likely to seek medical attention for atypical symptoms of coronary artery disease. (18)

As another example, observational studies have also consistently shown that antioxidant vitamins are associated with lower cardiovascular risk, but large randomized controlled trials have found no such effect (see Figure 10.3 in Chapter 10). (19) Therefore, clinicians can be guided by observational studies of treatment effects when there are no randomized trials to rely on, but should maintain a healthy skepticism.

STANDARDS FOR REPORTING RANDOMIZED CONTROLLED TRIALS

In order to determine whether the results of a randomized controlled trial are credible, one must be provided complete information on the design, conduct, analysis, and interpretation of the trial. An international group of clinical trialists, statisticians, epidemiologists, and biomedical editors have proposed standards for reporting, under the name CONSORT (CONsolidated Standards Of Reporting Trials). (20) Table 8.3 summarizes the basic elements of the CONSORT statement.

There remains a gap between these standards and actual reporting. For example, in a review of 122 trials of selective serotonin reuptake inhibitors for depression, only one paper described randomization adequately, according to CONSORT criteria. (21)

TABLE 8.3 ▪ **Standards for Reporting a Randomized Controlled Trial (Modified from the CONSORT Statement).**

Background

Scientific background and rationale

Design

Participants	Eligibility criteria and setting from which data were collected
Interventions	Details of interventions for each group and how the interventions were administered
Objectives	Research questions and hypotheses
Outcomes	Primary and secondary outcome measures
Sample size	How justified
Randomization	Methods used to generate random allocation sequence and implementation
Blinding	Participants who were blinded to group assignment and how success was evaluated
Statistical methods	Methods used to compare groups for primary outcomes and for additional analyses

Conduct

Participant flow	Flow of participants through each stage: randomly assigned, received intended treatment, completed study, analyzed for primary outcome
Recruitment	Dates of recruitment and follow-up

Analysis and Results

Baseline data	Baseline characteristics for each group
Number analyzed	Number of participants in each group and whether analysis was by intention-to-treat
Outcomes	Results for each group
Estimation	Estimated effect size and precision[a]
Ancillary analyses	Number of analyses and whether they were specified in advance[b]
Adverse events	Adverse events and side effects for each study group
Interpretation	**Interpretation of results, taking into account original hypotheses, bias, and chance**
Generalizability	External validity of trial findings
Overall evidence	Results in the context of current evidence

[a]See Chapter 10. Chance for a discussion of statistical precision
[b]See Chapter 10. Chance for a discussion of the significance of examining many subgroups without specifying which is of main importance in advance
(Source: Moher D, Schulz KF, Altman DG, for the CONSORT Group. The CONSORT statement: Revised recommendations for improving the quality of parallel-group randomized trials. Ann Intern Med 2001;134:657–662.)

PHASES OF STUDIES OF TREATMENT

For studies of drugs, it is customary to define three phases of trials in the order they are undertaken. **Phase I** trials are intended to identify a dose range that is well tolerated and safe (at least for high-frequency, severe side effects) and include very small numbers of patients (perhaps a dozen), without a control group. **Phase II** trials provide preliminary information on whether the drug is efficacious and the relationship between dose and efficacy; these tri-

als may be controlled but include too few patients in treatment groups to detect any but the largest treatment effects. **Phase III** trials are randomized trials and can provide definitive evidence of efficacy and rates of common side effects. They include enough patients, often dozens to thousands, to detect clinically important treatment effects and are usually published in biomedical journals.

Phase III trials are not large enough to detect differences in the rate, or even the existence, of uncommon side effects (see discussion of statistical power in Chapter 10). For this, it is necessary to follow up with very large numbers of patients after a drug is in general use, a process called **postmarketing surveillance.**

REVIEW QUESTIONS

Read the following and choose the best response.

_____ **8.1.** A randomized controlled trial compares angioplasty with fibrinolysis for the treatment of acute myocardial infarction. The authors state that "analysis was by intention to treat." An advantage of this approach is that

A. It describes the effects of treatments that patients have actually received.

B. It is not affected by patients dropping out of the study.

C. It is unlikely to underestimate treatment effect.

D. It describes the consequences of offering treatments whether or not they are actually taken.

E. It describes whether treatment can work under ideal circumstances.

_____ **8.2.** In a randomized trial, patients with meningitis who were treated with corticosteroids had lower rates of death, hearing loss, and neurologic sequelae. You have a patient with meningitis and want to know whether patients with her characteristics are at least as likely to benefit as patients in the trial as a whole. Which of the following is a randomized comparison?

A. Patients who took the drug compared with those who did not.

B. Patients who responded to the drug versus those who did not.

C. Patients who, at the time of randomization, were severely affected by the disease versus those only mildly affected.

D. Patients who experienced other interventions versus those who did not.

E. Patients who remained in the trial versus those who dropped out after randomization.

_____ **8.3.** You are reviewing a randomized controlled trial and wonder whether stratified randomization, which the trial used, was likely to improve internal validity. This approach might be particularly helpful if

A. One of the baseline variables is strongly related to prognosis.

B. The study includes many patients.

C. Many patients are expected to drop out.

D. Assignment to treatment group is not blinded.

E. An intention-to-treat analysis is planned.

_____ **8.4.** A patient asks for your advice about whether to begin an exercise program to reduce his risk of sudden death. You look for randomized controlled trials but find only observational studies of this question. Some are cohort studies comparing sudden death rates in exercisers with rates of sudden death in sedentary people; others are case-control studies comparing exercise patterns in people who had experienced sudden death and matched controls. Observational studies of treatment effects are likely to have all of the following advantages over randomized controlled trials except

A. Generalizability to more ordinary, real-world settings.

B. Reported effects are for patients who have actually experienced the intervention.

C. Treatment groups would have had a similar prognosis except for treatment itself.

D. It may be possible to carry out these studies using existing data, collected for other purposes.

E. A large sample size is easier to achieve.

_____ **8.5.** In a randomized controlled trial of a program to reduce lower extremity problems in patients with diabetes mellitus, patients were excluded if they were <40 years old, were diagnosed before becoming 30 years old, took medication for hyperglycemia, had other serious illness or disability, or were not compliant with prescribed treatment during a run-in period. This approach is likely to:

A. Improve the generalizability of the study.
B. Make it possible to do an intention-to-treat analysis.
C. Make an effectiveness trial possible.
D. Avoid selection bias.
E. Improve the internal validity of the study.

Read the following statement and mark the responses as True or False.

In a randomized controlled trial, a beta-blocker drug is found to be more effective than placebo for stage fright. Patients taking the beta-blocker tended to have a lower pulse rate and to feel more lethargic, which are known effects of this drug. In this situation, blinding is possible for which of the following:

_____ **8.6.** The investigators who assigned patients to treatment groups

_____ **8.7.** The patient in the trial

_____ **8.8.** The patients' physicians

_____ **8.9.** The investigators who assess outcome

Answers are in Appendix A.

REFERENCES

1. Schwab RS, England AC Jr, Poskanzer DC, Young RR. Amantadine in the treatment of Parkinson's disease. JAMA 1969;208:1168–1169.
2. EC/IC Bypass Study Group. Failure of extracranial-intracranial arterial bypass to reduce the risk of ischemic stroke. N Engl J Med 1985;313:1191–1200.
3. Allen C, Glasziou P, Del Mar C. Bed rest: A potentially harmful treatment needing more careful evaluation. Lancet 1999;354:1229–1233.
4. Opie on the heart [Editorial]. Lancet 1980;1:692.
5. Hawkins G, McMahon AD, Twaddle S, Wood SF, Ford I, Thomson NC. Stepping down inhaled corticosteroids in asthma: Randomized controlled trial. BMJ 2003;326:1115–1121.
6. Yusef S, Collins R, Peto R. Why do we need some large, simple randomized trials? Stat Med 1984;3:409–420.
7. Gillespie LD, Gillespie WJ, Robertson MC, Lamb SE, Cummings RG, Rowe BH. Interventions for preventing falls in elderly people. Cochrane Database Syst Rev 2001;(3):CD000340.
8. Cauley JA, Robbins J, Chen Z, Cummings SR, Jackson RD, LaCroix AZ, et al. Effects of estrogen plus progestin on risk of fracture and bone mineral density: The Women's Health Initiative randomized trial. JAMA 2003;290:1729–1738.
9. Hayden FG, Osterhaus AD, Treanor JJ, Fleming DM, Aoki FY, Nicholson KG, et al. Efficacy and safety of the neurominidase inhibitor zanamivir in the treatment of influenza infections. GG167 Influenza Study Group. N Engl J Med 1997; 337:874–880.
10. Devereaux PJ, Manns BJ, Ghali WA, Quan H, Lacchetti C, Montoni VM, et al. Physician interpretations and textbook definitions of blinding terminology in randomized controlled trials. JAMA 2001;285:2000–2003.
11. Mossad SB, Macknin ML, Medendorp SV, Mason P. Zinc gluconate lozenges for treating the common cold. A randomized, double-blind, placebo-controlled study. Ann Intern Med 1996;125:81–88.
12. Byington RP, Curb JD, Mattson ME. Assessment of double-blindness at the conclusion of the beta-blocker Heart Attack Trial. JAMA 1985;253:1733–1736.
13. Guyatt G, Sackett D, Taylor DW, Chong J, Roberts R, Pugsley S. Determining optimal therapy—Randomized trials in individual patients. N Engl J Med 1986;314:889–892.
14. Winawer SJ, Zauber AG, Ho MN, O'Brien MJ, Gottlieb LS, Sternberg SS, et al. Prevention of colorectal cancer by colonoscopic polypectomy. N Engl J Med 1993;329:1977–81.
15. Ball AJ, Feneley RCL, Abrams PH. The natural history of untreated "prostatism." British J Urology 1981;53:613–616.
16. Benson K, Hartz AJ. A comparison of observational studies and randomized controlled trials. N Engl J Med 2000;342:1878–1886.
17. Writing Group from the Women's Health Initiative Investigators. Risks and benefits of estrogen plus progestin in healthy postmenopausal women: Principal results from the Women's Health Initiative Randomized Controlled Trial. JAMA 2002;288:321–333.
18. Col NF, Pauker SG. The discrepancy between observational studies and randomized trials of menopausal hormone therapy: Did expectations shape experience? Ann Intern Med 2003;139:923–929.
19. The Heart Outcomes Prevention Evaluation Study Investigators. Vitamin E supplementation and cardiovascular events in high-risk patients. N Engl J Med 2000;342:154–160.
20. Moher D, Schulz KF, Altman DG for the CONSORT Group. The CONSORT statement: Revised recommendations for improving the quality of parallel-group randomized trials. Ann Intern Med 2001;134:657–662.
21. Hotopf M, Lewis G, Normand C. Putting trials on trial—the costs and consequences of small trials in depression: A systematic review of methodology. J Epidemiol Community Health, 1977;51:354–358.

CHAPTER **9**

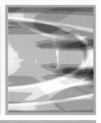

Prevention

KEY WORDS

Preventive care	Primary prevention	Interval cancers
Periodic health examination	Secondary prevention	Detection method
Immunizations	Tertiary prevention	Incidence method
Screening	Prevalence screen	Labeling effect
Behavioral counseling	Incidence screen	False-positive screening test
Lifestyle changes	Lead time bias	result
Chemoprevention	Length-time bias	Pseudodisease
Prevention	Compliance bias	Overdiagnosis

Live sensibly—among a thousand people, only one dies a natural death, the rest succumb to irrational modes of living.

— *Maimonides, A.D. 1135–1204*

Most doctors are attracted to medicine because they look forward to curing disease. But all things considered, most people would prefer never to contract a disease in the first place—or, if they cannot avoid an illness, they prefer that it be caught early and stamped out before it causes them any harm. To accomplish this, people without specific complaints undergo interventions to identify and modify risk factors, to avoid the onset of disease, or to find disease early in its course so that early treatment prevents sickness. When these interventions take place in clinical practice, the activity is referred to as **preventive care** or the **periodic health examination.** In the past, it was often called the "annual physical." Some patients think of a personal check-up in much the same way they view periodic tune-ups for their cars.

Preventive care constitutes a large portion of clinical practice. (1) Physicians should understand the conceptual basis and content of the periodic health examination. They should be prepared to answer questions from patients such as "Why do I have to get a Pap smear again this year, Doctor?" or "My neighbor gets a chest x-ray every year. Why aren't you ordering one for me?" or "I saw an ad for a total body MRI in the newspaper. Do you think I should get one?"

Much of the scientific approach to prevention in clinical medicine, particularly the principles underlying the use of diagnostic tests, disease prognosis, and effectiveness of interventions, has already been covered in this book. This chapter expands on those principles and strategies as they specifically relate to prevention.

POPULATION AND CLINICAL PREVENTION

Although this chapter concentrates on prevention activities clinicians undertake with individual patients, prevention at the community level can also be effective. Immunization requirements for students, no-smoking regulations in public buildings, and legislation restricting the sale of firearms are examples of community-wide prevention. For some problems, such as injury from firearms, community prevention works best. For others, such as colorectal cancer, screening in clinical settings works best. For still others, clinical efforts can complement community-wide activities. In smoking prevention efforts, clinicians help individual patients stop smoking and public education, regulations, and taxes prevent teenagers from starting to smoke.

In the clinical setting, preventive care activities often can be incorporated into the ongoing care of patients, as when a doctor checks the blood pressure in a patient complaining of a sore throat. At other times, a special visit just for preventive care is scheduled; thus the terms annual physical or periodic health examination.

Types of Clinical Prevention

There are four major types of clinical preventive care: immunizations, screening, behavioral counseling (sometimes referred to as lifestyle changes) and chemoprevention. All four apply throughout the life span.

Immunization

Childhood **immunizations** to prevent diseases such as diphtheria, tetanus, pertussis, measles, mumps, rubella, and pneumococcal disease largely determine visit schedules to the pediatrician in the first 18 months of life. Adult immunizations such as DPT boosters, influenza, and pneumococcal vaccinations are also effective.

Screening

Screening is the identification of asymptomatic disease or risk factors. Screening tests start in the prenatal period (as in alpha-fetoprotein testing) and continue throughout life (for example, when inquiring about hearing in the elderly). Much of this chapter discusses scientific principles of screening.

Behavioral Counseling (Lifestyle Changes)

Clinicians can give effective **behavioral counseling** to motivate **lifestyle changes,** ranging from encouraging parents of a newborn to purchase an infant seat for the car to encouraging moderation of alcohol consumption among problem drinkers. It is important to have evidence that counseling by clinicians is effective and to use protocols that have been found to be effective before spending time and effort on this approach to prevention (see Levels of Prevention below).

Chemoprevention

Chemoprevention is the use of drugs to prevent disease. It is used early in life (for example, ocular antibiotic prophylaxis of all newborns to prevent gonococcal ophthalmia neonatorum) but is more common in adults (for example, folate for women of childbearing age, aspirin prophylaxis for myocardial infarction, and statin treatment for hypercholesterolemia). This type of clinical prevention is growing rapidly.

LEVELS OF PREVENTION

Webster's dictionary defines **prevention** as "the act of preventing" and to prevent, "to keep from happening." (2) With these definitions in mind, almost all activities in medicine could be defined as prevention. After all, clinicians' efforts are aimed at preventing the untimely occurrences of the five Ds: death, disease, disability, discomfort, dissatisfaction, and destitution (discussed in Chapter 1). However, in clinical medicine, the definition of prevention is usually restricted, as outlined below.

Depending on when in the course of disease interventions are made, three levels of prevention are possible (Figure 9.1).

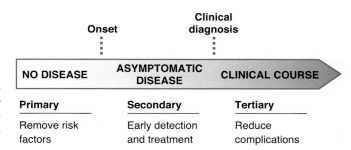

FIGURE 9.1 ■ Levels of prevention. Primary prevention prevents disease from occurring. Secondary prevention detects and cures disease in the asymptomatic phase. Tertiary prevention reduces complications of disease.

Primary Prevention

Primary prevention keeps disease from occurring at all by removing its causes. Examples of primary prevention include administering folic acid to prevent neural tube defects, giving immunizations for many communicable diseases, and counseling patients to adopt healthy lifestyles (such as helping patients to stop smoking, to eat foods low in saturated fats and cholesterol, to exercise appropriately, and to engage in safe sexual practices).

Primary prevention is often accomplished outside the health-care system at the community level. Examples include chlorination and fluoridation of the water supply and laws mandating seatbelt use in automobiles and helmet use on motorcycles. Certain primary prevention activities occur in specific occupational settings (use of ear plugs or dust masks), in schools (immunizations), or in specialized health settings (use of tests to detect hepatitis B or HIV in blood banks).

Secondary Prevention

Secondary prevention detects early disease when it is asymptomatic and when treatment can stop it from progressing. Pap smears, mammograms, and fecal occult blood tests are examples. Most secondary prevention is done in clinical settings, and all types of clinicians, especially those providing general care, undertake secondary prevention.

As pointed out earlier, screening is the identification of an unrecognized disease or risk factor by history taking (e.g., asking if the patient smokes), physical examination (e.g., a blood pressure measurement), laboratory test (e.g., a serum cholesterol-level determination), or other procedure (e.g., a sigmoidoscopy) that can be applied reasonably rapidly to asymptomatic people. Screening tests sort out apparently well persons who have a disease or a risk factor for a disease from people who do not. Screening tests are part of many primary and all secondary prevention activities. Sometimes the distinction is blurred, as when a clinician detects an early colon cancer (secondary prevention) during colonoscopy but also removes a precancerous adenoma, which strictly speaking, is primary prevention.

A screening test is not intended to be diagnostic and rarely is. If the clinician is not committed to further investigation of abnormal results and treatment, if necessary, the screening test should not be performed at all.

Tertiary Prevention

Tertiary prevention refers to those clinical activities that prevent further deterioration or reduce complications after a disease has declared itself. An example is the use of beta-blocking drugs to decrease the risk of death in patients who have recovered from myocardial infarction. The boundaries of tertiary prevention blend into curative medicine, but well-performed tertiary prevention goes beyond treating the problems patients present with. For example, in diabetic patients, tertiary prevention requires more than good control of blood glucose; patients need regular ophthalmologic examinations for early diabetic retinopathy, education for routine foot care, searches for and treatment of other cardiovascular risk factors, and monitoring for urinary protein so that angiotensin-converting enzyme inhibitors can be used to prevent renal failure.

There are few, if any, tertiary prevention programs outside the health-care system, but many health-care professionals in addition to physicians are active in these programs.

Tertiary prevention is particularly important in the management of patients having a fatal disease. The goal here is not to prevent death but to maximize the amount of high-quality time a patient has left.

EXAMPLE

Presently, there is no specific therapy for patients with amyotrophic lateral sclerosis, a neurologic condition causing progressive paralysis leading to respiratory failure. But careful medical management can lead to early intervention with a gastrostomy for administering food and liquids to prevent dehydration and weakness from starvation; a tracheostomy for better suctioning to prevent pneumonia for as long as possible; and, if the patient wishes, a portable respirator to rest respiratory muscles. With such a proactive approach toward tertiary prevention, the patient may avoid acute respiratory failure resulting from the combined effects of the underlying disease, dehydration, and pneumonia and preserve a more decent quality of life for as long as possible.

APPROACH TO CLINICAL PREVENTION

When considering what to do routinely for patients without specific symptoms for a given disease, the clinician must first decide which medical problems or diseases he or she should try to prevent. This statement is so clear and obvious that it would seem unnecessary to mention. But the fact is that many preventive procedures, especially screening tests, are performed without a clear understanding of what is being sought. For instance, physicians performing routine checkups on their patients frequently order a urinalysis. However, a urinalysis might be used to search for any number of medical problems, including diabetes, asymptomatic urinary tract infections, and renal disease. It is necessary to decide which, if any, of these conditions is worth screening for before undertaking the test.

Three criteria are important when deciding what condition to include in a periodic health examination (Table 9.1):

1. The burden of suffering caused by the condition.
2. The quality of screening test if one is to be performed.

TABLE 9.1 ▪ Criteria for Deciding Whether a Medical Condition Should Be Included in Preventive Care

1. How great is the burden of suffering caused by the condition in terms of:

Death	Discomfort
Disease	Dissatisfaction
Disability	Destitution

2. How good is the screening test, if one is to be performed, in terms of:

Sensitivity	Labeling effects
Specificity	Safety
Simplicity	Acceptability
Cost	

3. A. For primary prevention, how good is the intervention in terms of:

   Effectiveness
   Safety
   Cost-effectiveness

   or

   B. For secondary prevention, if the condition is found, how good is the ensuing treatment in terms of:

   Effectiveness
   Safety
   Early treatment after screening being more effective than later treatment without screening
   Cost-effectiveness

---

3. The quality (effectiveness, safety, and cost) of the intervention for primary prevention or the effectiveness of treatment for secondary prevention after the condition is found through screening.

BURDEN OF SUFFERING

Is prevention justified by the severity of the medical condition in terms of the mortality, morbidity, and suffering caused by the condition? Only conditions posing threats to life or health (the five Ds in Chapter 1) should be included in preventive care. The severity of the medical condition is determined primarily by the risk it poses or its prognosis (discussed in Chapters 5 and 7). For example, except during pregnancy and before urologic surgery, the health consequences of asymptomatic bacteriuria are not clear, even though it is common, especially in young girls. Whether or not it causes renal failure or hypertension is unknown. Even so, asymptomatic bacteriuria is frequently sought in periodic health examinations.

Burden of suffering also takes into account the frequency of a condition. A particular condition may cause great suffering for individuals who are unfortunate enough to get it, but may occur too rarely—especially in the individual's particular age group—for screening to be considered. Breast cancer and colorectal cancer are two such examples. Although both can occur in much younger people, they primarily occur in persons older than 50 years of age. For 20-year-old women, breast cancer incidence is about 1 in 100,000 (one-fifth the rate for men in their early 70s). (3) Although breast cancer should be sought in preventive care for older women, it is too uncommon in 20-year-old women and 70-year-old men for screening. Screening for very rare diseases means not only that, at most, very few people will benefit, but also results in false-positive tests in some people who may go on to experience labeling and further diagnostic evaluation (see below).

A particularly difficult dilemma faced by clinicians and patients is the situation in which a person is known to be at high risk for a condition, but the evidence regarding effectiveness of prevention is unclear. What should the physician and patient do?

EXAMPLE

People with Barrett's esophagus (a condition in which the squamous mucosa in the distal esophagus is replaced by columnar epithelium) run a thirtyfold to fortyfold greater risk of developing esophageal cancer than persons without Barrett's esophagus, with an annual risk of about 0.5–1.0%. However, the effectiveness of surgical prophylaxis is unknown. A randomized controlled trial evaluated medical versus surgical therapies for people with gastroesophageal reflux (including those with Barrett's esophagus). Nine to 10 years later, more people in the surgical group had died, a majority of patients in the surgical group continued to take antireflux medicines (although fewer than in the medical treatment group), and there was no significant difference in the development of esophageal cancer. (Few participants developed esophageal cancer at all, so an effect might have been missed.) Thus, even after long-term follow up, it is not clear whether or not definitive antireflux surgery is protective. (4)

There is no easy answer to the dilemma of a patient at high risk for a condition with little evidence for a protective intervention. But if physicians remember that screening will not help the patient unless early therapy is effective, they can weigh carefully the evidence about therapy with the patient. If the evidence is against effectiveness, they may hurt rather than help the patient by preventive activities.

SCREENING TESTS IN PREVENTIVE CARE

Screening tests are similar to diagnostic tests; often, the same test is used in both situations. However, when used in a screening situation, several special features become important that do not apply when the test is used for diagnosis. These include the difference between prevalence and incidence screens and three biases that can occur in screening studies: lead-time, length-time, and compliance biases. Lead-time and length-time biases are especially important in cancer screening.

Prevalence and Incidence Screens

The yield of screening decreases as screening is repeated over time. Figure 9.2 demonstrates why this is true. The first time that screening is carried out—the **prevalence screen**—cases of the medical condition will have been present for varying lengths of time. During the second round of screening, most cases found will have had their onset between the first and second screening. (A few will have been missed by the first screen.) Therefore, a second (and subsequent) screening is called an **incidence screen**. Figure 9.2 illustrates how, when a group of people are periodically rescreened, the number of cases of disease present in the group drops after the prevalence screen. This means that the positive predictive value for test results will decrease after the first round of screening.

Special Biases in Screening

As discussed in Chapter 8, the best way to establish the efficacy of treatment is with a randomized controlled trial. This is true for all interventions but especially for early treatment after screening.

Round of screening

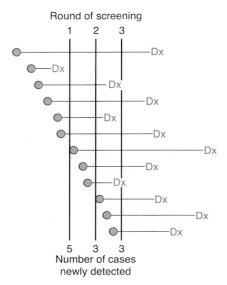

FIGURE 9.2 ■ The decreasing yield of a screening test after the first round of screening. The first round (prevalence screening) detects prevalent cases. The second and third rounds (incidence screenings) detect incident cases. In the figure, it is assumed that the test detects all cases and that all people in the population are screened. When this is not so, cases missed in the first round are available for detection in subsequent rounds—and the yield would be higher. O = onset of disease; Dx = diagnosis time, if screening were not carried out.

Typically, it takes years to establish that a preventive intervention is effective, and it requires large numbers of people to be studied. For example, early treatment after colorectal cancer screening can decrease colorectal cancer deaths by approximately one third. But to show this effect, a study of 45,000 people with 13 years of follow-up was required. (5) A "clinical impression" of the effect of screening simply does not suffice in this situation.

Careful studies are also necessary to avoid biases that are specific to studies of the effectiveness of screening programs.

Lead-Time Bias

Lead time is the period of time between the detection of a medical condition by screening and when it ordinarily would be diagnosed because a patient experiences symptoms and seeks medical care (Figure 9.3). The amount of lead time for a given disease depends on the biologic rate of progression of the disease and how early the screening test can detect the disease. When lead time is very short, as is presently the case with lung cancer, treatment of medical conditions picked up on screening is likely to be no more effective than treatment after symptoms appear. On the other hand, when lead time is long, as is true for cervical cancer (it takes approximately 30 years for it to progress from carcinoma in situ into a clinically invasive disease), treatment of the medical condition found on screening can be very effective.

How can lead time cause biased results in a study of the efficacy of early treatment? As Figure 9.3 shows, because of screening, a disease is found earlier than it would have been after the patient developed symptoms. As a result, people who are diagnosed by screening for a deadly disease will, on average, survive longer from the time of diagnosis than people who are diagnosed after they get symptoms, even if early treatment is no more effective than treatment

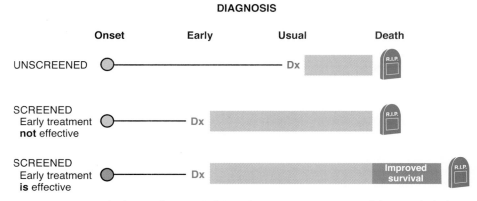

FIGURE 9.3 ■ How lead time affects survival time after screening; O = onset of disease. Shaded areas indicate length of survival after diagnosis (Dx).

TABLE 9.2 ■ Avoiding Bias in Screening

Bias	Effect	How to Avoid
Lead time	Appears to improve survival time but actually increases "disease" time after disease detection.	Use mortality rather than survival rates.
Length time	Outcome appears better in screened group because more cancers with a good prognosis are detected.	Compare outcomes in RCT with control group and one offered screening. Count *all* outcomes regardless of method of detection.
Compliance	Outcome in screened group appears better due to compliance, not screening.	Compare outcomes in RCT with control group and one offered screening. Count *all* outcomes regardless of compliance.

at the time of clinical presentation. In such a situation, screening would appear to help people live longer, spuriously improving survival rates when, in reality, they would have been given not more "survival time" but more "disease time."

An appropriate method of analysis to avoid lead-time bias is to study both a screened group of people and a control group of similar people who do not get screened, and compare age-specific mortality rates rather than survival rates from the time of diagnoses (Table 9.2). Early diagnosis and treatment of colorectal cancer are known to be effective because studies have shown that mortality rates of screened persons are lower than those of a comparable group of unscreened people.

Length-Time Bias

Length-time bias (see Figures 9.4 and 9.5) occurs because the proportion of slow-growing lesions diagnosed during screening is greater than the proportion of those diagnosed during usual medical care. As a result, length-time bias makes it seem that screening and early treatment are more effective than usual care.

Length-time bias occurs in the following way: Screening works best when a medical condition develops slowly. Most types of cancers, however, demonstrate a wide range of growth rates. Some cancers grow slowly, some very fast. Screening tests are likely to find mostly slow-growing tumors because they are present for a longer period of time before they cause symptoms. Fast-growing tumors are more likely to cause symptoms that lead to diag-

nosis in the interval between screening examinations. Screening, therefore, tends to find tumors with inherently better prognoses. As a result, the mortality rates of cancers found through screening may be better than those not found through screening, but screening is not protective in this situation.

Compliance Bias

The third major type of bias that can occur in effectiveness studies of presymptomatic treatment, **compliance bias**, is the result of the extent to which patients follow medical advice. Compliant patients tend to have better prognoses regardless of screening. If a study compares disease outcomes among

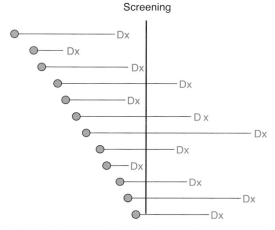

FIGURE 9.4 ■ Length-time bias. Cases that progress rapidly from onset (O) to symptoms and diagnosis (Dx) are less likely to be detected during a screening examination.

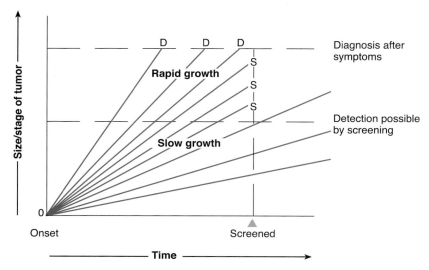

FIGURE 9.5 ■ Relationship between length-time bias and speed of tumor growth. Rapidly growing tumors come to medical attention before screening is performed, whereas more slowly growing tumors allow time for detection. *D* = diagnosis after symptoms; *S* = detection after screening.

volunteers for a screening program with outcomes in a group of people who did not volunteer, better results for the volunteers might not be the result of screening and early treatment but rather factors related to high compliance.

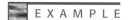

E X A M P L E

In a study of the effect of a periodic health examination program, one group of patients was invited for an annual examination and a comparable group was not invited. (6)

Over the years, however, some of the control group requested periodic examinations. As seen in Figure 9.6, those patients in the control group who actively sought out the examinations had better mortality rates than the patients who were invited for screening. The latter group contained not only compliant patients but also ones that had to be persuaded to participate or that refused.

Biases due to length time and patient compliance can be avoided by relying on studies that have concurrent screened and control groups that are

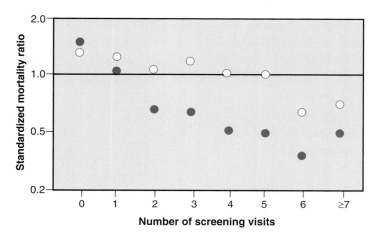

Number of screening visits

FIGURE 9.6 ■ Effect of patient compliance on the results of a screening program. The control group of patients (●) had a lower standardized mortality ratio (observed: expected deaths, standardized for age) than the study group (○) offered screening; but the control group included only patients who requested screening, whereas the study group included all patients offered screening, both those who wanted it and those who did not. (Redrawn from Friedman GD, Collen MF, Fireman BH. Multiphasic health checkup evaluation: A 16-year follow-up. J Chron Dis 1986;39:453–463.)

comparable. In each group, all people experiencing the outcomes of interest must be counted, regardless of the method of diagnosis or degree of participation (Table 9.2). Randomized trials are the strongest design because patients who are randomly allocated will have comparable numbers of slow- and fast-growing tumors and, on average, comparable levels of compliance. These groups then can be followed over time with mortality rates, rather than survival rates, to avoid lead-time bias. If a randomized trial is not possible, results of population-based studies can be valid. In such cases, the screened and control groups must be made up of similar populations, the control population should not have access to screening, and both populations must have careful follow-up to document all cases of the outcome being studied.

Because randomized controlled trials and prospective, population-based studies are difficult to conduct, take a long time, and are expensive, investigators sometimes try to use other kinds of studies, such as cohort studies (Chapter 5) or case control studies (Chapter 6), to investigate preventive maneuvers.

EXAMPLE

To test whether periodic screening with sigmoidoscopy reduces mortality from colorectal cancer within the reach of the sigmoidoscope, Researchers investigated the frequency of screening sigmoidoscopy over the previous 10 years among patients dying of colorectal cancer and among well patients, matched for age and sex. (7) To deal with lead-time and length-time biases, they investigated screening only in people who were known to have died (case group) or not to have died (control group) from colorectal cancer. To deal with compliance bias, they adjusted their results for the number of general periodic health examinations each person had. They also adjusted the results for the presence of medical conditions that could have led to both increased screening and increased likelihood of colorectal cancer. Patients dying of colorectal cancer in the rectum or distal sigmoid (where tumors could have been detected by sigmoidoscopy) were less likely to have undergone a screening sigmoidoscopy in the previous 10 years (8.8%) than those in the control group (24.2%). The investigators found that sigmoidoscopy followed by early therapy prevented almost 60% of deaths resulting from colorectal cancer arising in the distal colon or rectum. Also, by showing that there was no protection for colorectal cancers above the level reached by the sigmoidoscope, the authors suggested that "it is difficult to conceive of how such anatomical specificity of effect could be explained by confounding."

Case series, in which a group of people participating in a screening program are followed over time, is a common but inappropriate method of evaluating the effectiveness of screening programs because they are subject to all the biases discussed in Chapter 7 as well as lead time, length time, and compliance bias.

CRITERIA FOR A GOOD SCREENING TEST

The following criteria for a good screening test apply to all types of screening tests, whether they are history, physical examination, laboratory tests, or procedures.

High Sensitivity and Specificity

The very nature of searching for a disease in people without symptoms means that prevalence is usually very low, even among high-risk groups who were selected because of age, sex, and other characteristics. A good screening test must, therefore, have a high sensitivity, so that it does not miss the few cases of disease present. It must also be sensitive early in the disease when the subsequent course can still be altered. If a screening test is sensitive only for late-stage disease, which has progressed too far for effective treatment, the test would be useless. A screening test should also have a high specificity to reduce the number of people with false-positive results who require diagnostic evaluation.

Sensitivity and specificity are determined for screening tests much as they are for diagnostic tests, with one major difference. As discussed in Chapter 3, the sensitivity and specificity of a diagnostic test are determined by comparing the results to another test (the gold standard, which at times is a rather "tarnished gold" standard). In screening, the gold standard for the presence of disease is not only another test but also a period of follow-up. The gold standard test is routinely applied only to people with positive screening test results, to differentiate between true- and false-positive results. A period of follow-up is applied to all people who have a negative screening test result, in order to differentiate between true and false-negative test results.

Follow-up is particularly important in cancer screening, where the **interval cancers**, cancers subsequently discovered over the follow-up period, occur. A key challenge is to choose a correct period of follow-up. If the

---

TABLE 9.3 ■ Calculating Sensitivity of a Cancer Screening Test According to the Detection Method and the Incidence Method

---

Theoretical Example

A new screening test is introduced for pancreatic cancer. In a screening group, cancer is detected in 200 people; over the ensuing year, another 50 who had negative screening tests are diagnosed with pancreatic cancer. In a concurrent control group with the same characteristics and the same size, members did not undergo screening; 100 people were diagnosed with pancreatic cancer during the year.

Sensitivity of the Test Using the Detection Method

$$\text{Sensitivity} = \frac{\text{Number of screen-detected cancers}}{\text{Number of screen-detected cancers plus number of interval cancers}}$$
$$= \frac{200}{(200 + 50)}$$
$$= .80 \text{ or } 80\%$$

Sensitivity of the Test Using the Incidence Method

$$\text{Sensitivity} = 1 - (\text{interval rate in the screening group/ incidence rate in the control group})$$
$$= 1 - \left(\frac{50}{100}\right) = .50 \text{ or } 50\%$$

---

follow-up period is too short, disease missed by the screening test might not have a chance to make itself obvious and may overestimate the test's sensitivity. On the other hand, if the follow-up period is too long, disease not present at the time of screening might be found, resulting in a falsely low estimation of the test's sensitivity.

E X A M P L E

As noted above, screening for colorectal cancer was found to decrease mortality from that disease in a large randomized controlled trial of fecal occult blood tests. The sensitivity of the program of annual testing was determined by the ratio of the number of colorectal cancers detected by screening (confirmed histologically with a follow-up colonoscopy and biopsy) to the number of colorectal cancers detected by screening *and* the number discovered during the year after each screen. The assumption was that any cancer diagnosed during the year following a negative screen was an interval cancer present at screening but missed and the test result was false-negative. In the study, 178 cancers were detected at the time of screening, and 21 cancers became evident during the subsequent year in people who tested negative. Thus, sensitivity was calculated as 178 divided by (178 + 21), or 89.4%. (8)

Detection and Incidence Methods for Calculating Sensitivity

Calculating sensitivity by counting cancers detected during screening as true positives and interval cancers

as false negatives is sometimes referred to as the **detection method** (Table 9.3). The method works well for many screening tests, but there are two difficulties with it for some cancer screening tests. First, as already pointed out, it requires that the appropriate amount of follow-up time for interval cancers be known; often, it is not known and must be guessed. The detection method also assumes that the abnormalities detected by the screening test would go on to cause trouble if left alone. This second issue is a problem in screening for several cancers, particularly prostate cancer.

E X A M P L E

Histologic prostate cancer is common in older men. (It is estimated that 25% of 50-year-old men have histologic foci of prostate cancer, and that by the age of 90, virtually all men do). Screening tests can find such cancers in many men, but for most, the cancer will never become invasive. Thus, when the sensitivity of prostate cancer tests such as prostate-specific antigen (PSA) is determined by the detection method, the test may look quite good, because the numerator includes all cancers found, not just those with malignant potential.

To get around this problem, the **incidence method** calculates sensitivity by using the incidence in persons not undergoing screening and the interval cancer rate in persons who are screened (Table 9.3). The rationale for this approach is that the sensitivity of a test should affect interval cancer rates but not disease incidence. For prostate cancer, the incidence method defines sensitivity of the test as 1 minus the ratio of the interval prostate cancer rate in a group of men undergoing periodic screening to the incidence of prostate cancer in a group of men not undergoing screening (control group). The incidence method of calculating sensitivity gets around the problem of counting "benign" prostate cancers, but it may underestimate sensitivity because it excludes cancers with long lead times. True sensitivity of a test is, therefore, probably between the estimates of the two methods.

High Positive Predictive Value

Because of the low prevalence of most diseases, the positive predictive value of most screening tests is low, even for tests with high specificity. (The reverse is true for negative predictive value; because when prevalence is low, the negative predictive value is likely to be high.) Clinicians who perform screening tests on their patients must accept the fact that they will have to work up many patients who have positive screening test results but do not have disease. However, they can minimize the problem by con-

centrating their screening efforts on people with a higher prevalence for disease.

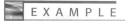
EXAMPLE

The incidence of breast cancer increases with age, from approximately 1 in 100,000/year at age 20 to 1 in 200/year over age 70. Also, sensitivity and specificity are better in older women. Therefore, a lump found during screening in a young woman's breast is more likely to be nonmalignant than a lump in an older woman. In a large study on breast cancer screening, finding cancer after an abnormal mammogram varied markedly according to the age of women; in women in their early 40s, about 57 women without cancer experienced further workup for every woman who was found to have a malignancy (Figure 9.7) with a positive predictive value of 1.7%. (9) But for women in their 80s, the number dropped to about 10, with a positive predictive value of 9.5%.

Simplicity and Low Cost

An ideal screening test should take only a few minutes to perform, require minimum preparation by the patient, depend on no special appointments, and be inexpensive.

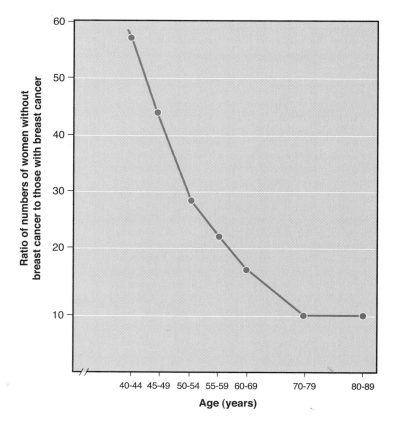

FIGURE 9.7 ▦ Yield of abnormal screening mammograms according to patients' age. Number of women without breast cancer for each woman diagnosed with breast cancer among women having an abnormal mammogram when screened for breast cancer. (Source: Carney PA, Miglioretti DL, Yankaskas BC, Kerlikowske K, Rosenberg R, Rutter CM, et al. Individual and combined effects of age, breast density, and hormone replacement therapy use on the accuracy of screening mammography. Ann Intern Med 2003; 138:168–175.)

Simple, quick examinations such as blood pressure determinations are ideal screening tests. Conversely, tests such as colonoscopy, which are expensive and require an appointment and bowel preparation, are best suited for diagnostic testing in patients with symptoms and clinical indications. They may be less acceptable as screening tests, especially if they must be repeated frequently. Nevertheless, screening colonoscopy is becoming more and more common in the United States. Other tests, such as visual field testing for the detection of glaucoma and audiograms for the detection of hearing loss, fall between these two extremes.

The financial "cost" of the test depends not only on the cost of (or charge for) the procedure itself but also on the cost of subsequent evaluations performed on patients with positive test results. Thus sensitivity, specificity, and predictive value affect cost. Cost is also affected by whether the test requires a special visit to the physician. Screening tests performed while the patient is seeing his or her physician for other reasons (as is frequently the case with blood pressure measurements) are much cheaper for patients than tests requiring special visits, extra time off from work, and additional transportation. Cost also is determined by how often a test must be repeated.

Taking all these issues into account at once sometimes leads to surprising conclusions.

EXAMPLE

Several different tests can be used to screen for colorectal cancer. They include fecal occult blood tests, sigmoidoscopy, colonoscopy, and barium enema. The tests vary greatly in their upfront costs, ranging from a few dollars for fecal occult blood tests to as much as $1,000 for screening colonoscopy. However, the cost per year of life saved by screening is not very different for these tests; all are in an acceptable range by U.S. standards. This is true for several reasons. First, the simpler, cheaper tests have to be done more often. Fecal occult blood tests are recommended yearly, whereas colonoscopy is recommended every 10 years. The cheaper tests also produce more false-positive results that lead to more testing (and therefore more costs). Finally, they produce more false-negative results and miss patients who actually have cancer. This leads to costs for care of patients with more advanced cancer. (10)

Safety

It is reasonable and ethical to accept a certain risk for diagnostic tests applied to sick patients seeking help for specific complaints. The patient comes asking for help, sometimes with a problem about which little is known. The physician cannot postpone action, especially when the patient is severely ill, and does his or her best. It is quite another matter to subject presumably well people to risks. In such circumstances, the procedure should be especially safe. This is partly because the chances of finding disease in healthy people are so low. Thus, although colonoscopy is hardly thought of as a dangerous procedure when used on patients with gastrointestinal complaints, some are concerned about its use as a screening procedure because of the possibility of bowel perforation. In fact, when colonoscopy, with a rate of two perforations per thousand examinations, is used to screen for colorectal cancer in people in their 50s, almost two perforations occur for every cancer found. For people in their 70s, the ratio is reversed, because colorectal cancer is so much more common.

Acceptable to Patients and Clinicians

If a screening test is associated with discomfort, it usually takes several years to convince large percentages of patients to obtain the test. This has been true for Pap smears, mammograms, and colorectal cancer screening.

The acceptability of the test to clinicians is a criterion usually overlooked by all but the ones performing it. Clinician acceptance is especially relevant for screening tests that involve clinical skill, such as mammography, sigmoidoscopy, or colonoscopy. Performing a procedure repeatedly can be tiring when the vast majority of results are normal. Screening can cause stress with the increasing number of associated malpractice suits. Because of these problems, clinician shortages in certain fields may develop. Even a screening test as well accepted as mammography became more difficult to obtain as more and more mammography facilities closed between 2000 and 2003 and radiologists did not want to specialize in breast imaging. (11)

Labeling

Studies suggest that test results can sometimes have important psychological effects on patients. The psychological impact of a test is called a **labeling effect.** A good screening test result produces either no labeling effect or a positive labeling effect.

Labeling can either help or hurt patients. A positive labeling effect may occur when a patient is told that all the screening test results were normal. Most clinicians have heard such responses as, "Great, that means I can keep working for another year." If being given a clean bill of health promotes a positive attitude toward one's daily activities, a positive labeling effect has occurred.

On the other hand, being told that the screening test result is abnormal and more testing is necessary may have an adverse psychological effect. This is especially true in cancer screening. If a screening test ultimately leads to a newly diagnosed cancer, it is natural to expect that the patient will be upset and will suffer a negative labeling effect.

However, studies have found that some people with abnormal screening tests who subsequently are found *not* to have cancer (that is, after they experience false-positive test results) also have a negative labeling effect, even after being told everything is normal. Because there are always many more patients with false-positive results in screening than true positive test results, and because this is a group of people *without* disease, negative labeling effects are particularly worrisome ethically. In such situations, screening efforts might promote a sense of vulnerability instead of health and might do more harm than good.

 E X A M P L E

A study of women with abnormal mammograms who, on subsequent evaluation were determined not to have cancer, found that several months later almost half reported mammography-related anxiety (47%) and worries about breast cancer (41%); 17% said the worries affected their daily function. (12) Most other studies also found that women continued to worry about breast cancer after having a "mammography scare." Anxiety occurs after abnormal screening results for other cancers too, as well as with blood pressure screening. In sum, people do not respond well when told, "Your screening test result was not quite normal, and we need to do more tests."

Labeling effects are sometimes unpredictable.

 E X A M P L E

An autosomal dominant gene has been identified for Huntington's disease, a neurological condition usually striking in middle age and causing mental deterioration leading to dementia, chorea, and death. Relatives of affected individuals can be tested to see if they carry the gene. Such a test may help people who wonder whether they should marry and have children, but it is reasonable to be concerned about the psychological reaction of people testing positive for the deleterious gene. A study of

reactions after genetic testing found that psychological health improved in people who tested negative for the gene; that is, they experienced a positive labeling effect. Moreover, those who were found to carry the deleterious gene also had (slightly) improved psychological health scores, perhaps because they were no longer dealing with uncertainty. (13) Studies of women being tested for genetic mutations that increase their risk for breast and ovarian cancer have also found that women for whom the test found no mutation experience improved psychological well-being, while those testing positive for the mutation experience little or no deterioration.

POSSIBLE ADVERSE EFFECTS FROM SCREENING

Adverse effects of screening tests include discomfort during the test procedure (the majority of women undergoing mammography say that the procedure is painful, although usually not so severe that patients refuse the test), long-term radiation effects after exposure to radiographic procedures (thus, pregnant women are excluded from radiographic screening tests), false-positive test results, and overdiagnosis (or pseudodisease). The last two will be discussed in the following section.

Risk of False-Positive Result

A **false-positive screening test result** is an abnormal result in a person without disease. As already pointed out, tests with low predictive values (resulting from low prevalence of disease, poor specificity of the test, or both) are likely to lead to a higher frequency of false positives. False-positive results, in turn, can lead to negative labeling effects, inconvenience, and expense in obtaining follow-up procedures.

False-positive results account for only a small minority of screening test results (only about 10% of screening mammograms are false-positives). But even so, they can affect large percentages of people who get screened. This happens in two ways. First, most clinicians do not perform only one or two tests on patients presenting for routine checkups. Modern technology, and perhaps the threat of lawsuits, has fueled the propensity to "cover all the bases." Automated blood tests allow physicians to order several dozen tests with a few checks in the appropriate boxes.

When the measurements of screening tests are expressed on interval scales (as most blood tests are),

TABLE 9.4 ■ Relation Between Number of Different Screening Tests Ordered and Percentage of Normal People with at Least One Abnormal Test Result [a]

Number of Tests	People with at Least One Abnormality (Percent)
1	5
5	23
20	64
100	99.4

[a] From Sackett DL. Clinical diagnosis and the clinical laboratory. Clin Invest Med 1978;1:37–43.

and when *normal* is defined by the range covered by 95% of the results (as is usual), the more tests the clinician orders, the greater the risk of a false-positive result. In fact, as Table 9.4 shows, if the physician orders enough tests, "abnormalities" will be discovered in virtually all healthy patients. (A spoof titled "The Last Well Person" was published on this phenomenon). (14)

Another reason that many people may experience a false-positive screening test result is that most screening tests are repeated at regular intervals. With each repeat screen, the patient is at risk for a false-positive result.

E X A M P L E

A study followed 1,200 women to determine the 10-year risk of a false-positive screening mammogram. Twenty-four percent experienced at least one false-positive result over the 10 years. Adjusting for the number of mammograms received, it was estimated that about half the women receiving annual mammograms for 10 years would have at least one false-positive mammogram. (15)

Risk of Pseudodisease (Overdiagnosis) in Cancer Screening

The underlying thesis behind screening for cancer is that the earlier a cancer is found, the better the chance of cure. Therefore, the thinking goes, it is always better to find cancer as early as possible. This thesis is being challenged by modern screening tests that are finding cancer earlier and earlier. The use of these tests can be accompanied by an increase in cancer incidence when screening

becomes widespread. A temporary increase in incidence is to be expected because a screening test moves the time of diagnosis forward and therefore adds early cases to the usual number of cancers being diagnosed without screening. But the temporary bump in incidence should come down after a few years. With some cancers, however, incidence remains increased once widespread screening is established. This has occurred with both prostate and breast cancer. It is as if screening causes more cancers. How could this be?

Some cancers are so slow-growing, and some even regress, that they do not cause any trouble for the patient. If such cancers are found through screening, they are called **pseudodisease**; the process leading to their detection is called **overdiagnosis** because finding them does not help the patient. Discovery of such cancers cause the apparent increase in cancer incidence. Overdiagnosis is an extreme example of length-time bias (Figure 9.8). The lesions found have such a good prognosis that they would never become evident without screening technology.

E X A M P L E

Neuroblastoma, a tumor of neurologic tissue near the kidney, is the second most common tumor occurring in children. Prognosis depends on the stage of the disease and is better when the tumor is diagnosed during infancy. Treatment involves surgery and chemotherapy. A simple urine test for catecholamine metabolites can be used to screen for the tumor. Japanese studies showed improved survival rates after screening, but lead time and a historical control group could have biased the results. Also, there was no population-based registry of childhood cancers in Japan to ensure ascertainment of all neuroblastoma cases. Finally, at least some cases of neuroblastomas regress without treatment, which raised the possibility of overdiagnosis.

Two population-based studies were therefore undertaken in Germany (16) and Quebec, (17) in which screening was offered for all infants in certain areas, while infants in other areas were not screened and acted as concurrent controls. In both studies, existing tumor registries were used to track all cases of and deaths due to neuroblastoma. In both studies, mortality rates from neuroblastoma over the subsequent five years were equivalent in the screened groups and the unscreened groups. However, the incidence of neuroblastoma doubled among the screened group in both studies. It appeared that the screening test primarily detected tumors with a favorable prognosis, many of which would have regressed if undetected. Meanwhile, highly invasive disease was often missed. Investigators of both studies concluded that screening infants for neuroblastoma leads to overdiagnosis but does not reduce mortality from neuroblastoma.

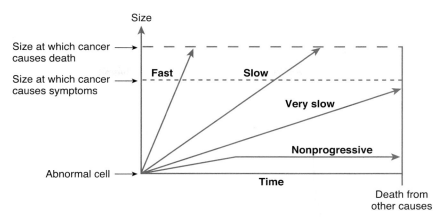

FIGURE 9.8 ▩ Mechanism of overdiagnosis in cancer screening. Note that nonprogressive, as well as some very slow growing, cancers will never cause clinical harm. When these cancers are found on screening, overdiagnosis has occurred. Overdiagnosis is an extreme form of length-time bias. (Reprinted from Welsh HG. Should I Be Tested for Cancer? Maybe Not and Here's Why. Berkeley and Los Angeles, California: University of California Press, 2004.)

There is evidence that at least some overdiagnosis occurs in screening for other cancers as well, especially prostate, breast, cervical, and lung cancer. As genetics research unravels the development of cancer, it appears that a sequence of genetic changes accompany pathogenesis from normal tissue to malignant disease. At each step, only some lesions go on to the next stage of carcinogenesis. It is likely that overdiagnosis occurs because lesions early in the chain are being picked up by newer screening tests. Pseudodisease is a particularly difficult issue because such lesions cannot always be distinguished from lesions destined to develop into invasive cancer, which are the reason for screening. The challenge is to differentiate those early lesions that will go on to cause morbidity and mortality from those that will lie dormant throughout life. So far, screening technology is not able to do this. To determine if and to what degree overdiagnosis occurs, it is necessary to determine disease-specific mortality rates (not survival rates) and to compare a screened group with a similar unscreened group.

EFFECTIVENESS OF TREATMENT

"Treatments" in *primary* prevention are immunizations, drugs, and behavioral counseling. Whatever the intervention, it should be efficacious (able to produce a beneficial result in ideal situations) and effective (able to produce a beneficial result under usual conditions, taking into account patient compliance). Because interventions for primary prevention are usually given to large numbers of healthy people, they also must be very safe.

Expert groups also consider cost when making recommendations that affect large segments of the population. Cost-effectiveness analysis formalizes this approach for policy makers, estimating all costs related to disease occurrence that might be saved as well as prevention costs.

EXAMPLE

Streptococcus pneumoniae is the leading bacterial cause of otitis media, pneumonia, bacteremia, and meningitis in infants and young children in the United States. A randomized controlled trial found that pneumococcal conjugate vaccine decreased these infections and saved lives when healthy infants were vaccinated at 2, 4, 6, and 12–15 months of age. A cost-effectiveness analysis was then performed. (18) The investigators estimated the medical costs, work-loss costs for parents, and future productivity costs associated with pneumococcal-associated disease events, as well as the costs of a vaccination program, using the list price for the vaccine. If instituted nationally, the investigators estimated that the vaccination program would prevent more than 12,000 cases of meningitis, which costs society $280,000 per case prevented; 53,000 cases of pneumonia, which costs $3,200 per case prevented; one million episodes of otitis media, which costs $160 per episode prevented; and 12,000 cases of bacteremia, which costs $15,000 per case prevented. An estimated 116 deaths would be prevented, at a cost of $80,000 per life-year saved. The cost per life-year saved puts pneumococcal vaccination at the high end of the range for current preventive measures. Expert groups recommend this vaccination for infants.

Efficacy and effectiveness are usually better documented for pharmaceuticals than they are for behavioral counseling. Federal laws require rigorous evidence of efficacy before pharmaceuticals are approved for use. However, the same is not true for behavioral counseling methods. Nevertheless, clinicians should require scientific evidence before incorporating routine counseling into health maintenance. Health behaviors are among the most important determinants of health in modern society; effective counseling methods could promote health more than most anything else a clinician can do, but counseling that does not work wastes time, costs money, and may harm patients.

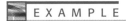

EXAMPLE

Smoking kills approximately 450,000 Americans each year. But, what is the evidence that advising patients to quit smoking gets them to stop? Are some approaches better than others? These questions were addressed by a panel that reviewed all studies done on smoking cessation, focusing on randomized trials. (19) They found 43 trials that assessed levels of counseling time and found a dose-response—the more contact time the better the abstinence rate (Figure 9.9). In addition, the panel found that randomized trials demonstrated that adding pharmacotherapy such as bupropion (a centrally acting drug that decreases craving), nicotine gum, nasal spray, or patches increased the smoking cessation rate still further. On the other hand, there was no effect of acupuncture, anxiolytics, or beta-blockers. By carefully evaluating behavioral counseling, with and without different drugs, analyses such as this are determining what approaches actually help patients stop smoking.

Treatments for *secondary* prevention are generally the same as treatments for curative medicine. Like interventions for symptomatic disease, they should be both efficacious and effective. In addition, it is

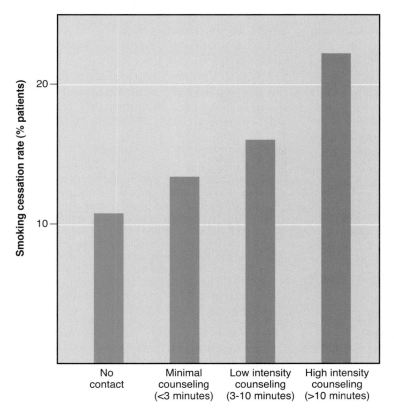

FIGURE 9.9 ■ Dose response of smoking cessation rates according to the effort clinicians make with patients. Combined results of 43 studies. (Source: Fiore MC, Bailey WC, Cohen SJ, Dorfman SF, Goldstein MG, Gritz ER, et al. Treating Tobacco Use and Dependence: Clinical Practice Guideline. Rockville, MD: U.S. Department of Health and Human Services. Public Health Service, June 2000.)

important to establish that treatment of early disease is superior to treatment of disease when it would be diagnosed in the usual course of events, when a patient seeks medical care for symptoms. If outcome in the two situations is the same, screening is not necessary.

E X A M P L E

Lung cancer is the leading cause of cancer-related death in the United States. Why, then, does no major professional medical group recommend screening for the disease? Several randomized trials begun in the 1970s and 1980s did not find screening protective. In one study of the use of chest x-rays and sputum cytology to screen for lung cancer, male cigarette smokers who were screened every 4 months and treated promptly when cancer was found did no better than those not offered screening and treated only when they presented with symptoms. Twenty years later, death rates from lung cancer were the same in the two groups—4.4 per 1,000 person-years in the screened men versus 3.9 per 1,000 persons-years in men not offered screening. (20) Early detection and treatment did not help patients with lung cancer more than treatment of people at the time they presented with symptoms. More modern screening techniques, particularly low-dose computed tomography, are being assessed with randomized controlled trials to determine whether their use will lower lung cancer mortality. (21)

CURRENT RECOMMENDATIONS

With progress in the science of prevention, current recommendations on health maintenance are quite different from those of the past. Several groups have recommended abandoning routine annual checkups in favor of a selective approach in which the tests to be done depend on a person's age, sex, and clinical characteristics (thereby increasing prevalence and positive predictive value). They also have turned their attention to the selection process for deciding what medical conditions should be sought. There is increasing concern for clear delineation of the criteria that tests should meet before they are incorporated into periodic health examinations. Groups with explicit criteria for selecting medical conditions are more conservative in their recommendations than groups without such criteria.

Because it is becoming clear that prevention has both good and harmful effects, and that different people might judge the balance differently, several groups making recommendations on clinical preventive care call for shared decision making between the patient and clinician. Before undertaking a health promotion procedure on a patient, especially when the procedure is controversial among expert groups, the clinician should discuss the pros (probability of known and hoped-for health benefits) and cons (probability of unintended effects) of the procedure with the patient. This must be done in ways that the patient can understand (see Risk Communication in Chapter 6).

E X A M P L E

Women want information about breast cancer screening from their physicians. For an individual woman to make an informed decision about screening mammography, or just to better understand the recommendation of her doctor, it is useful to demonstrate her risk of breast cancer as well as the benefits and possible harms resulting from screening. Figure 9.10 shows the risk of breast cancer for women ages 40 to 60 and the chances of experiencing a false-positive mammogram and a biopsy, breast cancer mortality with and without mammography screening, and of being diagnosed with ductal carcinoma in situ (a pre-invasive lesion that some investigators believe is associated with overdiagnosis). All the risks are shown in absolute terms (how often per 1,000 women over 10 years) so that the woman can have an idea of the likelihood of each outcome. (22) Such an approach not only is more honest with the patient but also helps clarify the situation for her so that her consent for whatever is chosen is truly informed.

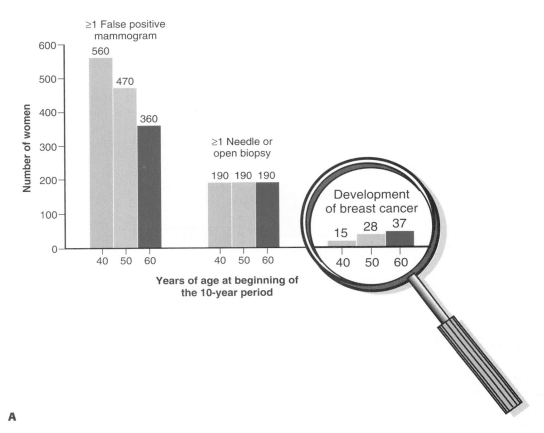

A

FIGURE 9.10 ▪ Type of information average-risk women should have when participating in shared decision making about screening mammography. Chances among 1,000 women who undergo annual screening mammography for 10 years: (A) of experiencing a false-positive mammogram, undergoing a breast biopsy, and developing breast cancer, and (B) being cured of breast cancer regardless of screening, being diagnosed with noninvasive breast ductal carcinoma in situ because of screening, and averting death from breast cancer because of screening mammography. (Reprinted from Fletcher SW, Elmore JG. Mammographic screening for breast cancer. N Engl J Med 2003;348:1672–1680.)

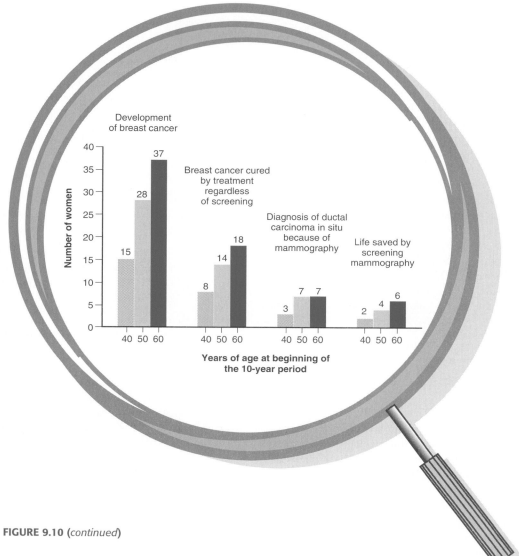

B

FIGURE 9.10 (*continued*)

REVIEW QUESTIONS

Read the scenario and answer the following questions.

A study was conducted to determine whether a fecal occult blood screening test reduced mortality from colorectal cancer. (5) People ages 50 to 60 years were randomized to the screening test or to a control group and followed for 13 years. Over this period of time, there were 323 cancer cases and 82 colorectal cancer deaths in the 15,570 people randomized to annual screening; there were 356 cancers and 121 colorectal cancer deaths in the 15,394 people randomized to the control group. Investigations of positive tests found that about 30% of the screened group had colon polyps. The sensitivity and specificity of the test for colon cancer were both about 90%.

9.1. Calculate the relative risk reduction of colorectal mortality in the screened group. How many patients would you need to screen over the next 13 years to prevent one death from colorectal cancer?

In a randomized controlled trial of screening chest x-rays and sputum cytology for lung cancer, approximately 9,000 men were randomized to screening or a control group. (20) After 20 years, the lung cancer mortality was the same in both groups (4.4/1,000 person-years in the screened group and 3.9/1,000 person-years in the control group). However, the median survival for early stage disease was 16 years in the screened group and only 5 years in the control group. Also, screening found more lung cancer—206 cancers were diagnosed in the screened group and 160 in the control group.

9.2. What are two possible biases that explain why these confusing results can occur in screening studies? How could they have happened in this study?

9.3. When assessing a new vaccine, state at least two questions for which you want answers before advising your patients?

9.4. What are the characteristics of a good screening test?

Read the following statements about diagnostic and screening tests and mark each one as True or False.

_____ **9.5.** A diagnostic test, but not a screening test, requires a gold standard.

_____ **9.6.** Disease prevalence for a diagnostic test is lower than that for a screening test.

_____ **9.7.** The incidence method can be used to calculate sensitivity for cancer screening tests.

_____ **9.8.** The positive predictive value of a test is an issue only with diagnostic tests.

_____ **9.9.** When a screening program is begun, more people with disease are found on the first round of screening than on later rounds.

Answers are in Appendix A.

REFERENCES

1. Cherry DK, Burt CW, Woodwell DA. National ambulatory medical care survey (2001 summary): Advance data from vital and health statistics. No. 337: National Center for Health Statistics, August 11, 2003. Available at: http://www.cdc.gov/nchs/data/ad/ad337.pdf. Last accessed November 19, 2004.
2. Agnes M (editor in chief). Webster's New World Dictionary, 4th Ed. Cleveland, Ohio: Wiley Publishing, Inc., 2002.
3. Ries LAG, Eisner MP, Kosary CL, Hankey BF, Miller BA, et al. SEER Cancer Statistics Review, 1975–2001, National Cancer Institute. Bethesda, MD. Available at: http://seer.cancer.gov/csr/1975_2001/. Last accessed November 19, 2004.
4. Spechler SJ, Lee E, Ahnen D, Goyal RK, Hirano I, Ramirez F, et al. Long-term outcome of medical and surgical therapies for gastroesophageal reflux disease: Follow-up of a randomized controlled trial. JAMA 2001;285:2331–2338.
5. Mandel JS, Bond JH, Church TR, Snover DC, Bradley M, Schuman LM, et al. (for the Minnesota Colon Cancer Control Study). Reducing mortality from colorectal cancer by screening for fecal occult blood. N Engl J Med 1993;328:1365–1371.
6. Friedman GD, Collen MF, Fireman BH. Multiphasic health checkup evaluation: A 16-year follow-up. J Chron Dis 1986;39:453–463.

7. Selby JV, Friedman GD, Quesenberry CP, Weiss NS. A case-control study of screening sigmoidoscopy and mortality from colorectal cancer. N Eng J Med 1992;326:653–657.

8. Church TR, Ederer F, Mandel JS. Fecal occult blood screening in the Minnesota study: Sensitivity of the screening test. J Natl Cancer Inst 1997;89:1440–1448.

9. Carney PA, Miglioretti DL, Yankaskas BC, Kerlikowse K, Rosenberg R, Rutter CM, et al. Individual and combined effects of age, breast density, and hormone replacement therapy use on the accuracy of screening mammography. Ann Intern Med 2003; 138:168–175.

10. Winawer SJ, Fletcher RH, Miller L, Godlee F, Stolar MH, Mulrow CD, et al. Colorectal cancer screening: Clinical guidelines and rationale. Gastroenterology 1997;112:594–642.

11. Chapter 3. Improving breast cancer screening services. In: Herdman R, Norton L, editors, Committee on New Approaches to Early Detection and Diagnosis. Saving women's lives: Strategies for improving breast cancer detection and diagnosis. Washington, D.C.: The National Academies Press; 2005.

12. Lerman C, Trock B, Rimer BK, Boyce A, Jepson C, Engstrom PF. Psychological and behavioral implications of abnormal mammograms. Ann Intern Med 1991;114:657–661.

13. Wiggins S, Whyte P, Huggins M, Adam S, Theilmann J, Bloch M, et al. The psychological consequences of predictive testing for Huntington's disease. Canadian collaborative study of predictive testing. N Engl J Med 1992;327:1401–1405.

14. Meador CK. The last well person. N Engl Med J 1994;330:440–441.

15. Elmore JG, Barton MB, Moceri VM, Polk S, Arena PJ, Fletcher SW. Ten-year risk of false positive screening mammograms and clinical breast examinations. N Engl J Med 1998;338:1089–1096.

16. Schilling FH, Spix C, Berthold F, Erttmann R, Fehse N, Hero B, et al. Neuroblastoma screening at one year of age. N Engl J Med 2002;346:1047–1053.

17. Woods WG, Gao R, Shuster JJ, Robison LL, Bernstein M, Weitzman S, et al. Screening of infants and mortality due to neuroblastoma. N Engl J Med 2002;346:1041–1046.

18. Lieu TA, Thomas RG, Black SB, Butler JC, Klein J, Breiman RF, et al. Projected cost-effectiveness of pneumococcal conjugate vaccination of healthy infants and young children. JAMA 2000;283:1460–1468.

19. Fiore MC, Bailey WC, Cohen SJ, Dorfman SF, Goldstein MG, Gritz ER, et al. Treating Tobacco Use and Dependence: Clinical Practice Guideline. Rockville, MD: U.S. Department of Health and Human Services. Public Health Service, June 2000.

20. Marcus PM, Bergstralh EJ, Fagerstrom RM, Williams DE, Fontana R, Taylor WF, et al. Lung cancer mortality in the Mayo Lung Project: Impact of extended follow-up. J Natl Cancer Inst. 2000;92:1308–1316.

21. Humphrey LL, Teutsch S, Johnson M. Lung cancer screening with sputum cytologic examination, chest radiography, and computed tomography: An update for the U.S. Preventive Services Task Force. Ann Intern Med. 2004;140:740–753.

22. Fletcher SW, Elmore JG. Mammographic screening for breast cancer. N Engl J Med 2003;348:1672–1680.

CHAPTER 10

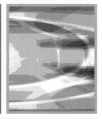

Chance

KEY WORDS

Hypothesis testing	Statistical testing	Statistical precision
Estimation	*P* value	Confidence interval
Statistically significant	Statistical tests	Sample size
Type I error (or α error)	Null hypothesis	Multiple comparisons
Type II error (or β error)	Statistical power	Secondary analyses
Inferential statistics	Point estimate	Multivariable modeling

> *Though . . . human beings are not unique in their responses to some treatment, there is no doubt that they are likely to be variable, and sometimes extremely variable. Two or three observations may, therefore, give, merely through the customary play of chance, a favorable picture in the hands of one doctor, an unfavorable picture in the hands of another.*
>
> *— Sir Austin Bradford Hill, 1971*

Learning from clinical experience, whether during formal research or in the course of patient care, is impeded by two processes: bias and chance. As discussed in Chapter 1, bias is systematic error, the result of any process that causes observations to differ systematically from the true values. In clinical research, a great deal of effort is aimed at avoiding bias whenever possible and controlling for and estimating its effects when bias is unavoidable.

On the other hand, random error, resulting from the play of chance, is inherent in all observations. It can be minimized but never avoided altogether. This source of error is called "random," because on average it is as likely to result in observed values being on one side of the true value as on the other.

Many clinicians tend to underestimate the importance of chance relative to bias when interpreting data. One might say, in essence, "If the statistical conclusions are strong, a little bit of bias can't do much harm." However, when data are biased, no amount of statistical elegance can save the day. As one scholar put it, perhaps taking an extreme position, "A well designed, carefully executed study usually gives results that are obvious without a formal analysis and if there are substantial flaws in design or execution a formal analysis will not help." (1)

In this chapter, chance is discussed in the context of a controlled clinical trial because it is a simple way of presenting the concepts. However, statistics are an element of all clinical research, whenever one makes inferences about populations based on information obtained from samples. Observations of samples, whether they are simple descriptions or comparisons, cannot be expected to represent the true situation exactly because of random variation. Statistical tests help estimate how well the observations approximate the true situation. Why not make measurements directly on the population and do away with this uncertainty? Research must ordinarily be conducted on a sample of patients and not all patients with the condition under study. As a result, there is always a possibility that the particular sample of patients in a study, even though selected in an unbiased way, might not be similar to the population of patients as a whole.

TWO APPROACHES TO CHANCE

Two general approaches are used to assess the role of chance in clinical observations. The first, called **hypothesis testing**, asks whether an effect (difference) is present or is not by using statistical tests to examine the hypothesis (the "null hypothesis") that there is no difference. This is the traditional way of assessing the role of chance and is associated with the familiar "P values." It has been popular since statistical testing was introduced at the beginning of the 20th century. The other approach, called **estimation**, uses statistical methods to estimate the range of values that is likely to include the true value. This approach has gained popularity recently and is now favored by most medical journals for reasons described below.

Bayes' theorem was introduced in Chapter 3 as the conceptual basis for the modern interpretation of diagnostic tests. Bayesian reasoning is also a way of understanding the role of chance in other kinds of clinical research.

Bayes' theorem will be mentioned again at the end of this chapter.

HYPOTHESIS TESTING

In the usual situation, the principal conclusions of a trial are expressed in dichotomous terms, such as a new treatment being better or not better than usual care, and the results are either "**statistically significant**"(unlikely to be purely by chance) or are not. There are four ways in which the statistical conclusions might relate to reality (Figure 10.1).

Two of the four possibilities lead to correct conclusions: (1) the new treatment really is better and that is the conclusion of the study; and (2) the treatments really have similar effects and the study concludes that a difference is unlikely.

False-Positive and False-Negative Statistical Results

There are also two ways of being wrong. The new treatment and usual care may actually have similar effects, but it is concluded that the new treatment is more effective. Error of this kind, resulting in a "false-positive" conclusion that the treatment is effective, is referred to as a **Type I error** or α *error*—the probability of saying that there is a difference in treatment effects when there is not. On the other hand, the new treatment might be more effective, but the study concludes that it is not. This "false-negative" conclusion is called a **Type II error** or β **error**—the probability of saying that there is no

		TRUE DIFFERENCE	
		Present	Absent
CONCLUSION OF STATISTICAL TEST	Significant	Correct	Type I (α) error
	Not significant	Type II (β) error	Correct

FIGURE 10.1 ▪ The relationship between the results of a statistical test and the true difference between two treatment groups. (*Absent* is a simplification. It really means that the true difference is not greater than a specified amount.)

difference in treatment effects when there is. "No difference" is a simplified way of saying that the true difference is unlikely to be larger than a certain size, which is considered too small to be of practical consequence. It is not possible to establish that there is no difference at all between two treatments.

Figure 10.1 is similar to the two-by-two table comparing the results of a diagnostic test to the true diagnosis (see Chapter 3). Here, the "test" is the conclusion of a clinical trial based on a statistical test of results from a sample of patients. Reality is the true difference in the treatments being compared—if it could be established, for example, by making observations on all patients with the illness or a large number of samples of these patients. Type I error is analogous to a false-positive and Type II error to a false-negative test result. In the absence of bias, random variation is responsible for the uncertainty of a statistical conclusion.

Because random variation plays a part in all observations, it is an oversimplification to ask whether chance is responsible for the results. Rather, it is a question of how likely random variation is to account for the findings under the particular conditions of the study. The probability of error due to random variation is estimated by means of **inferential statistics**, a quantitative science that, given certain assumptions about the mathematical properties of the data, is the basis for calculations of the probability that the results could have occurred by chance alone.

Statistics is a specialized field with its own jargon, such as null hypothesis, variance, regression, power, and modeling, that is unfamiliar to many clinicians. However, leaving aside the genuine complexity of statistical methods, inferential statistics should be regarded by the nonexpert as a useful means to an end. **Statistical testing** is a means by which the effects of random variation are estimated.

The next two sections discuss Type I and Type II errors and attempt to place hypothesis testing, as it is used to estimate the probabilities of these errors, in context. However, no attempt is made to deal with these subjects in a rigorous, quantitative fashion. For that, readers should consult any of a number of excellent textbooks on biostatistics.

Concluding That a Treatment Works

Most statistics encountered in the medical literature concern the likelihood of a Type I error and are expressed by the familiar **P value**. The P value is a quantitative estimate of the probability that differences in treatment effects in the particular study at hand could have happened by chance alone, assuming that there is in fact no difference between the groups. Another way of expressing this is that P is an answer to the question, "If there were no difference between treatments and the trial was repeated many times, what proportion of the trials would conclude that the difference between the two treatments was at least as big as that found in the study."

In this presentation, P value is called P_α to distinguish it from estimates of the other kind of error due to random variation, Type II error, which will be referred to as P_β. When a simple P is found in the scientific literature, it ordinarily refers to P_α.

The kind of error estimated by P_α applies whenever one concludes that one treatment more effective than another. If it is concluded that the P_α exceeds some limit (see below) and there is no statistical difference between treatments, then the particular value of P_α is not as relevant; in that situation, P_β (probability of Type II error) applies.

Dichotomous and Exact P Values

It has become customary to attach special significance to P values falling below 0.05 (1 in 20) because it is generally agreed that a chance less than 1 in 20 is a small enough risk of being wrong. A chance of 1 in 20 is so small, in fact, that it is reasonable to conclude that such an occurrence is unlikely to have arisen by chance alone. It could have arisen by chance, and there is a chance of 1 in 20 times that it will. But it is unlikely.

Differences associated with P_α less than 0.05 are statistically significant. However, setting a cutoff point at 0.05 is entirely arbitrary. Reasonable people might accept higher values or insist on lower ones, depending on the consequences of a false-positive conclusion in a given situation. For example, one might be willing to accept a higher chance of a false-positive statistical test if the disease is severe, there is no currently effective treatment, and the new treatment safe. On the other hand, one might be reluctant to accept a false-positive test if usual care is effective and the new treatment is dangerous. This reasoning is similar to that applied to the importance of false-positive and false-negative diagnostic tests (Chapter 3).

To accommodate various opinions about what is and is not unlikely enough, some researchers report the exact probabilities of *P* (e.g., 0.03, 0.07, 0.11, etc.), rather than lumping them into just two categories (≤ 0.05 or >0.05). Users are then free to apply their own preference for what is statistically significant. However, *P* values greater than 1 in 5 are usually reported as simply $P > 0.20$, because nearly everyone can agree that a probability of a Type I error greater than 1 in 5 is unacceptably high. Similarly, below very low *P* values (such as $p < 0.001$) chance is a very unlikely explanation for an observed difference, and little further information is conveyed by describing this chance more precisely.

Statistical Significance and Clinical Importance

A statistically significant difference, no matter how small the *P*, does not mean that the difference is clinically important. A *P* value of < 0.0001, if it emerges from a well-designed study, conveys a high degree of confidence that a difference really exists but says nothing about the magnitude of that difference or its clinical importance. In fact, trivial differences may be highly statistically significant if a large enough number of patients were studied.

EXAMPLE

The drug donepezil, a cholinesterase inhibitor, was developed for the treatment of Alzheimer's disease. In a randomized controlled trial to establish whether the drug produced worthwhile improvements, 565 patients with Alzheimer's disease were randomly allocated to donepezil or placebo. The statistical significance of some trial end points was impressive: Both the mini-mental state examination (MMSE) and the Bristol Activities of Daily Living Scale (BADLS) were statistically different at P<0.0001. However, the actual differences were small, 0.8 on a 30-point scale for the MMSE and 1 on a 60 point scale for the BADLS. Moreover, other outcomes, which more closely represented the burden of illness and care of these patients, were similar in the donepezil and placebo groups. These included entering institutional care and progression of disability (both primary end points) as well as behavioral and psychological symptoms, caregiver psychopathology, formal care costs, unpaid caregiver time, and adverse events or death. The authors concluded that the benefits of denepezil were "below minimally relevant thresholds" and that "more effective treatments . . . are needed for Alzheimer's disease." (2)

On the other hand, very unimpressive *P* values can result from studies showing strong treatment effects if there are few patients in the study.

Statistical Tests

Statistical tests are used to estimate the probability of a Type 1 error. The tests are applied to the data to give a test statistic, which in turn can be used to come up with a probability of error (Figure 10.2). The tests are of the **null hypothesis,** the proposition that there is no true difference in outcome between treatment groups. This device is for mathematical reasons, not because "no difference" is the working scientific hypothesis of the investigators conducting the study. One ends up rejecting the null hypothesis (concluding there is a difference) or failing to reject it (concluding that there is insufficient evidence in support of a difference). Note that not finding statistical significance is not the same as there being no difference. Statistical testing is not able to establish that there is no difference at all.

Some commonly used statistical tests are listed in Table 10.1. The validity of each test depends on certain assumptions about the data; a typical assumption is that the data have a normal distribution. If the data do not satisfy these assumptions, the resulting *P* value may be misleading. A discussion of how these statistical tests are derived and calculated and of the assumptions on which they rest can be found in any biostatistics textbook.

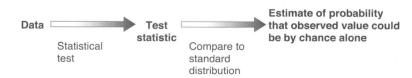

FIGURE 10.2 ▓ Statistical testing.

TABLE 10.1 ■ Some Statistical Tests Commonly Used in Clinical Research

To test the statistical significance of a difference

Chi square (χ^2)	Between two or more proportions (when there is a large number of observations)
Fisher's exact	Between two proportions (when there is a small number of observations)
Mann-Whitney U	Between two medians
Student t	Between two means
F test	Between two or more means

To describe the extent of association

Regression coefficient	Between an independent (predictor) variable and a dependent (outcome) variable
Pearson's r	Between two variables

To model the effects of multiple variables

Logistic regression	On a dichotomous outcome
Cox proportional hazards	On a time-to-event outcome

E X A M P L E

The chi square (χ^2) test for nominal data (counts) is more easily understood than most and so can be used to illustrate how statistical testing works. Consider the following data from a randomized trial of two ways of initiating anticoagulation with heparin: a weight-based dosing nomogram and standard care. (3) The outcome was a partial thromboplastin time (PTT) exceeding the therapeutic threshold within 24 hours of beginning anticoagulation. In the nomogram group, 60 of 62 (97%) did so; in the standard care group, 37 of 48 (77%).

Observed Rates

	PTT Exceeding Threshold		
	Yes	No	Total
Nomogram	60	2	62
Standard care	37	11	48
Total	97	13	110

How likely would it be for a study of this size to observe a difference in rates as great as this or greater if there was in fact no difference in effectiveness? That depends on how far the observed results depart from

what might have been expected if the treatments were of similar effectiveness and only random variation in the samples studied caused them to differ. If treatment had no effect on outcome, applying the success rate for the patients as a whole (97/110 = 88%) to the number of patients in each treatment group gives the expected number of successes in each group:

Expected Rates (Rounded to Nearest Integer)

	PTT Exceeding Threshold		
	Yes	No	Total
Nomogram	55	7	62
Standard care	42	6	48
Total	97	13	110

The χ^2 statistic, which quantifies the difference between the observed and expected numbers, is the sum for all four cells of:

$$\chi^2 = \sum \frac{(\text{Observed number} - \text{Expected number})^2}{\text{Expected number}}$$

The magnitude of the χ^2 statistic is determined by how different all of the observed numbers are from what would be expected if there were no treatment effect. Because they are squared, it does not matter whether the observed rates exceed or fall short of the expected. By dividing the squared difference in each cell by the expected number, the difference for that cell is adjusted for the number of patients in that cell.

The χ^2 statistic for these data is:

$$\frac{(60 - 55)^2}{55} + \frac{(2 - 7)^2}{7} + \frac{(37 - 42)^2}{42} + \frac{(11 - 6)^2}{6} = 8.79$$

This χ^2 is then compared to a table relating χ^2 values to probabilities (available in books and computer programs) for that number of cells, to obtain the probability of a χ^2 as that large or larger. It is intuitively obvious that the larger the χ^2, the less likely chance is to account for the observed differences. The result in this case is $P = 0.004$, which is the probability of a false-positive conclusion that the treatments had different effects.

Concluding That a Treatment Does Not Work

Some trials are unable to conclude that one treatment is better than the other. The risk of a false-negative result is particularly large in studies with relatively few patients. The question then arises, how likely is the result to have arisen by chance alone? Could the findings of such trials have misrepresented the truth because these particular studies had the bad luck to turn out in relatively unlikely ways? Specifically, how likely is a false-negative result (Type II or β error)?

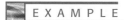

E X A M P L E

Does vitamin E supplementation reduce the risk of coronary heart disease? HOPE study investigators randomly assigned 9,541 people at increased risk for cardiovascular disease to vitamin E supplementation or a matching placebo. There were 1,511 primary outcome events (a composite of myocardial infarction, stroke, and death from cardiovascular causes). Of these, 16.2 percent occurred in patients assigned to vitamin E and 15.5 percent in those assigned to the placebo (relative risk 1.05). Adverse outcomes were more common in the vitamin E group, making the hypothesis that vitamin E was protective implausible. But how likely was this study to have missed a protective effect by chance when it was really present? The authors noted that the study was large enough to have a 90% chance of detecting a 13% relative reduction in risk for the primary outcome; alternatively, the study had a 10% chance of missing a difference this large or larger. Some professionals prefer a more visual impression of whether effects are present or not. Figure 10.3 shows the survival curve from the HOPE study. Treated and control patients had remarkably similar curves throughout follow-up, making a protective effect of vitamin E unlikely. (4)

Type II errors have received less attention than Type I errors for several reasons. They are more difficult to calculate. Also, most professionals simply prefer things that work and consider negative results unwelcome. Authors are less likely to submit negative studies to journals and when negative studies are reported at all, the authors may prefer to emphasize

subgroups of patients in which treatment differences are found, even when the differences are not statistically significant. Authors may also emphasize reasons other than chance to explain why true differences might have been missed. Whatever the reason for not considering the probability of a Type II error, it is the main question that should be asked when the results of a study indicate no difference.

The probability that a trial will find a statistically significant difference when a difference really exists is called the **statistical power** of the trial. In the example above, the statistical power was 90% for a 13% relative reduction in risk. Power and P_β are complementary ways of expressing the same concept.

$$\text{Statistical power} = 1 - P_\beta$$

Power is analogous to the sensitivity of a diagnostic test. One speaks of a study being powerful when it has a high probability of detecting differences when treatments really have different effects.

POINT ESTIMATES AND CONFIDENCE INTERVALS

The effect size that is observed in a particular study (such as treatment effect in a clinical trial or relative risk in a cohort study) is called the **point estimate** of the effect. It is the best estimate from the study of the true effect size and is the summary statistic usually given the most emphasis in reports of research.

However, the true effect size is unlikely to be exactly that observed in the study. Because of ran-

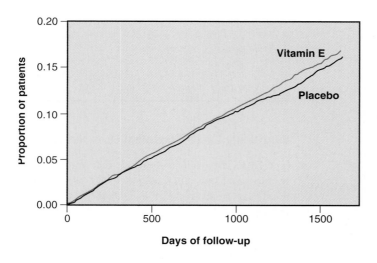

FIGURE 10.3 ■ Example of a "negative" trial. Effect of vitamin E supplements versus placebo on the proportion of high-risk patients who experienced the primary outcome of the HOPE trial—nonfatal myocardial infarction, stroke, and death from cardiovascular causes. (From The Heart Outcomes Prevention Evaluation Study Investigators. Vitamin E supplementation and cardiovascular events in high-risk patients. N Engl J Med 2000;342:154–160.)

dom variation, any one study is likely to find a result higher or lower than the true value. Therefore, a summary measure is needed for the **statistical precision** of the point estimate, which is the range of values likely to encompass the true effect size.

Statistical precision is expressed as a **confidence interval**, usually the 95% confidence interval, around the point estimate. Confidence intervals around an effect size are interpreted as follows: If the study is unbiased, there is a 95% chance that the interval includes the true effect size. The more narrow the confidence interval, the more certain one can be about the size of the true effect. The true value is most likely to be close to the point estimate, less likely to be near the outer limits of the interval, and could (5 times out of 100) fall outside these limits altogether. Statistical precision increases with the statistical power of the study.

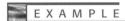

E X A M P L E

The Women's Heath Initiative included a randomized controlled trial of the effects of estrogen plus progestin on chronic disease outcomes in healthy postmenopausal women. Figure 10.4 shows relative risk and confidence intervals for four of these outcomes: stroke, hip fracture, breast cancer, and endometrial cancer. The four illustrate various possibilities for how confidence intervals are interpreted. Estrogen plus progestin was a risk factor for stroke; the best estimate of this risk is the point estimate, a relative risk of 1.41, but the data are consistent with a relative risk as low as 1.07 or as high as 1.85. The estrogen/progestin

protected against hip fracture, preventing as much as 65% and as little as 2% of fractures; that is, the data are consistent with very little benefit, though substantial benefit is likely. Although risk of breast cancer is likely to be increased, the data are consistent with no effect (the lower end of the confidence interval includes a relative risk of 1.0). Finally, the study is not very informative for endometrial cancer. Confidence intervals are very wide, so not only was there no clear risk or benefit but the estimate of risk was so imprecise that substantial risk or benefit remained possible. (5)

Confidence intervals contain the same information as statistical significance. If the value corresponding to no effect (that is, a relative risk of 1 or a treatment difference of 0) falls outside the 95% confidence intervals for the observed effect, the results are statistically significant at the 0.05 level. If the confidence intervals include this point, the results are not statistically significant.

Confidence intervals have advantages over P values. They put the emphasis where it belongs, on the size of the effect. Confidence intervals help the reader to see the range of plausible values and so to decide whether an effect size they regard as clinically meaningful is consistent with or ruled out by the data. (6) They also provide information about statistical power; if the confidence interval is relatively wide and barely includes the value corresponding to no effect, readers can see that low power might have been the cause of the negative result. In the HOPE study described in the preced-

OUTCOME

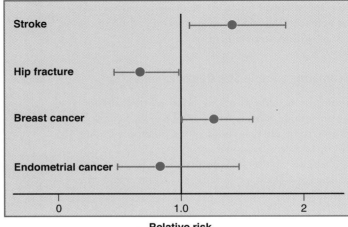

FIGURE 10.4 ■ Example of confidence intervals. The relative risk and confidence intervals for outcomes in the Women's Health Initiative: A randomized controlled trial of estrogen plus progestin in healthy postmenopausal women. Writing Group for the Women's Health Initiative Investigators. Risks and benefits of estrogen plus progestin in healthy postmenopausal women. JAMA 2002;288:321–333.

ing example, low power was not a problem because the confidence interval for the estimated relative risk of 1.05 was 0.95 to 1.16, suggesting that if vitamin E were better at all, it would only be by 5%.

Point estimates and confidence intervals are used to characterize the statistical precision of any rate (incidence and prevalence), comparisons of rates (relative and attributable risks), and other summary statistics. For example, studies have shown that 34% of U.S. adults have used unconventional therapy (95% confidence interval 31–37%), (7) that intensive treatment of insulin-dependent diabetes lowers the risk of development of retinopathy by 76% (95% confidence interval 62–85%) relative to conventional therapy, (8) and that the sensitivity of clinical examination for splenomegaly is 27% (95% confidence interval 19–36%). (9)

Confidence intervals have become the usual way of reporting the main results of clinical research because of their many advantages over the hypothesis testing (*P* value) approach. *P* values are still used because of tradition and as a convenience when many results are reported and it would not be feasible to include confidence intervals for all of them.

HOW MANY STUDY PATIENTS ARE ENOUGH?

Suppose you are reading about a clinical trial comparing a promising new treatment to usual care. You are aware that random variation can be the source of whatever differences are observed, and you wonder if the number of patients (sample size) in this study is large enough to make chance an unlikely explanation for what was found. How many patients would be necessary to make an adequate comparison of the effects of the two treatments?

Estimating Sample Size Requirements

From the hypothesis testing point of view, an adequate **sample size** depends on three characteristics of the study: the magnitude of the difference in outcome between treatment groups; P_α and P_β (the probability of the false-positive and false-negative conclusions you are willing to accept); and the nature of the study's data.

These are taken into account when the researcher plans a study, to ensure that the study will have enough statistical power to produce meaningful results.

Effect Size

Sample size depends on the magnitude of the difference to be detected. One is free to look for differences of any magnitude, and of course, the hope is to be able to detect even very small differences. But more patients are needed to detect small differences, everything else being equal. So, it is best to ask only what is a sufficient number of patients to detect the smallest degree of improvement that would be clinically meaningful. On the other hand, if one is interested in detecting only very large differences between treated and control groups (that is, strong treatment effects) then fewer patients need be studied.

Type I Error

Sample size is also related to the risk of a Type 1 error (concluding that treatment is effective when it is not). The acceptable probability for a risk of this kind is a value judgment; the risk could be as large as 1 or as small as 0. If one is prepared to accept the consequences of a large chance of falsely concluding that the treatment is effective, one can reach conclusions with relatively few patients. On the other hand, if one wants to take only a small risk of being wrong in this way, a larger number of patients will be required. As discussed earlier, it is customary to set P_α at 0.05 (1 in 20) or sometimes 0.01 (1 in 100).

Type II Error

The chosen risk of a Type 2 error is another determinant of sample size. An acceptable probability of this error is also a judgment that can be freely made and changed to suit individual tastes. Probability of P_β is often set at 0.20, a 20% chance of missing true differences in a particular study. Conventional Type 2 errors are much larger than Type 1 errors, reflecting a higher value usually placed on being sure an effect is really present when it is said to be.

Characteristics of the Data

The statistical power of a study is also determined by the nature of the data. When the outcome is expressed by counts or proportions of events or time-to-event, its statistical power depends on the rate of events: the larger the number of events, the greater the statistical power for a given number of people at risk. As Peto et al. put it,

> In clinical trials of time to death (or of the time to some other particular "event"— relapse, metastasis, first thrombosis, stroke, recurrence, or time to death from a particular

cause), the ability of the trial to distinguish between the merits of two treatments depends on how many patients *die* (or suffer a relevant event), rather than on the number of patients *entered*. A study of 100 patients, 50 of whom die, is about as sensitive as a study with 1,000 patients, 50 of whom die. (10)

If the data are continuous, such as blood pressure or serum cholesterol, power is affected by the degree to which patients vary among themselves. The greater the variation from patient to patient with respect to the characteristic being measured, the more difficult it is to be confident that the observed differences (or lack of difference) between groups is not because of this variation, rather than a true treatment effect. In other words, the larger the variation among patients, the lower the statistical power.

In designing a study, investigators choose the smallest treatment effect that is clinically important (larger treatment effects will be easier to detect) and the Type I and Type II errors they are willing to accept. They also obtain estimates of the data (outcome event rates or variation among patients). It is possible to design studies that maximize power for a given sample size, such as by choosing patients with a high event rate or similar characteristics—as long as they match the research question.

Interrelationships
The relationships among the four variables that together determine statistical power are summarized in Table 10.2. The variables can be traded off against one another. In general, for any given number of patients in the study, there is a trade-off between Type 1 and Type 2 errors. Everything else being equal, the more one is willing to accept one kind of error, the less it will be necessary to risk the other. Neither kind of error is inherently worse than the other.

Sample Size Depends on the Context

The consequences of accepting erroneous information depend on the clinical situation. When a better treatment is badly needed, such as when the disease is very dangerous and no satisfactory alternative treatment is available, and the proposed treatment is not dangerous, it would be reasonable to accept a relatively high risk of concluding a new treatment is effective when it really is not (large Type 1 error) to minimize the possibility of missing a valuable treatment (small Type 2 error). On the other hand, if the disease is less serious, alternative treatments are available, or the new treatment is expensive or dangerous, one might want to minimize the risk of accepting the new treatment when it is not really effective (low Type 1 error), even at the expense of a relatively large chance of missing an effective treatment (large Type 2 error). It is of course possible to reduce both Type 1 and Type 2 errors if the number of patients is increased, outcome events are more frequent, variability is decreased, or a larger treatment effect is sought.

For conventional levels of P_α and P_β, the relationship between the size of treatment effect and the number of patients needed for a trial is illustrated by the following examples. One represents a situation in which a relatively small number of patients was sufficient, and the other is one in which a very large number of patients was too small.

EXAMPLE

A small sample size that was adequate
Case series suggest that the nonsteroidal anti-inflammatory drug sulindac is active against colonic polyps. This possibility was tested in a randomized trial in which a total of 22 patients with familial adenomatous polyposis (an inherited condition in which patients develop hundreds of colonic

TABLE 10.2 ■ **Determinants of Sample Size**		
	Determined by	
	Investigator	**The Data**
N varies according to	$\dfrac{1}{\Delta, P_\alpha, P_\beta}$ and	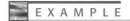

Where n = number of patients studied; Δ = size of difference in outcome between groups; P_α = probability of an α (Type I) error (i.e., false-positive results); P_β = probability of a β (Type II) error (i.e., false-negative result); V = variability of observations (for interval data); and P = proportion of patients experiencing outcome of interest (for nominal data)

adenomas, some of which progress to cancer) were randomized; 11 received sulindac and 11 placebo. (11) After 9 months, patients receiving sulindac had an average of 44% fewer polyps than those receiving placebo. This difference was statistically significant ($p = 0.014$). Because of the large effect size and the large number of polyps per patient, few patients were needed to establish that the effect was beyond chance. (In this analysis, it was necessary to assume that treatment affected polyps independently of which patient they occurred in—an unlikely, but probably not damaging, assumption.)

A large sample size that was inadequate

The Physicians' Health Study was a randomized controlled trial seeking to determine whether low-dose aspirin decreased cardiovascular mortality. Another aspect of the trial was to study the effect of β-carotene on the incidence of cancer. There were 22,071 participants, all of whom were physicians. The aspirin part of the trial was terminated earlier than planned, after an average follow-up of 60 months, in part because "no effect of aspirin on cardiovascular mortality could be detected in the trial [for at least another 12 years] because of the exceptionally low cardiovascular death rate among participating physicians" Also, at the time the trial was stopped the effect size was small; relative risk reduction in the aspirin group was 0.96, making a statistically significant effect even more difficult to detect if present. The study was therefore inconclusive on the main research question (effect on car-

diovascular mortality). However, myocardial infarction, a secondary end point, occurred frequently enough that the observed 44% reduction in risk in the aspirin group was statistically significant. There was also a twofold increase in risk of hemorrhagic stroke but too few of this secondary outcome event to rule out chance. (12)

For most of the therapeutic questions encountered today, a surprisingly large sample size is required. The value of dramatic, powerful treatments, such as insulin for diabetic ketoacidosis or surgery for appendicitis, could be established by studying a small number of patients. But such treatments come along rarely, and many of them are already well established. We are left with diseases, many of which are chronic and have multiple, interacting causes, for which the effects of new treatments are generally small. This makes it especially important to plan clinical studies that are large enough to distinguish real from chance effects.

Clinicians should be able to estimate the power of published studies for themselves. Figure 10.5 shows the relationship between sample size and treatment difference for several baseline rates for outcome events. It is apparent that studies involving

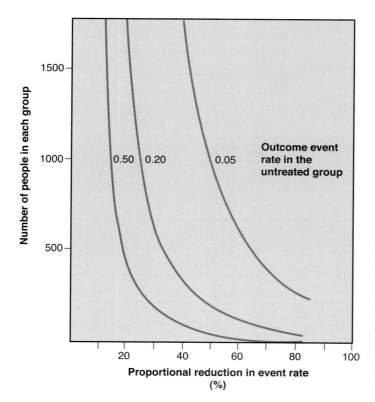

FIGURE 10.5 ■ The number of people required in each of two treatment groups (of equal size), for various rates of outcome events in the untreated group, to have an 80% chance of detecting a difference ($p = 0.05$) in reduction in outcome event rates in treated relative to untreated patients. (Calculated from formula in Weiss NS. Clinical epidemiology. The study of the outcome of illness. New York: Oxford University Press, 1986.)

fewer than 100 patients have a rather poor chance of detecting statistically significant differences of even large treatment effects. Looked at another way, it is difficult to detect effect sizes of less than 25%. In practice, statistical power can be estimated by means of readily available formulas, tables, nomograms, or computer programs.

Sample Size Based on Confidence Intervals

Confidence intervals can also be used to plan sample size. For example, one might want to plan a study of a diagnostic test performance or complication rate on the belief that a certain degree of statistical precision is necessary. One can then calculate the number of patients needed to produce confidence intervals of that width, based on assumptions about what the sensitivity or complication rate is likely to be.

Statistical Power After the Study Is Completed

Calculation of statistical power based on the hypothesis testing approach is done before a study is undertaken to ensure that enough patients will be entered to have a good chance of detecting a clinically meaningful effect if one is present. However, after the study is completed this approach is less relevant. (13) There is no longer need to estimate effect size, outcome event rates, and variability among patients because they are all known. Rather, attention should be directed to point estimates and confidence intervals. With them, one can see the range of values that are consistent with the results and whether the effect sizes of interest are within this range or are ruled out by the data.

EQUIVALENCE TRIALS

Some trials are intended to establish that two treatments have similar effects. This might be useful, for example, if a new treatment is safer, simpler, or cheaper than the current one. If the primary effects were similar, the new treatment would be better, all things considered.

No trial can establish that the effects of two treatments are the same. However, trials can establish that differences in effects are no greater than a specified size, below which the differences are not clinically important. A trial has established "equivalence" to the extent that its confidence interval for the difference in treatment effects excludes a clinically important effect. Such trials must have a good

chance of detecting this relatively small effect size and are likely to be larger than those that set out to establish a difference in effect. These trials require special care because many of the potential problems such as crossover, dropout, nonsystematic and misclassification of outcomes, will tend to bias the results toward finding no difference.

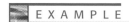

E X A M P L E

In India, amoxicillin has been used for nonsevere pneumonia in young children. The usual duration of treatment was 5 days, but some evidence suggested that 3 days might be as effective. To test this possibility, 2,188 children age 2 to 59 months with nonsevere pneumonia were randomly allocated to 3 or 5 day treatment with amoxicillin. (14) Clinical cure rates with 3 and 5 days of treatment were 89.5% and 89.9% respectively. The difference was a 0.4 percentage point, and the 95% confidence interval for the difference was −2.1 to 3.0. In other words, effectiveness of both treatments was within a narrow range, and the two could be said to be, for all intents and purposes, "equivalent." This trial provided a sound basis for avoiding the cost and difficulties associated with a longer course of treatment without fear that shorter treatment is inferior.

DETECTING RARE EVENTS

It is sometimes important to know how likely a study is to detect a relatively uncommon event (for example, 1/1,000), particularly if that event is severe, such as aplastic anemia or life-threatening arrhythmia. A great many people must be observed in order to have a good chance of detecting even one such event, much less to develop a relatively stable estimate of its frequency. For most clinical research, sample size is planned to be sufficient to detect main effects, the answer sought for the primary research question. Sample size is likely to be well short of the number needed to detect rare events such as uncommon side effects and complications. For that, a different approach, involving many more patients, is needed. An example is postmarketing surveillance of a drug, in which thousands of users are monitored for side effects.

Figure 10.6 shows the probability of detecting an event as a function of the number of people under observation. A rule of thumb is as follows: To have a good chance of detecting a $1/x$ event, one must observe $3x$ people. (15) For example, to detect at least one event if the underlying rate is a 1/1,000, one would need to observe 3,000 people.

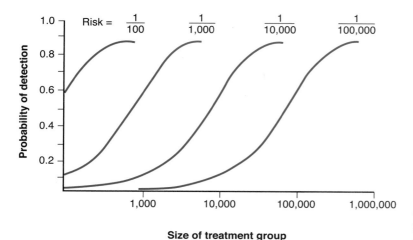

Size of treatment group

FIGURE 10.6 ▨ The probability of detecting one event according to the rate of the event and the number of people observed. (From Guess HA, Rudnick SA. Use of cost effectiveness analysis in planning cancer chemoprophylaxis trials. Control Clin Trials 1983; 4:89–100.)

MULTIPLE COMPARISONS

The statistical conclusions of research have an aura of authority that defies challenge, particularly by non-experts. But as many skeptics have suspected, it is possible to "lie with statistics" even if the research is well designed, the mathematics flawless, and the investigators' intentions beyond reproach.

Statistical conclusions can be misleading because the strength of statistical tests depends on the number of research questions considered in the study and when those questions were asked. If many comparisons are made among the variables in a large set of data, the P value associated with each individual comparison is an underestimate of how often the result of that comparison, among the others, is likely to arise by chance. As implausible as it might seem, the interpretation of the P value from a single statistical test depends on the context in which it is done.

To understand how this might happen, consider the following example:

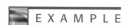

E X A M P L E

Suppose a large study has been done in which there are multiple subgroups of patients and many different outcomes. For instance, it might be a clinical trial of the value of a treatment for coronary artery disease for which patients are in 12 clinically meaningful subgroups (e.g., 1-, 2-, and 3-vessel disease; good and bad ventricular function; the presence or absence of arrhythmias; and various combinations of these), and four outcomes are considered (e.g., death, myocardial infarction, heart failure, and angina). In this example, we do not take into account combinations of these characteristics. Suppose also that there are no true associations between

treatment and outcome in any of the subgroups and for any of the outcomes. Finally, suppose that the effects of treatment are assessed separately for each subgroup and for each outcome—a process that involves a great many comparisons, in this case 12 subgroups multiplied by 4 outcomes = 48 comparisons. With a P_α = .05, 1 in 20 of these comparisons is likely to be statistically significant by chance alone. In the general case, if 20 comparisons are made, on average, one would be found to be statistically significant; if 100 comparisons are made, about five would be likely to emerge as significant, and so on. Thus, when a great many comparisons have been made, a few will be found that are unusual enough, because of random variation, to reach statistical significance even if no true associations between variables exist in nature. The more comparisons that are made, the more likely that one of them will be found to be statistically significant. As the saying goes, "if you torture the data long enough, they will confess!"

This phenomenon is referred to as the **multiple comparisons** problem. Because of this problem, the strength of evidence from clinical research depends on how focused its questions were at the outset.

Unfortunately, when the results of research are presented, it is not always possible to know how many comparisons really were made. Sometimes, interesting findings have been selected from a larger number of uninteresting ones that are not mentioned. This process of deciding what is and is not important about a mass of data after the fact can introduce considerable distortion of reality. Table 10.3 summarizes how this misleading situation arises.

How can the statistical effects of multiple comparisons be taken into account when interpreting research? Although ways of adjusting P values have been proposed, probably the best advice is to be aware of the

TABLE 10.3 ■ A Common Way in Which Multiple Comparisons Can Be Misleading
1. Make multiple comparisons within a study
2. Apply tests of statistical significance to each comparison
3. Find a few comparisons that are "interesting" (statistically significant)
4. Build an article around one of these interesting findings
5. Do not mention the context in the article (how many questions were examined and which was considered primary before the data were examined)
6. Construct a *post hoc* argument for the plausibility of the isolated finding

problem and to be cautious about accepting positive conclusions of studies in which multiple comparisons were made. As one statistician put it:

> If you dredge the data sufficiently deeply and sufficiently often, you will find something odd. Many of these bizarre findings will be due to chance. I do not imply that data dredging is not an occupation for honorable persons, but rather that discoveries that were not initially postulated as among the major objectives of the trial should be treated with extreme caution. Statistical theory may in due course show us how to allow for such incidental findings. At present, I think the best attitude to adopt is caution, coupled with an attempt to confirm or refute the findings by further studies. (16)

Investigators should look at all aspects of their data and share interesting findings with readers, but they should make it clear how extensively the data were searched.

SUBGROUP ANALYSIS

It is tempting to go beyond the main results of the study to examine results within subgroups of patients who have special characteristics or particular outcomes. Indeed, this is a responsible way to behave; it helps clinicians tailor their care as closely as possible to individual patients. Doing so, however, incurs some risks of being misled that are not present when examining the principal conclusions alone. These

risks should be taken into account when interpreting information from subgroups.

One danger in examining subgroups is the increased chance of finding effects in a particular subgroup that are not present, in the long run, in nature, that is, a false-positive finding. This arises because of multiple comparisons as discussed above.

A second danger is of a false-negative conclusion. Examining subgroups for example, defined by certain kinds of patients or specific kinds of outcomes, involves a great reduction in the data available, so it is frequently impossible to come to firm conclusions. Nevertheless, the temptation to look is there, and some tentative information can be gleaned. Some guidelines for deciding whether a finding in a subgroup is real are summarized in Table 10.4.

SECONDARY ANALYSES

Secondary analyses are ones that were not the main reason for the study, or perhaps not planned at all, when the study was conceived. They may involve examination of subgroups, as described in the earlier section, or of various outcomes, as in the following example.

TABLE 10.4 ■ Guidelines for Deciding Whether Apparent Differences in Effects Within Subgroups Are Real[a]
From the study itself
• Is the magnitude of the observed difference clinically important?
• How likely is the effect to have arisen by chance, taking into account: 　The number of subgroups examined? 　The magnitude of the *P* value?
• Was a hypothesis that the effect would be observed made before its discovery (or was justification for the effect argued for after it was found)?
• Was it one of a small number of hypotheses?
From other information
• Was the difference suggested by comparisons *within* rather than *between* studies?
• Has the effect been observed in other studies?
• Is there indirect evidence that supports the existence of the effect?
[a] Adapted from Oxman AD, Guyatt GH. A consumer's guide to subgroup analysis. Ann Intern Med 1992;116:78–84.

One of the reasons the Physicians' Health Study was stopped earlier than planned was because fewer myocardial infarctions occurred in the treated group than in the control group. The authors believed that the effect on myocardial infarction, although not the answer to a main study question at the outset, was real because it was biologically plausible, because it had been found in other studies, and because the chance of a false-positive conclusion was estimated to be very small (1/10,000). On the other hand, although the authors observed a small increase in risk of stroke in the treated group, they were unsure whether or not this effect was real because there were too few physicians having this end point. Thus, in a study that could not address the main research question, the authors interpreted the validity of findings for different outcomes (both positive and negative) in relation to the totality of information that might bear on the validity of these findings.

DESCRIBING ASSOCIATIONS

Statistics are also used to describe the degree of association between variables, such as the relationship between body mass and blood pressure. Familiar expressions of association are Pearson's product moment correlation (r) for interval data and Spearman's rank correlation for ordinal data. Each of these statistics expresses in quantitative terms the extent to which the value of one variable is associated with the value of another. Each has a corresponding statistical test to assess whether the observed association is greater than might have been expected by chance alone.

MULTIVARIABLE METHODS

Most clinical phenomena are the result of many variables acting together in complex ways. For example, coronary heart disease is the joint result of lipid abnormalities, hypertension, cigarette smoking, family history, diabetes, exercise, inflammation, coagulopathy, and perhaps personality. It is appropriate to try to understand these relationships by first examining relatively simple arrangements of the data, such as stratified analyses that examine whether the effect of one variable is changed by the presence or absence of one or more other variables. It is relatively easy to understand the data when they are displayed in this way.

However, as pointed out in Chapter 7, it is usually not possible to account for more than a few variables using this method, because there are not enough patients with each combination of characteristics to allow stable estimates of rates. For example, if 120 patients were studied, 60 in each treatment group, and just one additional dichotomous variable was taken into account, there would only be, at most, about 15 patients in each subgroup; if patients were unevenly distributed among subgroups, there would be even fewer in some.

What is needed then, in addition to tables showing multiple subgroups, is a way of examining the effects of several variables at a time. This is accomplished by **multivariable modeling**—or developing a mathematical expression of the effects of many variables taken together. It is "multivariable" because it examines the effects of multiple variables simultaneously. It is "modeling" because it is a mathematical construct, calculated from the data based on assumptions about characteristics of the data (for example, that the variables are all normally distributed or all have the same variance).

Mathematical models are used in two general ways in clinical research:

1. To study the independent effect of one variable on outcome while taking into account the effects of other variables that might confound or modify this relationship
2. To predict a clinical event by calculating the combined effect of several variables acting together

The basic structure of a multivariable model is:

$$\text{Outcome variable} = \text{constant} + (\beta_1 \times \text{variable}_1) + (\beta_2 \times \text{variable}_2) + \ldots$$

where β_1, β_2, . . . are coefficients determined by the data and variable$_1$, variable$_2$, . . . are the predictor variables that might be related to outcome. The best estimates of the coefficients are determined mathematically, based on assumptions about the distributions of the data, and are dependent upon on the powerful calculating ability of modern computers.

Modeling involves several steps:

1. Identify and measure variables that might be related to the outcome of interest.
2. Reduce the number of variables to be considered in the model to a manageable number, usually no more than several. Often this is

done by selecting variables that, when taken one at a time, are most strongly related to outcome. If a statistical criterion is used at this stage, it is usual to err on the side of including variables, e.g., by choosing all variables showing an association with the outcome of interest at a cutoff level of $p < 0.10$. Evidence for the biologic importance of the variable is also considered in making the selection.

3. Some variables may be strongly related to one another. If so, they might be excluded because both contain about the same information.

4. The remaining variables are entered in the model, with the strategy for the order in which they are tried determined by the research question. For example, if some are to be controlled for in a causal analysis, they are entered in the model first, followed by the variable of primary interest. The model will then identify the independent effect of the main variable. On the other hand, if the investigator wants to make a prediction based on several variables, the variables can be entered in order of the strength of their association to the outcome variable, as determined by the model.

Modeling is now a regular feature of the medical literature. Some commonly used kinds of models are logistic regression (for dichotomous outcome variables such as those that occur in case-control studies) and Cox proportional hazards models (for time-to-event studies).

Multivariable modeling is an essential part of many clinical studies. There is no other way to adjust for or to include many variables at the same time. However, this advantage comes at a price. Models tend to be black boxes, and it is difficult to "get inside" them and understand how they work. Their validity is based on assumptions about the data that may not be met. They are clumsy at recognizing different effects in different subgroups of patients. An exposure variable may be strongly related to outcome yet not appear in the model because it occurs rarely—and there is little direct information on the statistical power of the model for that variable. Finally, model results are easily affected by quirks in the data, the results of random variation in the characteristics of patients from sample to sample. It has been shown, for example, that a model frequently identified a different set of pre-

dictor variables and produced a different ordering of variables on different random samples of the same data set. (17) To protect against this possibility, there is a rule of thumb that there should be at least 10 outcome events for each predictor variable in the model.

For these reasons, the models themselves cannot be taken as a standard of validity and must be validated independently. Usually, this is done by observing whether or not the model predicts what is found in another, independent sample of patients (see Chapter 12). The results of the first model are considered a hypothesis that is to be tested by new data. If random variation is mainly responsible for the results of the first model, it is unlikely that the same random effects will occur in the validating data set, too. Other evidence for the validity of a model is its biologic plausibility and its consistency with simpler, more transparent analyses of the data, such as stratified analyses.

BAYESIAN REASONING

An altogether different approach to the information contributed by a study is based on Bayesian inference. We introduced this approach in Chapter 3 where we applied it to the specific case of diagnostic testing.

Bayesian inference begins with prior belief about the answer to a research question, analogous to pretest probability of a diagnostic test, which is based on everything known about the answer up to the point when new information was contributed by a study. Then, it asks how much the results of the new study change that belief.

Some aspects of Bayesian inference are compelling. Individual studies do not take place in an information vacuum; rather, they are in the context of all other information available at the time. Starting each study from the null hypothesis—that there is no effect—is a fiction because something is already known about the answer to the question before the study is even begun. Also, the extent to which results of individual studies change belief depends on their direction and magnitude, as well as their scientific strength. For example, if all preceding studies are negative and the next one is found to be positive, an effect is still unlikely. On the other hand, a weak prior belief might be reversed by a single strong study. Finally, with this approach, it is not important whether a small number of hypotheses are identified beforehand (nor are multiple comparisons a problem). Rather, prior belief depends on the plausibility of the assertion rather than whether the assertion was established before or after the study was begun.

While Bayesian inference is appealing, so far it has been difficult to apply because of poorly developed ways of assigning numbers to prior belief and to the information contributed by a study. An exception is in diagnostic testing, in which "belief" is prior probability and the new information is expressed as a likelihood ratio. However, Bayesian inference is the conceptual basis for qualitative thinking about cause (see Chapter 11), as well as for quantitative summaries of clinical trials (see Chapter 12).

REVIEW QUESTIONS

Read the following and circle the best answer from the options provided.

10.1. A randomized controlled trial of thrombolytic therapy versus angioplasty for acute myocardial infarction finds no difference in survival to discharge from the hospital, which is the main outcome event. The investigators explored whether this was also true for subgroups of patients defined by age, number of vessels affected, ejection fraction, comorbidity, and other patient characteristics. Which of the following is *not* true about these subgroup analyses?

   A. Examining subgroups increases the risk of a false-positive (misleading statistically significant) result in one of the comparisons

   B. Examining subgroups increases the chance of a false-negative finding in one of these subgroups, relative to the main outcome

   C. Subgroup analyses would be more credible if a limited number were identified beforehand

   D. Subgroup analyses are bad scientific practice and should not be done

   E. Reporting results in subgroups help clinicians tailor information in the study to individual patients

10.2. A new drug for hyperlipidemia was compared with placebo in a randomized controlled trial of 10,000 patients. Serum cholesterol, the primary outcome, was 240 mg% in the control group and 238 in the group receiving the new drug ($P < 0.001$). This low P value means that:

   A. Bias is unlikely to account for the observed difference

   B. The difference is clinically important

   C. A difference as big or bigger than observed would have arisen by chance one time in 1,000

   D. The results are generalizable to other patients with hypertension

   E. The statistical power of this study was inadequate

10.3. In a well-designed clinical trial of treatment of ovarian cancer, remission rate at 1 year is similar for a new drug and usual care. The P value is 0.4. This means that:

   A. Both treatments are effective

   B. Neither treatment is effective

   C. The statistical power of this study is 60%

   D. The best estimate of treatment effect size is 0.4

   E. It is not possible, given just this information, to decide whether one treatment is better than the other

10.4. In a cohort study, vitamin A intake was found to be a risk factor for hip fracture in women. The relative risk (highest quintile versus lowest quintile) was 1.48, and the 95% confidence interval was 1.05 to 2.07.

   A. The association is not statistically significant at the $P < 0.05$ level.

   B. A strong association between vitamin A intake and hip fracture was established.

   C. The statistical power of this study is 95 %.

D. There is a 95% chance that a range of relative risks as low as 1.05 and as high as 2.07 includes the true risk.

E. Bias is an unlikely explanation for this result.

10.5. A study reports that the effectiveness of two drugs is equivalent.

A. It is possible to establish that treatment effects are identical.

B. To claim equivalence, confidence interval should exclude a clinically important difference in effect.

C. Crossovers and dropouts tend to create differences between treatment groups.

D. Studies to establish equivalence require no bigger sample size than trials to establish effectiveness.

E. Equivalence is always associated with a very low *P* value.

Answers are in Appendix A.

REFERENCES

1. Johnson AF. Beneath the technological fix: Outliers and probability statements. J Chronic Dis 1985;38: 957–961.

2. AD2000 Collaborative Group. Long-term donepezil treatment in 565 patients with Alzheimer's disease (AD2000): Randomized double-blind trial. Lancet 2004;363:2105–2115.

3. Raschke RA, Reilly BM, Guidry JR, Fontana JR, Srinivas S. The weight-based heparin dosing nomogram compared with a "standard care" nomogram: A randomized controlled trial. Ann Intern Med 1993; 119:874–881.

4. The Heart Outcomes Prevention Evaluation Study Investigators. Vitamin E supplementation and cardiovascular events in high-risk patients. N Engl J Med 2000;342:154–160.

5. Writing Group for the Women's Health Initiative Investigators. Risks and benefits of estrogen plus progestin in healthy postmenopausal women. JAMA 2002;288:321–333.

6. Braitman LE. Confidence intervals assess both clinical significance and statistical significance. Ann Intern Med 1991;114:515–517.

7. Eisenberg DM, Kessler RC, Foster C, Norlock FE, Calkins DR, Delbanco TL. Unconventional medicine in the United States: Prevalence, costs, and patterns of use. New Engl J Med 1993;328:246–252.

8. Diabetes Control and Complications Trial Research Group. The effect of intensive treatment of diabetes on the development and progression of long-term complications in insulin-dependent diabetes mellitus. New Engl J Med 1993;329:977–986.

9. Grover SA, Barkun AN, Sackett DL. Rational Clinical Examination. Does the patient have splenomegaly? JAMA 1993;270:2218–2221.

10. Peto R, Pike MC, Armitage P, Breslow NE, Cox DR, Howard SV, et al. Design and analysis of randomized clinical trials requiring prolonged observation of each patient. I. Introduction and design. Br J Cancer 1976;34: 585–612.

11. Giardiello FM, Hamilton SR, Krush AJ, Piantadosi S, Hylind LM, Celano P, et al. Treatment of colonic and rectal adenomas with sulindac in familial adenomatous polyposis. New Engl J Med 1993;328: 1313–1316.

12. Steering Committee of the Physicians' Health Study Research Group. Final report on the aspirin component of the ongoing Physicians' Health Study. N Engl J Med 1989;321:129–135.

13. Goodman SN, Berlin JA. The use of predicted confidence intervals when planning experiments and the misuse of power when interpreting results. Ann Intern Med 1994;121:200–206.

14. ISCAP Study Group. Three-day versus five-day treatment with amoxicillin for nonsevere pneumonia in young children: A multicentre randomized controlled trial. BMJ 2004;328:791–794.

15. Sackett DL, Haynes RB, Gent M, Taylor DW. Compliance. In: Inman WHW, Ed. Monitoring for drug safety, Lancaster, UK: MTP Press, 1980.

16. Armitage P. Importance of prognostic factors in the analysis of data from clinical trials. Control Clin Trials 1981;1:347–353.

17. Diamond GA. Future imperfect: The limitations of clinical prediction models and the limits of clinical prediction. J Am Coll Cardiol 1989;14:12A–22A.

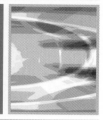

Cause

In what circumstances can we pass from [an] observed association to a verdict of causation? Upon what basis should we proceed to do so?

— Sir Austin Bradford Hill, 1965

Clinicians are confronted frequently with information about possible causal relationships. In fact, most of this book has been about methods used to establish cause, although we have not called special attention to the term.

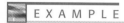

EXAMPLE

Some years ago, medical students were presented a study of the relationship between the cigarette smoking habits of obstetricians and the vigor of babies they delivered. Infant vigor is measured by an Apgar score; a high score (8–10) indicates that the baby is healthy, whereas a low score indicates the baby might be in trouble and require close monitoring. The study suggested that smoking by obstetricians (not in the delivery suite!) had an adverse effect on Apgar scores in newborns. The medical students were then asked to comment on what was

wrong with this study. After many suggestions, someone finally said that the conclusion simply did not make sense.

It was then acknowledged that, although the study was real, the "exposure" and "disease" had been altered for the presentation. Instead of comparing smoking habits of obstetricians with Apgar scores of newborns, the study, published in 1843 by Oliver Wendell Holmes (then professor of anatomy and physiology and later dean of Harvard Medical School), concerned hand washing habits by obstetricians and subsequent puerperal sepsis in mothers. The observations led Holmes to conclude that "The disease known as puerperal fever is so far contagious, as to be frequently carried from patient to patient by physicians and nurses." (1)

One mid-19th century response to Holmes's assertion about unwashed hands causing puerperal fever was remarkably similar to that of the medical students: The findings made no sense. "I prefer to attribute them [puerperal sepsis cases] to accident, or Providence, of which I can form a conception, rather than to contagion of which I cannot form any clear idea, at least as to this particular malady," wrote Dr. Charles D. Meigs, professor of midwifery and the diseases of women and children at Jefferson Medical College.

Holmes and Meigs were confronted with a question about cause. Holmes was convinced by his data that the spread of puerperal sepsis was caused by obstetricians not washing their hands between deliveries. He could not, however, supply the pathogenetic mechanism by which hand washing was related to the disease, as bacteria had not yet been discovered. Meigs, therefore, remained unconvinced that the cause of puerperal sepsis had been established (and presumably did not bother to wash his hands).

In this chapter, we review concepts of cause in clinical medicine. We then outline the different kinds of evidence that, when present, strengthen the likelihood that an association represents a causal relationship. We also briefly deal with a kind of research design not considered thus far in this book: studies in which exposure to a possible cause is known only for groups and not specifically for the individuals in the groups.

CONCEPTS OF CAUSE

Webster's defines **cause** as "anything producing an effect or a result." (2) In medical textbooks, cause is usually discussed under such headings as "etiology," "pathogenesis," "mechanisms," or "risk factors."

Cause is important to practicing physicians primarily because it guides their approach to three clinical tasks: prevention, diagnosis, and treatment. The clinical example at the beginning of this chapter illustrates how knowledge of cause-and-effect relationships can lead to successful preventive strategies. Likewise, when clinicians periodically check patients' blood pressure, they are reacting to evidence that hypertension causes morbidity and mortality and that treatment of hypertension prevents myocardial infarction, congestive heart failure, and stroke. The diagnostic process, especially in infectious disease, frequently involves a search for the causative agent. Less directly, the diagnostic process sometimes depends on information about cause when the presence of risk factors is used to iden-

tify groups of patients in whom disease prevalence is high (see Chapter 3). Finally, belief in a causal relationship underlies every therapeutic intervention in clinical medicine. Why give azithromycin for pneumococcal pneumonia unless one believes that it will result in a cure? Or why advise a patient with metastatic cancer to undergo chemotherapy unless one believes that the antimetabolite will cause a regression of metastases and a prolongation of survival, comfort, and/or ability to carry on daily activities?

By and large, clinicians are more interested in treatable or reversible than immutable causes. Researchers, on the other hand, might also be interested in studying causal factors for which no efficacious treatment or prevention exists, in hopes of developing preventive or therapeutic interventions in the future.

Single and Multiple Causes

In 1882, 40 years after the Holmes-Meigs confrontation, Koch set forth postulates for determining that an infectious agent is the cause of a disease. Basic to his approach was the assumption that a particular disease has one cause and a particular cause results in one disease. He stipulated that:

- The organism must be present in every case of the disease;
- The organism must be isolated and grown in pure culture;
- The organism must cause a specific disease when inoculated into an animal; and
- The organism must then be recovered from the animal and identified.

Interestingly, he did not consider the effect of treatment in establishing cause, something he might have been able to add a century later when effective treatments had become common for infectious diseases.

Koch's postulates contributed greatly to the concept of cause in medicine. Before Koch, it was believed that many different bacteria caused any given disease. The application of his postulates helped bring order out of chaos. They are still useful today. That a given organism causes a given disease was the basis for the discovery in 1977 that Legionnaire's disease is caused by a Gram-negative bacterium, the determination in the 1980s that the newly discovered HIV causes AIDS and the discovery in 2003 that a newly discovered coronavirus causes Severe Acute Respiratory Syndrome (SARS). (3)

For most diseases, however, cause cannot be established simply by Koch's postulates. Would that disease were so simple that there was always a one cause-one disease relationship. Smoking causes lung cancer, chronic obstructive pulmonary disease, peptic ulcers, bladder cancer, and coronary artery disease. Coronary artery disease has multiple causes, including cigarette smoking, hypertension, hypercholesterolemia, diabetes, inflammation, and heredity. It is also possible to have coronary artery disease without experiencing any of these known risk factors.

Usually, many factors act together to cause disease in what has been called the "**web of causation.**" (4) A causal web is well understood in conditions such as coronary artery disease, but is also true for infectious diseases, where presence of the organism is a **necessary cause** for disease to occur but not necessarily a **sufficient cause**. AIDS cannot occur without exposure to HIV, but exposure to the virus does not necessarily result in disease. For example, exposure to HIV rarely results in AIDS after needlesticks (3/1,000 or 4/1,000) because the virus is not nearly as infectious as, say, the hepatitis B virus.

Proximity of Cause to Effect

When biomedical scientists study cause, they usually search for the underlying pathogenetic mechanism or final common pathway of disease. Sickle-cell anemia is an example, with the genetic change associated with hemoglobin S (HbS) leading to polymerization and erythrocytic sickling when HbS gives up oxygen. More recently, work on the human genome led to discovery of the germ-cell genetic changes associated with some cancers. In cardiovascular disease pathogenesis, it is known that statins inhibit HMG CoA reductase and lead to lower serum LDL levels and improved cardiovascular outcomes.

Disease is also determined by less specific, more remote causes, or risk factors, such as people's behavior or characteristics of their environments. These factors may be even more important causes of disease than pathogenetic mechanisms. For example, a large proportion of cardiovascular and cancer deaths in the United States can be traced to behavioral and environmental factors such as cigarette smoking, diet, and lack of exercise; the spread of AIDS is due primarily to unsafe sexual behaviors and drug use; and deaths from violence and accidents are rooted in social conditions, access to

guns, intoxication while driving, and seatbelt use. To view cause in medicine exclusively as cellular and subcellular processes is to restrict the possibilities for useful clinical interventions.

Even when the pathogenetic mechanism is not clear, knowledge of strong risk factors may still lead to effective treatments and preventions. Thus, Holmes was right in his assertion that obstetricians should wash their hands, even though he had little notion of bacteria. A more modern example is that, despite the fact that for decades evidence was strong for a causal link between smoking and lung cancer, only in 1996 was a pathogenetic mechanism for it first documented. (5)

For many diseases, both pathogenetic mechanisms and nonspecific risk factors have been important in the spread and control of the diseases. Sometimes, the many different causes interact in complicated ways.

EXAMPLE

Koch's postulates were originally used to establish that tuberculosis is caused by inoculation of the acid-fast bacillus *Mycobacterium tuberculosis* into susceptible hosts. The final common pathway of tuberculosis is the invasion of host tissue by the bacteria. From a pathogenetic perspective, conquering the disease required antibiotics or vaccines that were effective against the organism. Through biomedical research efforts, both have been achieved.

However, the development of the disease tuberculosis is far more complex. Other important causes are the susceptibility of the host and the degree of exposure (Figure 11.1); these causes determine whether invasion of host tissue can occur.

Some clinicians would be hesitant to label host susceptibility and level of exposure as causes of tuberculosis, but these are very important components of cause. In fact, social and economic improvements influencing host susceptibility, such as less crowded living space and better nutrition, may have played a more prominent role in the decline in tuberculosis rates in developed countries than treatments created through the biomedical-pathogenetic research model. Figure 11.2 shows that the death rate from tuberculosis had dropped dramatically long before antibiotics were introduced (the vaccine came even later).

Between 1985 and 1992, the number of tuberculosis cases in the United States began to increase (Figure 11.3). (6) Why was this so? Sixty percent of the increase occurred in foreign-born persons. HIV

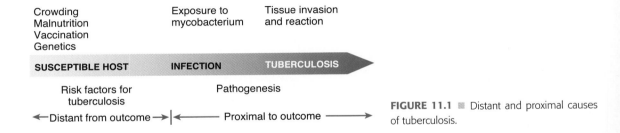

FIGURE 11.1 ▩ Distant and proximal causes of tuberculosis.

infection also was a factor, as AIDS weakens the immune system. These susceptible hosts were more likely than the general population to be exposed to tuberculosis, because both AIDS and tuberculosis are more common in economically depressed populations. Finally, changes occurred in the bacillus itself, with the evolution of multidrug resistant strains. To complicate the picture further, multidrug resistance also was caused by a web of circumstances. Genetic changes in the *Mycobacterium* are more likely to occur with medication noncompliance, which is more likely among intravenous drug users, an important risk group for AIDS. Changes in the bacterium's genetic makeup also may have been related to high replication rates in immunodeficient hosts. Thus, the interplay of environment, behavior, and subcellular biology may be incredibly complex when thinking about cause. To combat the new epidemic of tuberculosis, use of multidrug regimens (biologic efforts) and directly observing therapy to ensure compliance (behavioral efforts) both increased. The rate of tuberculosis began to decline

and was down to about 15,000 cases in 2003, the level that earlier projections had predicted reaching a decade earlier. (7)

Interaction of Multiple Causes

When more than one cause acts together, the resulting risk may be greater or less than would be expected by simply combining the effects of the separate causes. This interplay is called **interaction**. Clinicians call this phenomenon **synergism** when the joint effect is greater than the sum of the effects of the individual causes, and **antagonism** when it is less. Sometimes, the term **biologic interaction** is used to distinguish it from **statistical interaction**.†

---

† *Statistical interaction* is present when combinations of variables in a mathematical model add to the model's explanatory power after the net effects of the individual predictor variables have been taken into account. It is conceptually related to biologic synergy and antagonism but is a mathematical construct, not an observable phenomenon in nature.

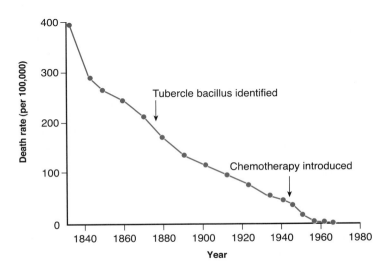

FIGURE 11.2 ▩ Declining death rate from respiratory tuberculosis in England and Wales over the past 150 years. Most of the decrease occurred before antibiotic therapy was available. (From McKeown T. The Role of Medicine: Dream, Mirage, or Nemesis. London: Nuffield Provincial Hospital Trust; 1976.)

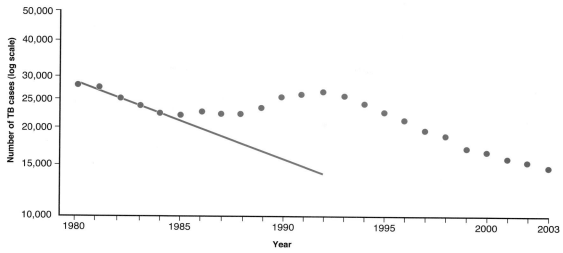

FIGURE 11.3 ▦ Tuberculosis cases in the United States, 1980–2003. The solid line shows the projected trend and the closed circles show the actual numbers. The numbers projected for 1993 were not reached until a decade later. (Data from CDC. Reported tuberculosis in the United States, 2002. Atlanta, GA: U.S. Department of Health and Human Services, CDC, September 2003, and Centers for Disease Control and Prevention. Trends in tuberculosis—United States, 1998–2003. MMWR 2004;53:209–214.)

E X A M P L E

Figure 11.4 shows the probability of developing coronary artery disease over a 5-year period among men aged 55. Men with normal systolic blood pressure, a normal ratio of total cholesterol to HDL cholesterol, no history of diabetes or left ventricular hypertrophy on EKG, and no history of smoking have a low chance (2.1%) of developing coronary heart disease over the next 5 years. Risk increases, up to 7.3%, when the various risk factors are present individually. But when all risk factors are present together, the absolute risk of developing coronary artery disease in the next 5 years (43.4%) is almost twice the sum of the individual risks. (8)

Elucidation of cause is more difficult when many factors play a part than when a single one predominates. However, when multiple causative factors are present and interact, it may be possible to make a substantial impact on a patient's health by changing only one cause, or just a few of them. Thus, in the previous example, getting patients to give up smoking and treating hypertension can substantially lower the risk of developing cardiovascular disease in men, even in the continuing presence of other causative factors.

Effect Modification

Interaction is often expressed as **effect modification** when the strength of the relationship between two variables is different according to the level of some third variable, called an **effect modifier**.

E X A M P L E

Several studies have found that alcohol consumption moderately increases the risk of breast cancer. An analysis was done to determine the effect of the vitamin folate on breast cancer risk related to drinking. For women who consumed more than one alcoholic drink a day, daily folate intake of at least 600 micrograms appeared to exert a protective effect, and there was an inverse dose response for lesser amounts (Figure 11.5). The study results suggested that a woman who takes a daily multivitamin containing 400 micrograms of folate and eats leafy vegetables could enjoy a moderate amount of daily alcoholic beverages without increasing her risk of breast cancer. (9)

ESTABLISHING CAUSE

In clinical medicine, it is not possible to prove causal relationships beyond any doubt, because understanding of the relationships are based on

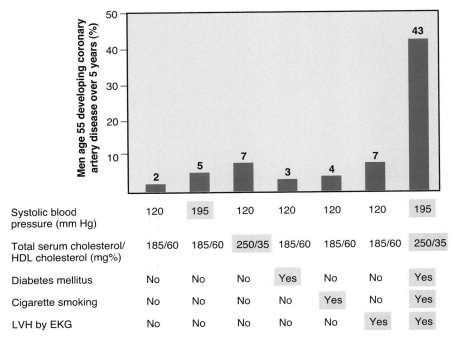

Systolic blood pressure (mm Hg)	120	195	120	120	120	120	195
Total serum cholesterol/ HDL cholesterol (mg%)	185/60	185/60	250/35	185/60	185/60	185/60	250/35
Diabetes mellitus	No	No	No	Yes	No	No	Yes
Cigarette smoking	No	No	No	No	Yes	No	Yes
LVH by EKG	No	No	No	No	No	Yes	Yes

FIGURE 11.4 ▪ Interaction of multiple causes of disease. The 5-year risk of developing coronary artery disease in 55-year-old men, according to the level of several risk factors alone and in combination. Abnormal values are in shaded boxes. LVH = left ventricular hypertrophy. (Calculated from coronary artery disease risk calculator from Anderson KM, Wilson PWF, Odell PM, Kannel WB. An updated coronary risk profile: A statement for health professionals. Circulation 1991;83:357–363.)

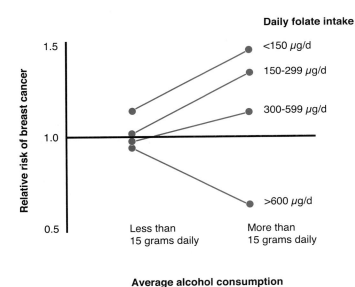

FIGURE 11.5 ▪ Example of effect modification: How the risk of breast cancer varies according to degree of alcohol consumption and by amount of daily folate ingestion. (Data from Zhang S, Hunter D, Hankinson SE, Giovannucci EL, Rosner BA, Colditz GA, et al. A prospective study of folate intake and the risk of breast cancer. JAMA 1999;281:1632–1637. Reprinted from Gansehow PS, Norlock FE, Jacobs EA, Marcus EA, eds. Breast Health and Common Breast Problems: A Practical Approach. Philadelphia, PA: American College of Physicians; 2004.)

empiric evidence and it is at least theoretically possible that new evidence could change our understanding. Therefore, it is only possible to increase
one's conviction of a cause-and-effect relationship
by means of empiric evidence to the point at which
for all intents and purposes, cause is established.
Conversely, evidence against a cause can be
mounted until a cause-and-effect relationship
becomes implausible. A postulated cause-and-effect
relationship should be examined in as many different ways as possible. This usually means that several
studies must be done to build evidence for or
against cause.

Association and Cause

Two factors—the suspected cause and the effect—
obviously must be associated if they are to be considered as causally related. However, not all associations are causal. Figure 11.6 outlines other reasons
for association that must be excluded. First, one
must ask if an apparent association between a
purported cause and an effect is real or is merely an
artifact of the study because of bias or random variation. Selection and measurement biases and chance
can give rise to apparent associations that do not
exist in nature. If these problems can be considered
unlikely, a true association exists. But before deciding that the association is causal, it is necessary to
know whether the association occurs indirectly,
through another (confounding) factor, or directly.
If confounding is not found, a causal relationship is
likely.

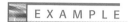

EXAMPLE

Several studies found that women fared worse than
men after coronary bypass surgery, and it was thought
that female sex caused a worse postoperative prognosis. On further study, the diameter of the midleft
anterior descending artery, which was associated with
patient gender and body size, was found to be an
important variable in predicting in-hospital mortality after
surgery, decreasing from 15.8% for 1.0 millimeter
vessels to 1.5% for 2.5–3.5 millimeter vessels. The
authors concluded "smaller coronary arteries explain
higher perioperative mortality with CABG . . . in women
and smaller people." (10) Gender was related to both
coronary artery diameter and postoperative prognosis,
and thus confounded the relationship.

Hierarchy of Research Designs

When considering a possible causal relationship, the
strength of the research design used to establish the
relationship is an important piece of evidence. However, the hierarchy of research designs is only a
rough guide, based on the extent of susceptibility to
bias. The manner in which an individual study is
performed can do a great deal to increase or decrease
its validity, regardless of the type of design used.

Of the research designs discussed so far in this
book, the best evidence for a cause-and-effect relationship come from well-conducted randomized
controlled trials, with adequate numbers of patients;
blinding of therapists, patients, and researchers;
limited or no loss to follow-up; and carefully standardized methods of measurement and analysis.

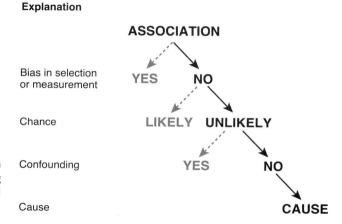

FIGURE 11.6 ■ Association and cause. Selection
and measurement biases; chance and confounding
should be excluded before concluding that a causal
association is likely.

Randomized controlled trials guard against differences in the groups being compared, both for factors already known to be important (a problem that can be overcome by other methods) and for unknown confounding factors (a problem that cannot be addressed with observational studies).

Clinicians ordinarily rely on randomized controlled trials to provide evidence about causal relationships for treatments and prevention. However, as pointed out in Chapter 7, randomized controlled trials are rarely feasible when studying risk factors (causes) of disease because it is not ethical to randomize interventions thought to be harmful. Observational studies must be used instead.

In general, the further one departs from randomized trials, the less the research design protects against possible biases and the weaker the evidence is for a cause-and-effect relationship. Well-conducted cohort studies are the next best design, because they can be performed in a way that minimizes known confounding, selection, and measurement biases. Case-control studies are vulnerable to selection bias and can be susceptible to confounding and measurement bias. Cross-sectional studies are weak because they provide no direct evidence of the sequence of events. True prevalence surveys—cross-sectional studies of a defined population—guard against selection bias but are subject to measurement and confounding biases. Weakest of all are case series, because they have no defined population and no comparison group.

ECOLOGICAL STUDIES

Until now in this book, we have discussed evidence for cause when exposure and disease status are known for each individual in the study. In a different kind of research, most often used for evaluating health services or for epidemiologic studies of large populations, exposure is known only for the groups, not for the individuals in the groups.

Studies in which exposure to a risk factor is characterized by the average exposure of the group to which individuals belong are called **aggregate risk studies**. Another term is **ecological studies**, because people are classified by the general level of exposure in their environment, which may or may not correspond to exposure of specific individuals.

EXAMPLE

What factors are associated with cardiac mortality in developed countries? Investigators gathered data on rates of ischemic heart disease mortality in 18 developed countries to explore the contribution of various economic, health services, and dietary variables. One finding that was not anticipated was a strong negative association between ischemic heart disease, death and wine consumption (Figure 11.7). (11)

This study raised the hypothesis that alcohol protects against ischemic heart disease. Since then, studies on individuals have shown that the association of alcohol consumption and mortality is a U-shape curve, with alcohol protecting against mortality with moderate consumption and increasing mortality with heavy consumption.

Aggregate risk studies are rarely definitive in and of themselves. The main problem is a potential bias called the **ecological fallacy**, in which affected individuals in a generally exposed group may not themselves have been the ones exposed to the risk factor. Also, exposure may not be the only characteristic that distinguishes people in the exposed group from those in the nonexposed group, that is there may be confounding factors. Thus, aggregate risk studies are most useful in raising hypotheses, which must then be tested with more rigorous research.

Time-Series Studies

Evidence from aggregate risk studies that a factor is actually responsible for an effect can be strengthened when observations are made at more than two points in time (before and after) and in more than one place. In a **time-series study**, the effect is measured at various points in time before and after the purported cause has been introduced. It is then possible to see whether or not the effect varies as expected. If changes in the purported cause are followed by changes in the purported effect, the association is less likely to be spurious. An advantage of a time-series analysis is that it can distinguish between changes occurring over time (secular trends) from the effects of the intervention.

EXAMPLE

Health insurance reforms in the United States increasingly involve cost-containment strategies. What is the effect of these efforts? Soumerai and colleagues studied

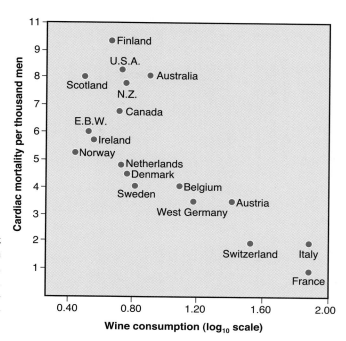

FIGURE 11.7 ■ Example of an aggregate risk study: Relationship between wine consumption and cardiac mortality in developed countries. (Drawn from St. Leger AS, Cochrane AL, Moore F. Factors associated with cardiac mortality in developed countries with particular reference to the consumption of wine. Lancet 1979;1:1017–1020.)

a natural experiment in New Hampshire in which Medicaid imposed a 3-prescription limit on reimbursement for drugs for 11 months. The researchers studied patients with chronic schizophrenia and found that the cap resulted in a 15% to 49% reduction in use of prescribed drugs but increased visits to mental health facilities and sharply increased emergency room visits (Figure 11.8). After the limit was lifted, these effects were reversed. Estimated increases in mental health care exceeded the savings in drug costs during the imposed limit. (12) This time-series study suggested that limiting drug prescriptions cost more money and resulted in poorer care for this group of patients.

Multiple Time-Series Studies

In a **multiple time-series study**, the suspected cause is introduced into several different groups at different times. Measurements are then made among the groups to determine whether the effect occurred in the same sequential manner in which the suspected cause was introduced. When an effect regularly follows introduction of the suspected cause at various times and places, there is stronger evidence for cause than when this phenomenon is observed only

once, because it is even more improbable that the same extraneous factor(s) occurred at the same time in relation to the intervention in many different places and times.

EXAMPLE

Because there were no randomized controlled trials of cervical cancer screening programs before they became widely accepted, their effectiveness had to be evaluated by means of observational studies. A multiple time-series study has provided some of the most convincing evidence of their effectiveness. (13) Data were gathered on screening programs begun in Canadian provinces at various times during a 10-year period in the 1960s and 1970s. Reductions in cervical cancer mortality regularly followed the introduction of screening programs regardless of time and location. With these data, it was concluded that "screening had a significant effect on reduction in mortality from carcinoma of the uterus."

EVIDENCE FOR AND AGAINST CAUSE

In all studies of cause, but especially when randomized controlled trials are not available, several fea-

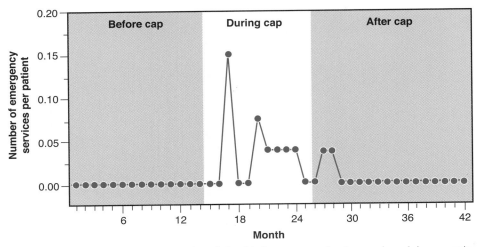

FIGURE 11.8 ▨ A time-series study of the relationship between capping the number of drug prescriptions for schizophrenic patients and the use of emergency health services at a mental health center. (Reprinted from Soumerai SB, McLaughlin TJ, Ross-Degnan D, Casteris CS, Bollini P. Effects of limiting Medicaid drug-reimbursement benefits on the use of psychotropic agents and acute mental health services by patients with schizophrenia. N Engl J Med 1994;331:650–655.)

tures increase the likelihood that an association is causal. In 1965, the British statistician Sir Austin Bradford Hill proposed a set of features that should be sought when deciding whether a relationship between some environmental factor and a sickness is causal or just an association. (14) His proposals for observational studies of risk have been widely used, sometimes with modifications (Table 11.1). We will review these elements mainly using the example of smoking as a risk factor for lung cancer. The individual elements in the list are not all of equal weight in deciding about cause.

Temporal Relationships Between Cause and Effect

Causes should obviously precede effects. This fundamental principle seems self-evident and is not an issue in the relationship between smoking and lung cancer. Sometimes, however, the principal can be overlooked when interpreting cross-sectional and case-control studies, in which both the purported cause and the effect are measured at the same point in time. It is sometimes assumed that one variable precedes another without actually establishing that this is so. In other cases, it may be difficult to establish which came first.

TABLE 11.1 ▨ **Evidence That an Association Is Cause and Effect**[a]

Criteria	Comments
Temporality	Cause precedes effect
Strength	Large relative risk
Dose-response	Larger exposures to cause associated with higher rates of disease
Reversibility	Reduction in exposure is followed by lower rates of disease
Consistency	Repeatedly observed by different persons, in different places, circumstances, and times
Biologic plausibility	Makes sense, according to biologic knowledge of the time
Specificity	One cause leads to one effect
Analogy	Cause-and-effect relationship already established for a similar exposure or disease

[a] Modified from Bradford Hill A. The environment and disease: Association and causation. Proc R Soc Med 1965;58:295–300.

It has long been noted that overweight persons are at higher risk of death, especially cardiovascular death, than people with normal weight. Thus, it is reasonable to assume that weight loss would be protective among overweight people. However, several cohort studies have found excess mortality among people who lose weight, even among people without any apparent preexisting disease. Also, there is a U-shaped curve relating weight to mortality, with mortality increased both among lean and overweight people. (15) These distressing findings may be explained if a subtle, preclinical effect of fatal illness is weight loss. (16) Thus, fatal conditions may precede and cause weight loss, not vice versa. This possibility could be excluded if it were known whether the weight loss was voluntary in those losing weight.

Although it is absolutely necessary for a cause to precede an effect—and, therefore, the lack of such a sequence is powerful evidence *against* cause—an appropriate temporal sequence alone is weak evidence *for* cause. Many things happen before an event that have nothing to do with the event.

Strength of the Association

A strong association between a purported cause and an effect, as expressed by a large relative or absolute risk, is better evidence for a causal relationship than a weak association. Thus, the tenfold higher incidence of lung cancer among male smokers compared to nonsmokers is much stronger evidence that smoking causes lung cancer than the finding that smoking is related to renal cancer, for which the relative risk is much smaller (1.47). (17) Similarly, a relative risk of more than 200 for the association of hepatitis B infection and hepatocellular cancer is strong evidence that the virus is a cause of liver cancer. (18) Unrecognized bias could account for small relative risks but is unlikely to result in large ones.

Dose-Response Relationships

A dose-response relationship is present if increasing the exposure to the purported cause is followed by a larger and larger effect. Demonstrating a dose-response relationship strengthens the argument for cause and effect, but its absence is relatively weak evidence against causation because not all causal associations exhibit a dose-response relationship. Figure 11.9 shows a clear dose-response curve when lung cancer death rates (responses) are plotted against the number of cigarettes smoked (doses).

Although a dose-response curve is good evidence for a causal relationship, especially when coupled with a large relative or absolute risk, its existence does not exclude confounding factors.

Both the strong association between smoking and lung cancer and the demonstrated dose-response relationship could be examples of confounding. According to this argument, an unknown variable may exist that both causes people to smoke and increases their risk of developing lung cancer. The more the factor is present, the more both smoking and lung cancer are found; hence,

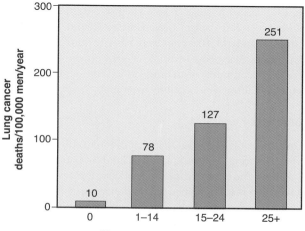

FIGURE 11.9 ▧ Example of a dose-response relationship: Lung cancer deaths in male physicians according to dose (number) of cigarettes smoked. (Drawn from Doll R, Peto R. Mortality in relation to smoking: 20 years' observations on male British doctors. Br Med J 1976;2: 1525–1536.)

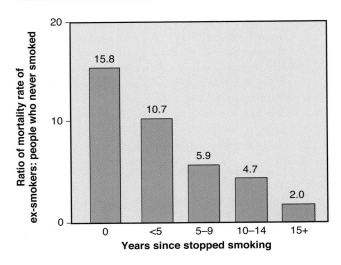

FIGURE 11.10 ■ Reversible association: Declining mortality from lung cancer in ex-cigarette smokers. The data exclude people who stopped smoking after getting cancer. (Drawn from Doll R, Petro R. Mortality in relation to smoking: 20 years' observations on male British doctors. Br Med J 1976;2:1525–1536.)

the dose-response relationship. Such an argument is a theoretically possible explanation for the association between smoking and lung cancer, although just what the confounding factor might be has never been clarified. Short of a randomized controlled trial (which would, on the average, allocate the people with the confounding factor equally to smoking and nonsmoking groups) the confounding argument is difficult to refute completely.

Reversible Associations

A factor is more likely to be a cause of disease whenever its removal results in a decreased risk of disease. An example is when the association between suspected cause and effect is reversible. Figure 11.10 shows that when people give up smoking they decrease their likelihood of getting lung cancer.

Reversible associations are strong, but not infallible, evidence of a causal relationship. Confounding could conceivably explain a reversible association. For example, Figure 11.10 is consistent with the (unlikely) explanation that people willing to give up smoking have smaller amounts of an unidentified confounding factor than those who continue to smoke.

Consistency

When several studies, conducted at different times in different settings and with different kinds of patients, all come to the same conclusion, evidence for a causal relationship is strengthened. Causation is particularly supported when studies using several different research designs, with complementary strengths and weaknesses, all lead to the same result because studies using the same design can all make the same mistake. For the association of smoking and lung cancer, no randomized trial has ever been conducted. But many cohort, case-control, and time-series studies have shown that increased tobacco use is followed by increased lung cancer incidence, in both sexes, in various ethnic groups, and in different countries.

It is often the case that different studies produce different results. Lack of consistency does not necessarily mean that the results of a particular study are invalid. One good study should outweigh several poor ones. Also, different results of studies may be related not to a varying quality of research methods but to the different kinds of patients or slight variations in treatment. These differences could be pointing to important new refinements of a causal association.

Biologic Plausibility

The assertion that cause and effect is consistent with our knowledge of the mechanisms of disease, as it is currently understood, is often given considerable weight when causation is being assessed. When one has absolutely no idea how an association might have arisen, one tends to be skeptical that the association is real. Such skepticism often serves us well. For example, the substance Laetrile was touted as a cure for cancer in the early 1980s. However, the scientific community was not convinced, mainly because it could think of no biologic reason why an extract of apricot pits that was not chemically related to compounds with known anticancer activity should be effective against cancer cells. To nail down the issue, researchers finally submitted Laetrile to a clinical trial in which it was shown that the substance was, in fact, without activity against the cancers studied. (19)

It is important to remember, however, that what is considered biologically plausible depends on the state of medical knowledge at the time. In Meig's day, contagious diseases were biologically implausible. Today, a biologically plausible mechanism for puerperal sepsis, the effects of streptococcal infection, has made it easier today to accept Holmes's observations. In another example, as pointed out earlier, a possible mechanism by which smoking causes lung cancer was identified decades after studies demonstrated a strong association.

Sometimes, new findings from clinical and epidemiological studies stimulate work that identifies biological mechanisms.

EXAMPLE

To many scientists in the Western world, the suggestion that sticking needles into the body and twirling them can decrease pain and control vomiting seems biologically implausible. However, randomized controlled trials of acupuncture among cancer patients receiving chemotherapy have found acupuncture effective. One carefully done trial included a group with sham acupuncture to deal with the possibility of a placebo effect. During chemotherapy treatment, the mean number of emesis episodes per patient was 6.29 in the acupuncture group, 10.73 in the sham acupuncture group, and 13.41 in the control group, which was a highly significant difference. (20) A search for possible biomedical mechanisms of the effect suggest that acupuncture might work through components of the emetic reflex and opiate receptors.

In sum, biologic plausibility, when present, strengthens the case for causation. When it is absent, other evidence for causation should be sought. If the other evidence is strong, the lack of biologic plausibility may indicate the limitations of medical knowledge, rather than the lack of a causal association.

Specificity

Specificity—one cause, one effect—is more often found for acute infectious diseases (such as polio-

myelitis and tetanus) and for genetic diseases (such as familial adenomatous polyposis, ochronosis, and phenylketonuria). Chronic, degenerative diseases often have many causes for the same effect or many effects from the same cause. Lung cancer is caused by cigarette smoking, asbestos, and radiation. Cigarettes cause not only lung cancer but also bronchitis, peptic ulcer disease, periodontal disease, and wrinkled skin. The presence of specificity is strong evidence for cause, but the absence of specificity is weak evidence against a cause-and-effect relationship.

Analogy

The argument for a cause-and-effect relationship is strengthened when examples exist of well-established causes that are analogous to the one in question. Thus, if a slow virus is known to cause a chronic, degenerative central nervous system disease (such as subacute sclerosing panencephalitis), it is easier to accept that another virus might cause degeneration of the immunologic system (such as acquired immunodeficiency syndrome). In the smoking-lung cancer association, it is known that other environmental toxins such as asbestos, arsenic, and uranium cause lung cancer. In general, however, analogy is weak evidence for cause.

WEIGHING THE EVIDENCE

When determining cause, one must consider the evidence from all available studies. After examining the research design and quality of studies and the elements for and against cause, the case for causality can be strengthened or eroded. This calls for a good deal of judgment, especially when the evidence from different studies is conflicting. In such cases, clinicians must decide where the weight of the evidence lies.

Figure 11.11 summarizes the different types of evidence for and against cause, depending on the research design, and features that strengthen or weaken the evidence for cause. The figure roughly indicates relative strengths in helping to establish or discard a causal hypothesis. Thus, a carefully done cohort study showing a strong association and a dose-response relationship that is reversible is strong evidence for cause, while a cross-sectional study finding no effect is weak evidence against cause.

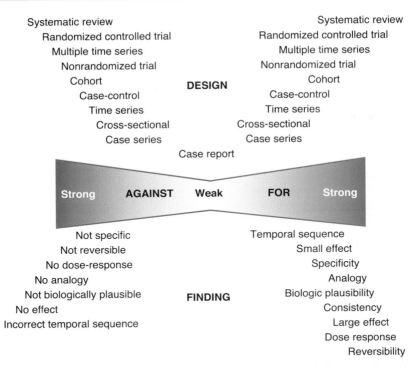

FIGURE 11.11 ■ Relative strength of evidence for and against a causal effect. Note that with study designs, the strength of evidence *for* a causal relationship is a mirror image of that *against.* With findings, evidence *for* a causal effect does not mirror evidence *against* an effect.

Grading the Quality of the Evidence

Increasingly, when evaluating evidence for a possible causal association, a literature search is undertaken. All relevant studies are reviewed according to specific criteria, most commonly criteria about the kind of research design and methods used. This **systematic review** is then used to determine the strength of the evidence for the causal relationship (see Chapter 12).

Often a **quality of evidence grade** is assigned.

E X A M P L E

The U.S. Preventive Services Task Force makes recommendations for preventive services that should be done in clinical practice. Since its inception, the Task Force has graded the quality of scientific evidence used for making the recommendations (which are also graded). Over time, the grading system has evolved to take into account more and more factors. Table 11.2 shows that grades are given both for research design and for how well a study using a particular design was carried out. Then a final grade is given, generally according to the highest level of

scientific evidence available among all studies relating to a particular preventive practice, as well as the generalizability of the findings and how directly the evidence is linked to an important clinical outcome. For example, if several well-done studies were available on a particular question, including a randomized trial and several cohort and case-control studies, the grade assigned would be for the randomized trial, not the studies with weaker research designs. (21)

REVIEW QUESTIONS

Read the following statements and circle all the correct answers for 11.1–11.3.

11.1. A patient comes to you because she has read that cell phones cause brain cancer, and she wants to know your opinion. You discover that the incidence of malignant brain tumors is increasing in the United States. What is the most important reason a randomized controlled trial (RCT) can-

---

TABLE 11.2 ■ Grading the Strength of Evidence for a Clinical Cause: Approach of the U.S. Preventive Services Task Force

The Task Force assigns each study two separate grades: one for study design and one for how well the study was done (internal validity). A grade is then given for overall quality of all evidence from all studies, considering the quality of studies as well as the generalizeability and how direct the link is between prevention and outcome.

Grades for the Research Design of Individual Studies

• I	Evidence obtained from at least one properly randomized controlled trial
• II-1	Evidence obtained from well-designed controlled trials without randomization
• II-2	Evidence obtained from well-designed cohort or case-control analytic studies, preferably from more than one center or research group
• II-3	Evidence obtained from multiple time-series with or without the intervention.Dramatic results from uncontrolled trials (such as the results of the introduction of penicillin treatment in the 1940s) could also be regarded as this type of evidence.
• III	Opinions of respected authorities, based on clinical experience, descriptive studies and case reports, or reports of expert committees

Grades for the Internal Validity of Individual Studies

• Good

• Fair

• Poor

Criteria to determine the validity of each type of study, as outlined in this book, are applied. A grade of I-good is given to a well-performed randomized controlled trial. A grade of II-2-fair means the study was a fair cohort or case-control study.

Grades for the Overall Quality of Evidence for Each Preventive Service

• Good:	Evidence includes consistent results from well-designed, well-conducted studies in representative populations that directly assess effects on health outcomes.
• Fair:	Evidence is sufficient to determine effects on health outcomes, but the strength of the evidence is limited by the number, quality, or consistency of the individual studies, generalizability to routine practice, or indirect nature of the evidence on health outcomes.
• Poor:	Evidence is insufficient to assess the effects on health outcomes because of limited number or power of studies, important flaws in their design or conduct, gaps in the chain of evidence, or lack of information on important health outcomes.

(From Harris RP, Woolf SH, Lohr KN, Mulrow CD, Teutsch SM, Atkins D, for the Methods Work Group, Third U.S. Preventive Services Task Force. Current methods of the U.S. Preventive Services Task Force: A review of the process. Am J Prev Med 2001; 20(3S):21–35.)

---

not be done to determine whether or not cell phones cause brain cancer?

A. An RCT would cost too much
B. People would not agree to participate
C. It would be unethical
D. It would take too long
E. An RCT is a research method that cannot answer the question

11.2. You discover that case-control studies have been done to determine whether or not cell phone use is associated with the development of brain cancer. In one, patients with brain cancer and matched controls without brain cancer were asked about cell-phone use.(22) The estimated relative risk for at least 100 hours of use compared to no or rare use was 1.0 for all types of brain tumors combined (95% confidence interval, 0.6 to 1.5). This finding is consistent with:

A. Use of cell phones increases the incidence of brain tumors 50%

B. Use of cell phones protect against brain tumors

C. Use of cell phones is not associated with protection of development of brain tumors

D. Specific types of brain tumors might be associated with cell phone use

11.3. You know that case-control studies are not a strong research design when evaluating a possible cause-and-effect relationship. Which of the following would strengthen your sense that cell phones are or are not related to brain tumors?

A. A dose-response was sought.

B. Different measures of "dose" were explored.

C. Analysis was made according to which side the tumor occurred and telephone was used.

11.4. Is the study adequately powered? Explain your answer.

11.5. Given the information above, what is a possible major bias in this case-control study?

11.6. Using the first two parts of the grading system of the U.S. Preventive Services Task Force (Table 11.2), what grade would you give this study?

11.7. List at least three other types of studies that would be feasible to study the possible relationship between cell phone use and brain cancer, then grade each one.

Answers are in Appendix A.

REFERENCES

1. Holmes OW. On the contagiousness of puerperal fever. Med Classics 1936;1:207–268. [Originally published, 1843.]

2. Agnes M, editor in chief. Webster's New World Dictionary, 4th Ed. Cleveland, Ohio: Wiley Publishing, Inc., 2002.

3. Fouchier RA, Kuiken T, Schutten M, van Amerongen G, van Doornum GJ, van den Hoogen BG, et al. Koch's postulates fulfilled for SARS virus. Nature 2003;423:240.

4. MacMahon B, Pugh TF. Epidemiology: Principles and Methods. Boston: Little, Brown & Co., 1970.

5. Denissenko MF, Pao A, Tang M, Pfeifer GP. Preferential formation of benzo[a]pyrene adducts at lung cancer mutational hotspots in P53. Science 1996;274: 430-432.

6. Cantwell MF, Snider DE, Cauthen GM, Onorato IM. Epidemiology of tuberculosis in the United States, 1985 through 1992. JAMA 1994;272:535–539.

7. Centers for Disease Control and Prevention. Trends in tuberculosis: United States, 1998–2003. MMWR 2004;53:209–214.

8. Anderson KM, Wilson PWF, Odell PM, Kannel WB. An updated coronary risk profile: A statement for health professionals. Circulation 1991;83:357–363.

9. Zhang S, Hunter D, Hankinson SE, Giovannucci EL, Rosner BA, Colditz GA, Speizer FE, Willett WC. A prospective study of folate intake and the risk of breast cancer. JAMA 1999;281:1632–1637.

10. O'Conner NJ, Morton JR, Birkmeyer JD, Olmstead EM, O'Connor GT. Effect of coronary artery diameter in patients undergoing coronary bypass surgery. Circulation 1996;93:652–655.

11. St. Leger AS, Cochrane AL, Moore F. Factors associated with cardiac mortality in developed countries with particular reference to the consumption of wine. Lancet 1979;1:1017–1020.

12. Soumerai SB, McLaughlin TJ, Ross-Degnan D, Casteris CS, Bollini P. Effects of limiting Medicaid drug-reimbursement benefits on the use of psychotropic agents and acute mental health services by patients with schizophrenia. N Engl J Med 1994;331:650–655.

13. Cervical Cancer Screening Programs. I. Epidemiology and natural history of carcinoma of the cervix. Can Med Assoc J 1976;114:1003–1012.

14. Bradford Hill A. The environment and disease: Association or causation? Proc R Soc Med 1965;58:295–300.

15. Calle EE, Thun MJ, Petrelli JM, Rodriguez C, Heath CW. Body-mass index and mortality in a prospective cohort of U.S. adults. N Engl J Med 1999;341: 1097–1105.

16. Kuller L, Wing R. Weight loss and mortality. Ann Intern Med 1993;119:630–632.

17. Centers for Disease Control and Prevention. Smoking and health: A national status report (A report to

Congress). Rockville, MD: DHHS Publication No. (CDC) 87-8396, 1990.

18. Beasley RP, Lin CC, Hwang LY, Chien CS. Hepato-cellular carcinoma and hepatitis B virus. Lancet 1981;2:1129–1133.

19. Moertel CG, Fleming TR, Rubin J, Kvols LK, Sarna G, Koch R, et al. A clinical trial of amygdalin (Laetrile) in the treatment of human cancer. N Engl J Med 1982;306:201–206.

20. Shen J, Wenger N, Glaspy J, Hays RD, Albert PS, Choi C, Shekelle PG. Electroacupuncture for control of myeloablative chemotherapy-induced emesis: A randomized controlled trial. JAMA 2000;284:2755–2761.

21. Harris RP, Woolf SH, Lohr KN, Mulrow CD, Teutsch SM, Atkins D, for the Methods Work Group, Third U.S. Preventive Services Task Force. Current methods of the U.S. Preventive Services Task Force: A review of the process. Am J Prev Med 2001;20(3S):21–35.

22. Inskip PD, Tarone RE, Hatch EE, Wilcosky TC, Shapiro WR, Selker RG, Fine HA, Black PM, Loef-fler JS, Linet MS. Cellular-telephone use and brain tumors. N Eng J Med 2001;344:79–86.

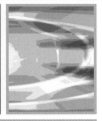

Systematic Reviews

KEY WORDS

Systematic reviews	Funnel plots	Fixed-effect model
CONSORT	Forest plot	Random-effects model
STARD	Meta-analysis	Cumulative meta-analysis
Publication bias	Homogeneity	QUOROM

Where is the wisdom we have lost in knowledge?
Where is the knowledge we have lost in information?

— *T.S. Eliot*

Clinical decisions are based on the weight of evidence bearing on a question. Sometimes, large studies are so compelling that they eclipse all studies that preceded them. More often, however, clinicians depend on the accumulation of evidence from many less definitive studies. When examining an individual study, clinicians should question the context of that one piece of evidence by asking, "Have there been other good studies of the same question?" and "If so, what have they shown?" Also, "Is this study the only one to show an effect, or does it confirm many others that have reached more or less the same conclusion?"

PROVIDING THE CONTEXT FOR INDIVIDUAL STUDIES

If the authors of a research article are doing their job appropriately, they will provide information about results of previous studies, specifically in the Introduction and Discussion sections. Sometimes, commentaries are published in conjunction with the research article. Review articles are the main way in which the evidence as a whole is summarized.

Reviews are done in many different ways, and each has its strengths and weaknesses. In this chapter, we will briefly describe traditional reviews and then take up in more detail a powerful approach called *systematic reviews*. In the final chapter we will describe additional ways to manage information, including feasible approaches to finding the best clinical research results and judging their validity and generalizability.

TRADITIONAL REVIEWS

In traditional "review articles," a senior expert in the field summarizes evidence and recommendations. Usually, the reviews address broad-gauged questions, such as "management of the diabetic patient" and take up a range of management issues, such as diagnostic criteria, blood glucose control and monitoring, cardiovascular risk factor modification, and complications. There may be information about compliance and cost-effectiveness. Clinicians need guidance on such a range of questions. Experts are in a good position to provide it because they know both the pertinent literature and how it should affect actual practice.

But the lack of structure of traditional reviews may hide important threats to validity. Original research may be cited without a clear account of how articles were found, raising the danger that they might be selectively quoted to support a point of view. Personal experience and conventional wisdom are often included and may be difficult to distinguish from bedrock evidence. The strength of the original research may not be carefully critiqued, but instead be suggested by shorthand indicators of quality, such as the prestige of the journal, eminence of the author, currency of the study, number of articles for and against a given point, and perhaps, general research design. The review may imply, for example, that randomized trials are good without regard for how well they were executed. Also, there may be no rationale for why one research finding is valued over another.

SYSTEMATIC REVIEWS

Systematic reviews are rigorous reviews of specific clinical questions. They are "systematic" because they summarize the original research bearing on the question following a scientifically based plan that has been decided in advance and made explicit at every step. As a result, readers can see the strength of the evidence for whatever conclusions are reached and, in principle, check the validity for themselves. Sometimes, it is possible to combine studies, giving a more precise estimate of effect size.

When Are Systematic Reviews Appropriate?

Systematic reviews are especially useful in addressing a single, focused question such as whether angiotensin-converting enzyme inhibitors reduce the death rate in patients with congestive heart failure or whether skin adhesives are better than sutures for superficial lacerations. For a systematic review to be useful, strong studies of the question should be available but not so much in agreement with one another that the question is already answered. There should not be so few studies of the question that one could just as well critique the individual studies directly and dispense with the review. The study results should disagree or at least leave the question open; if all the studies agree with one another, there is nothing to reconcile in a review.

Although systematic reviews most often summarize randomized controlled trials, the same methods are used to summarize studies of risk, such as the risk of breast cancer related to alcohol consumption, and studies of diagnostic test performance, such as the sensitivity and specificity of Pap smears for cervical cancer.

The elements of a systematic review are summarized in Table 12.1 and will be taken up, one at a time, in the rest of this chapter.

Finding All Relevant Studies

The first step in a systematic review is to find all the studies that bear on the question at hand. The reader wants to be sure that the review has included all the best studies of the question, not just a biased sample of studies that happen to have come to attention. Clinicians who review topics less formally (for colleagues for rounds, morning report, and journal clubs, for example) face a similar challenge and should use similar methods, although the process will rarely be so exhaustive.

How can one be reasonably sure that the reviewer has found all the best studies, considering that the

TABLE 12.1 ■ **Elements of a Systematic Review**

1. Define the clinical question.

2. Identify all completed studies of the question, published and unpublished.

3. Select the studies that meet high standards for scientific validity.

4. Look for evidence of bias in the studies selected.

5. Describe the scientific quality of the studies.

6. Ask whether the quality is systematically related to results of the studies.

7. Describe the studies with a figure (forest plot).

8. Decide whether the studies are similar enough to justify combining them.

9. If they are similar enough to combine, calculate a summary measure of effect and confidence interval.

medical literature is vast and widely dispersed? No one method of searching is sufficient for this task, so multiple approaches are used (Table 12.2).

MEDLINE, the National Library of Medicine's comprehensive electronic database of published articles, is a good place to start. However, even in the best hands the sensitivity of MEDLINE searches is far from perfect. An expert in searching, using the best available search terms, found only 93% of randomized trials and 80% of studies of diagnostic test performance. (1) Most reviewers, who may not be experts in searching, are likely to do worse. Another limitation of a MEDLINE search alone is that MEDLINE does not include all the world's journals. MEDLINE includes articles from nearly 4,500 journals in more than 70 countries and is heavily weighted toward English-language journals in North America and Europe. But with tens of thousands of medical journals in the world, MEDLINE is bound to leave out some good articles.

Other ways of finding the right articles make up for what a MEDLINE search might have missed (Table 12.2). Recent reviews and textbooks are other sources. In addition, experts in the content area (e.g., rheumatic heart disease or salmonella infection) may recommend studies that were not turned up by the other approaches. References cited in articles already found are another possibility. The Cochrane Library, found online at http://www.cochrane.org, includes the Cochrane Database of Systematic Reviews and publishes searches of the world's literature on treatment effectiveness; participants search by all available means, including examining local journals in person. There are a growing number of registries of clinical trials that can be used to find unpublished results.

The goal of consulting all these sources is to avoid missing any important article, even at the expense of inefficiency. In diagnostic test terms, the reviewer uses multiple parallel tests to increase the sensitivity of the search, even at the expense of many false-positive results (that is, unwanted or redundant citations), which need to be weeded out by examining the studies themselves.

Besides exercising due diligence in finding articles, authors of systematic reviews should have explicitly described the search strategy in their review, including MEDLINE search terms. In this way, readers can see the extent to which the reviewer took into account all the important information that was available at the time.

Systematic Reviews Are Limited to Scientifically Strong Studies

To be included in a systematic review, studies must meet a threshold for scientific strength. The assumption is that only the relatively strong studies should count. How is that threshold established? Various expert groups have proposed criteria for adequate scientific strength. Among these are the **CONSORT** criteria for reporting randomized controlled trials

TABLE 12.2 ■ **Approaches to Finding All the Studies Bearing on a Question**

Search MEDLINE.

Read recent reviews and textbooks.

Seek the advice of experts in the content area.

Consider articles cited in the articles already found by other approaches.

Consult databases of articles such as the Cochrane Database of Systematic Reviews.

Review registries of clinical trials (to detect publication bias, if present).

(2) and the **STARD** criteria for studies of diagnostic test performance. (3)

Usually only a small proportion of studies are selected from a vast number of potential articles on the topic (Table 12.3). Many articles describe the biology of disease and are not ready for clinical application. Others communicate opinions or summaries of existing evidence, not original clinical research. Much original clinical research is not strong, and the information contained in it is eclipsed by stronger studies. Therefore, relatively few articles address the clinical question directly

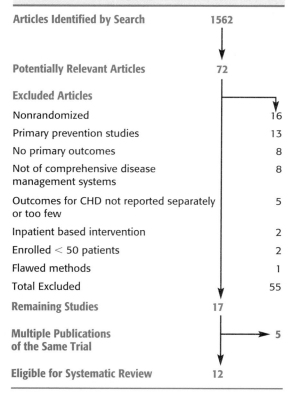

TABLE 12.3 ■ **Systematic Reviews Include Only a Small Proportion of Articles on a Question. Selection of Articles for a Systematic Review of Randomized Trials of Secondary Prevention Programs for Coronary Heart Disease (CHD).**

Articles Identified by Search	1562
Potentially Relevant Articles	72
Excluded Articles	
Nonrandomized	16
Primary prevention studies	13
No primary outcomes	8
Not of comprehensive disease management systems	8
Outcomes for CHD not reported separately or too few	5
Inpatient based intervention	2
Enrolled < 50 patients	2
Flawed methods	1
Total Excluded	55
Remaining Studies	17
Multiple Publications of the Same Trial	5
Eligible for Systematic Review	12

(Data from McAlister FA, Lawson FME, Teo KK, Armstrong PW. Randomized trials of secondary prevention programmes in coronary heart disease: Systematic review. BMJ 2001;323: 957–962.)

and are both scientifically strong and clinically relevant.

Publication Bias

The articles cited in systematic reviews should include every scientifically strong study of the question. The reviewer should have guarded against several biases in selecting the studies and should tell the reader how the selection was done.

Publication bias is the tendency for published studies to be systematically different from all completed studies of a question. Some completed studies are never published, and they are systematically different from the rest. In general, published studies are more likely to be "positive" (that is, they find an effect), because of a pervasive preference for positive results. Investigators are less likely to complete studies that may end up negative and less likely to submit them to journals. (4) For their part, journal editors may be less likely to find negative studies interesting news and publish them. (5) To get around these problems, some reviewers make a concerted effort to find unpublished studies, including those that were funded and started but not completed. They are aided in this effort by public registries of all studies that have been started.

Industry sponsorship of research can also lead to distortions in the scientific record. Almost two thirds of clinical research in the United States is funded by industry. Studies sponsored by industry (usually drug companies) are more likely to have outcomes favoring the sponsor's product than those with other funding sources. (6) One possible reason is that industry sponsors sometimes require, as a condition of funding research, that they approve the resulting articles before they are submitted to journals. Sometimes industry sponsors have blocked publication of research they have funded that has not, in their opinion, found the "right" result.

E X A M P L E

A leading manufacturer of a levothyroxin (thyroid hormone) preparation had long claimed that its drug was better than other preparations because the drug was more bioavailable; that is, more reliably absorbed, dose for dose, than the others. To support this claim, the manufacturer funded a study comparing the bioavailability of its product and three competitors. When the study showed that the four were in fact bioequivalent, the manufacturer "waged an energetic campaign to discredit the study and prevent publication." (12) The investigators' university found the study sound, and a report of the study was accepted by a leading journal after review by five outside experts. However, the investigator withdrew the report, citing "impending legal action" based on the fact the she had signed a legal document stating that she could not publish the results of the study unless the sponsor agreed. The U.S. Food and Drug Administration and the popular press became involved and the article was finally published 7 years after the study was completed and 2 years after the journal had accepted it. (7) U.S. medical schools are making joint efforts to eliminate contracts with funding entities that constrain publication of research results.

Other factors can bias the selection of articles in systematic reviews. Reviewers tend to be aware of articles in their own language (most often English) more often than those written in other languages. Europeans tend to cite European articles, and North Americans tend to cite North American articles. Large studies that result in several publications are more readily noticed than small ones.

Funnel plots are a way of detecting bias in the selection of studies for systematic reviews. (8) The main results of each study are plotted against sample size, with one point for each trial (Figure 12.1). In the absence of bias, small studies (plotted at the bottom of the figure) are more likely to vary in reported effect size because of statistical imprecision, and so be spread out at the bottom of the figure, surrounding the true effect size (Figure 12.1A). On the other hand, large trials (plotted at the top of the figure) yield more precise estimates and should be more closely grouped around the true effect size. The result, in the absence of bias, is a symmetrical, peaked distribution (an inverted funnel).

Bias shows up as asymmetry in the funnel plot (Figure 12.1B).

EXAMPLE

A systematic review of the effectiveness of Glucosamine and Chondroitin for osteoarthritis identified 15 double-blind, randomized, placebo-controlled trials of more than 4 weeks duration. Could these 15 studies have been a biased selection of all strong studies of this question? The authors prepared a funnel plot (Figure 12.1B). The plot shows asymmetry, with relatively few studies having both small sample size and small (or no) treatment effect. The authors interpreted this as strong evidence of publication bias. (9)

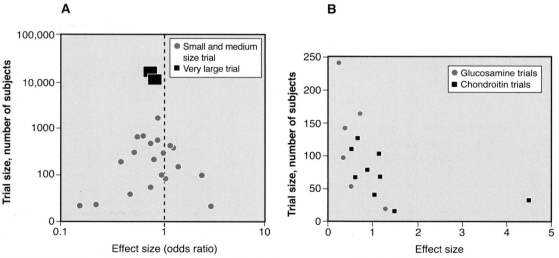

FIGURE 12.1 ▦ Funnel plots to detect publication bias. A shows a symmetrical plot of trials of streptokinase for acute myocardial infarction, suggesting no bias. Circles indicate odds ratios for small and medium-sized trials, and the squares indicate odds ratios with 95% confidence intervals for very large trials. B shows an asymmetrical funnel plot for trials of glucosamine and chondroitin sulfate for osteoarthritis. Effect size is based on a scale in which 0.8 reflects a large effect, 0.5 a moderate effect, and 0.2 a small effect. (Adapted from Egger M, Smith GD. Misleading meta-analysis: Lessons from "an effective, safe, and simple" intervention that wasn't. BMJ 1995;310:752–754; and McAlindon TE, LaValley MP, Gulin JP, Felson DT. Glucosamine and chondroitin for treatment of osteoarthritis: A systematic quality assessment and meta-analysis. JAMA 2000;283:1469–1475.)

How Good Are the Best Studies?

Clinicians need to know just how good the best studies of a question are so that they will know how seriously to take the conclusions. Are the studies so strong that it would be irresponsible to discount them? Or are they weak, suggesting that it is not unreasonable to not follow their lead?

E X A M P L E

In a meta-analysis of randomized trials of glucosamine and chondroitin for osteoarthritis, each trial was graded on 14 aspects of clinical trial conduct and was assigned an overall quality score expressed as a percentage of the maximum possible score for all these elements. The investigators reported that "only one provided sufficient information to determine that allocation concealment [whether the investigators assigning patients to treatments knew which treatment each patient would get] had been adequate . . . only 2 articles reported an intent-to-treat analysis . . . and 7 studies did not present dropout rates." The mean quality score was 35% (range 12% to 55%). Because the strength of the research evidence is far from perfect, responsible clinicians are free to recommend these drugs for osteoarthritis or not." (9)

The same criteria for quality used to select articles can be used to describe differences in quality among those selected. Table 12.4 summarizes one of the simplest sets of criteria for studies of whether or not treatment is effective. Other lists differ mainly in the number of items included.

TABLE 12.4 ■ **A Simple Scale for Measuring the Quality of Randomized Controlled Trials**

Questions

1. Was the study described as randomized?

2. Was the study described as double-blind?

3. Was there a description of withdrawals and dropouts?

Scoring

Give a score of 1 point for each "yes" and 0 points for each "no." There are no in-between marks.

(From: Jaded AR, Moore RA, Carroll D, Jenkinson C, Reynolds DJ, Govaghan DJ, et al. Assessing the quality of reports of randomized controlled trials: Is blinding necessary? Controlled Clinical Trials 1996;17:1–12.)

Is Scientific Quality Related to Research Results?

An underlying assumption of clinical epidemiology is that the results of scientifically strong studies, according to the criteria described throughout this book, will come closer to the truth than weaker studies. Is there empiric evidence for this belief?

Many studies have shown that one or another attribute of quality, such as randomization, concealment of treatment assignment, or blinding, are systematically related to study results. However, studies of the relationship between overall study quality and results, among studies selected for systematic reviews, have not shown a clear pattern. (10, 11, 12)

Why might this be? First, the component studies in systematic reviews are already highly selected and so might not differ much from one another in quality. Second, instruments to measure quality typically add up scores for the presence or absence of each element of quality and there is no reason to believe that each element makes an equal contribution to the overall validity of the study. It is not difficult to imagine, for example, weakness in one aspect of a study being so damaging that it renders the entire study invalid, even though all the other aspects of quality are perfect.

E X A M P L E

In a randomized, placebo-controlled trial, women with unexplained fatigue but no anemia had less fatigue after taking an iron supplement. The effect was small, only about 1 point on a 10-point scale for fatigue, but statistically significant. Most aspects of the study such as randomization, allocation concealment, sample size, and follow-up were strong. The iron and placebo pills were visually identical. However, iron causes characteristic side effects (such as dark stools and constipation) that could have prompted the women to recognize whether they were taking iron or placebo. Also, fatigue is a relatively "soft" outcome that might be influenced by beliefs about the effectiveness of iron supplements. Even if all other aspects of the study were beyond reproach (and the overall quality score was excellent), this one aspect of quality—patients being aware of which treatment they were taking coupled with an outcome easily influenced by this knowledge—could have accounted for the small, observed difference, rather than a true treatment effect. (13)

What is the bottom line? Quality check lists and scores have a place but are no substitute for critically examining the individual studies in a systematic review, with an eye toward how much any imperfections they do have might have influenced their results.

Summarizing Results

The results of a systematic review are typically displayed as a **forest plot** showing the point estimate and confidence interval for each of the studies. Figure 12.2 shows an example, a synthesis of studies of anticholinergic drugs for overactive bladder. (14) The measure of effectiveness in this example is change in the frequency of urination in 24 hours. The origins of the name "forest plot" are uncertain, but are variously attributed to a researcher's name or the appearance, resembling a "forest of lines." (15) We believe they help readers "see the forest and the trees."

Forest plots summarize a tremendous amount of information for the reader, information that would have required great effort to find on their own. Six kinds of information are especially useful.

1. The number of the studies meeting stringent criteria for quality. In the example, there are seven strong studies.

2. References to publications of the component studies so that readers can see how old the studies are and where they can be found. (References to studies are not shown in Figure 12.2 but are included in the article).

3. The pattern of effect sizes. Do they mostly favor the experimental treatment or placebo? Are they consistent with one another, or do they disagree? In the example, 6 of the 7 studies report an effect size favoring treatment.

4. The number of studies that are statistically significant. It may be, as shown in the figure, that most studies would have been reported as "negative" (not statistically significant or, alternatively, confidence intervals including no effect) because they were not large enough to detect a clinically-important effect. This would give the impression, in a simple accounting of the number of "positive" and "negative" studies, that treatment is not effective even though it may be effective. In the example, 4 of 7 studies did not report a statistically significant effect, even though 3 of the 4 favored treatment.

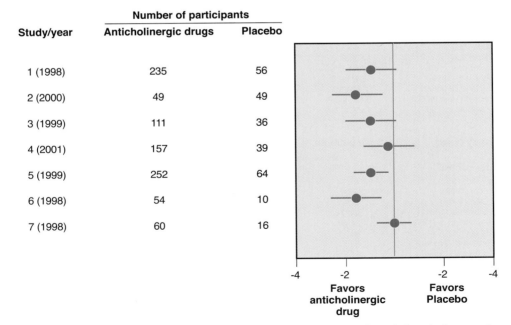

FIGURE 12.2 ▨ Forest plot of randomized controlled trials. Effectiveness of anticholinergic drugs on the number of urinations per 24 hours in patients with overactive bladder. (Redrawn from Hrebison P, Hay-Smith J, Ellis G, Moore K. Effectiveness of anticholinergic drugs compared with placebo in the treatment of overactive bladder: Systematic review. BMJ 2003;326:1–7.)

5. What do the large, statistically precise studies show relative to the smaller ones? Often, the large studies show an effect beyond chance while the small ones do not because of wide confidence intervals. In the example, the confidence interval for 1 of the 2 most precise studies (#5) excludes no effect and the other (#7) includes it.

6. The order in which studies are listed, usually chronological, shows how the results of individual studies changed over time and when the big ones were done.

In these ways, a single picture conveys in a glance a lot of basic information about the very best studies of a question.

Summarizing Observational and Diagnostic Test Studies

Systematic reviews of observational and diagnostic test studies also can be summarized by figures. Figure 12.3 shows a summary of observational studies of passive smoking and the risk of coronary heart

disease. (16) All of the cohort studies found increased risk, although results from 8 of the 10 were not statistically significant. The largest study, with the narrowest confidence intervals, showed a statistically significant result. It was difficult for the individual studies to rule out chance effects because the relative risk was small, only about 1.2, but by combining the results of all studies, the systematic review found a statistically significant association (see below for a discussion of when combining studies is justified). Case-control study results were consistent with those for cohort studies.

Studies of diagnostic tests can also be summarized in systematic reviews. Figure 12.4 shows an ROC curve summarizing data points for each of 62 studies of the sensitivity and specificity of Pap smear for cervical cancer. (17) The figure shows how sensitivity and specificity varied from study to study and defines the general shape of it as a trade-off between the two. Of course, other factors, such as patient selection and methods of sample collection, also could have accounted for some of the differences across studies.

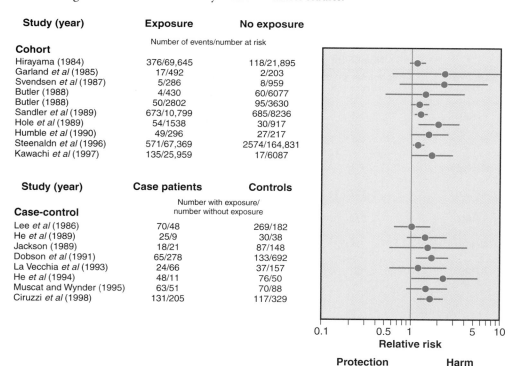

FIGURE 12.3 ■ A systematic review of observational studies of risk. A forest plot of 18 observational studies of passive smoking and relative risk of coronary heart disease. (Adapted from He J, Vipputuri S, Allen K, Prerost MS, Hughes J, Welton PK. Passive smoking and the risk of coronary heart disease—a meta-analysis of epidemiologic studies. New Engl J Med 1999;340:920–926.)

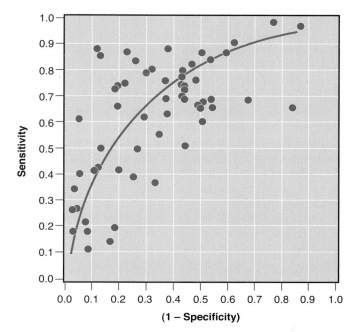

FIGURE 12.4 ■ A systematic review of diagnostic test performance. An ROC curve based on 62 studies of the sensitivity and specificity of Pap smear screening for cervical cancer. The solid line shows the summary for all studies. (From Fahey MT, Irwig L, Macaskill P. Meta-analysis of Pap test accuracy. Am J Epid 1995;141:680–689.)

COMBINING STUDIES IN META-ANALYSES

Meta-analysis is the practice of combining the results of individual studies (or patients in these studies) provided the studies are similar enough to be combined. When appropriate, meta-analyses provide more precise estimates of effect sizes than are available in any of the individual studies.

Are the Studies Similar Enough to Justify Combining?

It makes no sense to pool the results of very different studies—studies of altogether different kinds of patients, interventions, follow-ups, and outcomes. Treating "apples and oranges" as if they are all just fruits discards useful information. But reasonable people might disagree on how similar studies must be to justify combining them.

EXAMPLE

A systematic review of screening for colorectal cancer using the fecal occult blood test (FOBT) identified four randomized trials of FOBT screening that had reported colorectal cancer deaths as an outcome. Relative risks for the individual studies ranged from .86 to .67 (corresponding to relative risk reductions of 14% to 33 %). A

summary relative risk reduction for people allocated to screening, the weighted average of these 4, was 16%.

However, the studies differed substantially in the specific question they were asking. Some were of FOBT screening every year, and others were of screening every two years. Some were of rehydrated samples (rehydration increases sensitivity and decreases the specificity of the test) and others were not. Follow-up ranged from 8 to 13 years. The pattern of results matched what would be expected, given the "dose" of the screening intervention. Studies of every other year, nonrehydrated FOBT (the apparently weaker intervention) reported reduction in colorectal cancer death rates of 12% to 18%, whereas the study of yearly, rehydrated FOBT (the apparently stronger intervention) reported a reduction nearly twice as big, or 33%. The reviewers in this case were willing to combine the results of the four trials despite these differences. (18) Others have thought that the more important questions concern how the study results *differed* in relation to their conditions. For example, how much mortality reduction was lost by stretching the interval between screening tests from 1 to 2 years or by not rehydrating the sample (that is, using a less sensitive test)?

Two general approaches are used to decide whether it is appropriate to pool study results. One is a statistical test for **homogeneity**, the extent to which the trial results are similar. A statistical test is applied to the study results to see whether they differ beyond what might have been expected by chance alone. Failing to reject the null hypothesis of no difference among the studies may seem reassuring, but there is a problem. Most meta-analyses are of relatively few studies and so of limited statistical power. The risk of a false-negative result, a conclusion that the studies are homogeneous when they are not, is typically high. Power is also affected by the number of patients in these studies and how evenly they are distributed among the studies. (19) If one of the component studies is much larger than the others, it contributes most of the information bearing on the question and it may be more useful to examine it carefully, then contrast it with the others.

A second approach is to make an informed judgment about whether the patients, interventions, follow-up, and outcomes are similar enough to constitute studies of the same (or reasonably similar) question. Thus, regardless of the results of a statistical test, one might be reluctant to pool studies of the effectiveness of vitamins E, A, and C on the grounds that they are all "antioxidants." On the other hand, some trials are so similar to one another that it seems totally reasonable to combine them.

EXAMPLE

A meta-analysis of the effectiveness of thyroid hormone suppressive therapy for benign solitary thyroid nodules was restricted to 6 randomized trials involving 346 patients. Each study met stringent criteria: ". . . solitary nodule proven benign by fine needle aspiration, follow-up of at least 6 months, documented suppression of thyroid-stimulating hormone, and measurements by ultrasound." (20) The relative risk was 1.9 (favoring treatment), but even for the combined data confidence intervals were wide—0.95 to 3.81. So, up to the point in time when that meta-analysis was done, it seemed likely but not certain that thyroid hormone had a small effect on benign thyroid nodule size. It would seem that the strict selection criteria produced a homogeneous set of trials. It might be argued, however, that homogeneity remains in question because many different diseases produce benign thyroid nodules, and they might differ in their response to thyroid hormone.

What Is Combined—Studies or Patients?

Until now, the discussion has been about how *studies* are combined, which is the usual way meta-analyses are done. But an even more powerful approach is to obtain data on each individual *patient* in each of the

component studies and to pool these data to produce, in effect, a single large study. Relatively few meta-analyses are done this way because of the difficulties in obtaining all these data from the investigators. However, when it can be done it becomes possible to look for effects in clinically important subgroups of patients such as the severely affected, the elderly, or those with other diseases. The numbers of patients in these subgroups are likely to be too small in the individual studies to produce stable estimates of effects, but the pooled numbers may be sufficient.

EXAMPLE

The Antithrombotic Trialists' Collaboration studied the effects of antiplatelet therapy on vascular events in patients at high risk of cardiovascular disease. The investigators identified 195 strong randomized controlled trials of this question. They asked the authors of trials that had included at least 200 patients to provide data on individual patients. Overall, allocation to antiplatelet therapy reduced the rate of any serious vascular event by about one quarter. With meta-analyses of patient-level data, investigators were able to show that antiplatelet therapy prevented vascular events in patients who had acute myocardial infarction, stable angina, atrial fibrillation, and cardiac valve surgery. This information was not available in the individual trials and became available only after combining patient-level data from all of the trials. (21)

How Are the Results Summarized?

When studies are summarized, those that contribute large amounts of information are weighted more heavily than those that make small contributions. Each individual study contributes to the summary effect size in relation to its size (strictly speaking, the inverse of its variance).

Two kinds of mathematical models are used to summarize studies in a meta-analysis. (22) These models differ in what is being summarized and in how conservative they are in estimating overall confidence intervals (Figure 12.5). We summarize the concepts involved but not the mathematics.

With the **fixed-effect model**, it is assumed that each of the studies is of exactly the same question so that the results of the studies differ only by chance. This model is called "fixed effect" because only one underlying effect size is assumed, although the results of the individual studies do differ from one another because of the play of chance. The main problem with this approach is that, on the face of it, the studies rarely

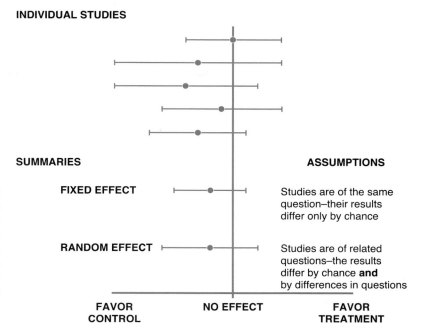

INDIVIDUAL STUDIES

SUMMARIES

FIXED EFFECT

RANDOM EFFECT

ASSUMPTIONS

Studies are of the same
question–their results
differ only by chance

Studies are of related
questions–the results
differ by chance **and**
by differences in questions

**FAVOR
CONTROL**   **NO EFFECT**   **FAVOR
TREATMENT**

FIGURE 12.5 ▪ Two ways to summarize studies in a meta-analysis: Fixed-effect and random-effects models. Studies are represented by point estimates and confidence intervals. Estimates of effect size are similar for the two methods. The confidence intervals are narrower for the summaries than for individual studies but wider for the random- than for fixed- effect model.

resemble one another so closely in terms of patients, interventions, follow-up, and outcomes that they can be considered simple replications of one another. Should aspirin, sulfinpyrazone, and clopidogrel really be considered simply examples of "antiplatelet drugs," even though they have different biochemical structures and mechanisms of action? Or are they different enough from one another that they might have different effects? To the extent that the study questions differ somewhat, the width of confidence intervals calculated by the fixed-effect model tends to imply a greater degree of precision than is actually the case. Also, by combining dissimilar studies one loses useful information that might have resulted from contrasting them. An example is the combining for FOBT studies, described above.

The **random-effects model** assumes that the studies address somewhat different questions and that they form a closely related family of studies of a similar question. The studies are taken to be a random sample of all studies bearing on the question. Even if a statistical test for homogeneity fails, it may still be reasonable to combine studies using a random-effects model, as long as the studies are similar enough to one another (obviously a value judgment). Random-effects models produce wider confidence intervals than fixed-effect models and for this

reason are thought to be more realistic. However, it is uncertain how the family of similar studies is defined and whether the studies are really a random sample of all such studies of a question. Nevertheless, because random-effects models at least take heterogeneity into account, and are less likely to overestimate precision, they are the model most often used in recent years.

Displaying the Summary Effect

When an overall effect size is calculated, it is usually displayed as a point estimate and confidence interval at the bottom of the forest plot of component studies. Figure 12.6 shows an example from a systematic review of lipid-lowering drugs for the primary prevention of coronary heart disease. (23) The summary is often displayed as a diamond, to distinguish it from the individual studies. The summary effect is a more precise and formalized presentation of what might have been concluded from the pattern of results available in the forest plot.

Cumulative Meta-analysis

Usually the studies in a forest plot are represented separately in chronological order. Another way to

	Number events/number subjects	
Study/year	**Treated group**	**Control group**
1 (1984)	68/1906	71/1900
2 (1987)	45/2051	42/2030
3 (1995)	106/3302	135/3293
4 (1998)	152/3304	145/3301
Total	**371/10,563**	**393/10,524**

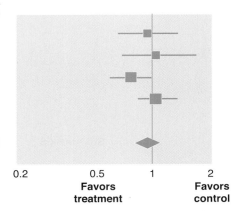

0.2   0.5   1   2

Favors treatment   Favors control

FIGURE 12.6 ▪ A forest plot showing summary effect and confidence interval. The effect of lipid-lowering drugs on coronary heart disease mortality in patients with no known coronary heart disease. (Data form Pignone M, Phillips C, Mulrow C. Use of lipid-lowering drugs for primary prevention of coronary heart disease: Meta-analysis of randomized trials. BMJ 2000;321:986–990.)

look at the same information is to present a **cumulative meta-analysis**. A new summary effect size and confidence interval is calculated each time the results of a new study become available. The figure, therefore, represents a running summary of all the studies up to each point in time.

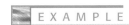

E X A M P L E

Figure 12.7 is a cumulative meta-analysis of 21 randomized controlled trials of antibiotic prophylaxis for colorectal surgery published between 1969 and 1987. Most of the studies were relatively small (the mean sample size was 73), and all were "negative" trials; that is, none was statistically significant. However, a cumulative meta-analysis shows that it was clear from about 1975, after 603 patients had been randomized, that antibiotic prophylaxis was protective. Subsequent studies merely narrowed the confidence interval of the estimated effect size. (24)

Cumulative meta-analyses make apparent the point in time when the studies as a whole had answered the question conclusively (beyond chance) and how studies after that time have narrowed the statistical precision of the summary effect size. The columns show the cumulative number of patients randomized as time passed, and the rows show the years in which the various studies were done. Cumulative meta-analyses have provided insights into the state of the science concerning some questions that were not apparent to experts in the field, who had relied on less formal summaries of the same information.

What Are the Advantages and Risks of Combining Studies?

The distinct advantage of pooling is that it improves statistical power. Looked at another way, it produces more precise estimates of effect size.

E X A M P L E

None of the individual studies summarized in Figure 12.7 was statistically significant, yet the results of 17 of the 21 studies favored treatment. Confidence intervals for most of the studies were wide, suggesting that none was, by itself, of sufficient size to answer the question. But taken together, in the meta-analysis, there was more than enough power to conclude that antibiotics worked for this purpose.

This advantage extends to subgroups. Most studies are planned to be only large enough to answer the main research question. But when study results are combined, it may be possible to find effects in clinically important subgroups, as illustrated for antiplatelet drugs and cardiovascular disease earlier in this chapter. Combining studies provides a more precise estimate of effect size than is available from each of the individual studies. This may make it possible to decide whether the effect is likely to be big enough to be clinically important or that a clinically important effect has been ruled out.

The advantage also extends to the detection of rare events, such as uncommon side effects of

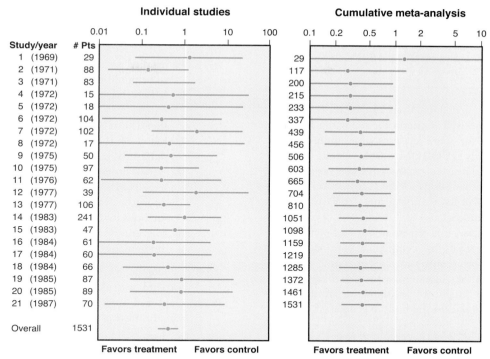

Individual studies

Cumulative meta-analysis

FIGURE 12.7 ▦ A cumulative meta-analysis. Reduction in perioperative deaths (oddsratios) by antibiotic prophylaxis for colorectal surgery. On the left are studies in chronological order; on the right is a cumulative meta-analysis. (From Lau J, Schmid CH, Chalmers TC. Cumulative meta-analysis of clinical trials builds evidence for exemplary medical care. J Clin Epid 1995;48:45–57.)

treatment. Most clinical trials are, by design, not large enough to detect an increased rate of uncommon side effects, even if they are severe. Postmarketing surveillance of much larger numbers of people taking a drug is used to identify these effects. But pooling studies, each of which reported only a handful of these outcome events, might make it possible to detect a difference in rare event rates in the intervention and control groups. These effects can be established with a lot more rigor in randomized trials than is possible in postmarketing surveillance, an observational approach.

The main disadvantage of meta-analyses is that they can give the misleading impression that results are known with a high degree of precision when in fact many assumptions underlie the main results. Also, pooling draws attention away from differences in study results that may provide insights into clinically important differences in effects, such as the differences in various types of fecal occult blood testing for colorectal cancer, described earlier. Another disadvantage is that meta-analyses usually report pooled

effects as estimated relative risks (odds ratios) because of the mathematical models they are based on, whereas effectiveness might differ according to level of baseline risk. Clinicians need information on the underlying outcome event rates (risk difference).

When Meta-analyses and Large Trials Disagree

The results of meta-analyses and large randomized trials usually agree. Indeed, larger trials receive the most weight in meta-analyses. There have been, however, disconcerting examples of meta-analyses of small trials disagreeing with the results of a subsequent large trial of the same question.

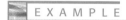

EXAMPLE

In the combined results of small trials, magnesium reduced mortality during acute myocardial infarction. In contrast, a megatrial (>10,000 patients), which was undertaken in part because of effectiveness reported in smaller trials, showed no evidence of effect. The difference between results of meta-analysis and megatrial was explained by differences in the baseline event rate, differences in study design, or publication bias. The best evidence favored the results of the megatrial in this case. (25)

Of course, a meta-analysis can be misleading if it is not done well. Criteria for reporting have been proposed for meta-analyses of randomized controlled trials **QUOROM** (26) as well as diagnostic tests. (27) The Meta-analysis of Observational Studies in Epidemiology (MOOSE) Group has suggested a plan for reporting meta-analyses of observational studies. (28)

In any case, it is unwise to think of meta-analyses and large trials as competing with each other. Rather, both contribute information. The main issue when they disagree is why they disagree, which should be sought by examination of the studies themselves, not the methods in general.

REVIEW QUESTIONS

Read the following and circle the best response.

12.1. A systematic review of observational studies of antioxidant vitamins to prevent cardiovascular disease combined the results of 12 studies to obtain a summary effect size and confidence interval. Which of the following would be the strongest rationale for combining studies results?

  A. You wish to obtain a more generalizable conclusion.
  B. A statistical test shows that the studies are heterogeneous.
  C. Most of the component studies are statistically significant.
  D. The component studies have different, and to some extent complementary, biases.
  E. A more precise estimate of effect size is needed than the individual studies provide.

12.2. You are asked to critique a review of the literature on whether alcohol is a risk factor for breast cancer. You see that the reviewer has searched MEDLINE and found several

observational studies of this question. All of the following are limitations of this search strategy except

  A. Studies with negative results tend not to be published.
  B. MEDLINE searches typically miss some articles even when they are included in the MEDLINE database.
  C. Many of the world's studies are not published in MEDLINE.
  D. Some articles are found by asking experts in this field, looking up recent review articles, and following up on citations in the articles you have found.
  E. The studies you have found are not randomized controlled trials.

12.3. Systematic reviews of antiplatelet agents for cardiovascular disease prevention have combined individual patients, not trials. An advantage of this approach is:

  A. It is more efficient for the investigator.
  B. It is possible to obtain more precise estimates of effect in clinically important subgroups of patients.
  C. Flaws in study design can be overcome.
  D. It is not necessary to choose between fixed- and random-effects models when combining data.
  E. Publication bias is less likely.

Read the statements below and mark each one True or False.

You are aware of growing evidence that aspirin is effective for the primary prevention of cardiovascular disease. You find a cumulative meta-analysis of this question in the Cochrane Database of Systematic Reviews. The following are advantages of this graphic summary:

_____ 12.4. You can see when and how each new trial has changed the overall evidence of effectiveness.

_____ 12.5. The summary effect size is the best available estimate of the true effect size for similar patients.

_____ 12.6. You can be confident that all of the trials studied exactly the same research question.

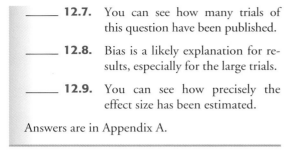

12.7. You can see how many trials of this question have been published.

12.8. Bias is a likely explanation for results, especially for the large trials.

12.9. You can see how precisely the effect size has been estimated.

Answers are in Appendix A.

REFERENCES

1. Haynes RB, Wilczynski N, McKibbon KA, Walker CJ, Sinclair JC. Developing optimal search strategies for detecting clinically sound studies in MEDLINE. J Am Med Informatics Assoc 1994;1:447–458. (Also in Sackett DL, Straus SE, Richardson WS, Rosneberg W, Haynes RB. Evidence-Based Medicine: How to Practice and Teach EBM. 2nd Ed. New York:Churchill Livingstone, 2000.)

2. Moher D, Schulz KF, Altman DG, for the CONSORT Group. The CONSORT statement: Revised recommendations for improving the quality of parallel-group randomized trials. Ann Intern Med 2001; 134:657–662.

3. Bossuyt PM, Reitsma JB, Bruns DE, Gatsonis CA, Glaszion PP, Irwig LM, et al. Toward complete and accurate reporting of studies of diagnostic accuracy: The STARD Initiative. Ann Intern Med 2003;138: 40–44.

4. Easterbrook PJ, Berlin JA, Gopalan R, Matthews DR. Publication bias in clinical research. Lancet 1991;337: 867–872.

5. Dickersin K, Min Y-I, Meinert CL. Factors influencing publication of research results. JAMA 1992;267: 374–378.

6. Lexchin J, Bero LA, Djulbegovic B, Clark O. Pharmaceutical industry sponsorship and research outcome and quality: Systematic review. BMJ 2003;326: 1167–1170.

7. Rennie D. Thyroid storm. JAMA 1997;277:1238–1243.

8. Egger M, Smith GD, Schneider M, Minder C. Bias in meta-analysis detected by a simple, graphical test. BMJ 1997;315:629–634.

9. McAlindon TE, LaValley MP, Gulin JP, Felson DT. Glucosamine and chondroitin for treatment of osteoarthritis: A systematic quality assessment and meta-analysis. JAMA 2000;283:1469–1475.

10. Balk EM, Bonis PA, Moskowitz H, Schmid CH, Ioannidis JP, Wang C, et al. Correlation of quality measures with estimates of treatment effect in meta-analyses of randomized controlled trials. JAMA 2002; 287:2973–2982.

11. Juni P, Witschi A, Bloch R, Egger M. The hazards of scoring quality of clinical trials for meta-analyses. JAMA 1999; 282:1054–1060.

12. Moher D, Pham B, Jones A, Cook DJ, Jadad AR, Moher M, et al. Does quality of reports of randomized trials affect estimates of intervention efficacy reported in meta-analyses? Lancet 1998;352:609–613.

13. Verdon F, Burnaud B, Stubi CLF, Graff CBM, Michaud M, Bischoff T, et al. Iron supplementation for unexplained fatigue in nonanemic women: Double-blind, randomized, placebo controlled trial. BMJ 2003;326:1124–1228. [In EB Practice]

14. Herbison P, Hay-Smith J, Ellig, Moore K. Effectiveness of anticholinergic drugs compared with placebo in the treatment of overactive bladder: Systematic review. BMJ 2003;326:841–844.

15. Lewis S, Clarke M. Forest plots: Trying to see the woods and the trees. BMJ 2001;322:1479–1480.

16. He J, Vipputuri S, Allen K, Prerost MR, Hughes J, Welton PK. Passive smoking and the risk of coronary heart disease—a meta-analysis of epidemiologic studies. New Engl J Med 1999;340:920–926.

17. Fahey MT, Irwig L, Macaskill P. Meta-analysis of Pap test accuracy. Am J Epid 1995;141:680–687.

18. Towler B, Irwig L, Glasziou P, Kewenter J, Weller D, Silagy C. A systematic review of the effects of screening for colorectal cancer using the faecal occult blood test, Hemoccult. BMJ 1998;317:559–565.

19. Hardy RJ, Thompson SG. Detecting and describing heterogeneity in meta-analysis. Statistics in Medicine 1998;17:841–856.

20. Castro MR, Carabello PJ, Morris JC. Effectiveness of thyroid hormone suppressive therapy in benign solitary thyroid nodules: A meta-analysis. J Clin Endocrinol Metab 2002;87:4154–4159.

21. Antithrombotic Trialists' Collaboration. Collaborative meta-analysis of randomized trials of antiplatelet therapy for prevention of death, myocardial infarction, and stroke in high risk patients. BMJ 2002;324: 71–86.

22. Lau J, Ioannidis JPA, Schmid CH. Summing up the evidence: One answer is not always enough. Lancet 1998;351:123–127.

23. Pignone M, Phillips C, Mulrow C. Use of lipid-lowering drugs for primary prevention of coronary heart disease: A meta-analysis of randomized trials. BMJ 2000;321:983–986.

24. Lau J, Schmid CH, Chalmers TC. Cumulative meta-analysis of clinical trials builds evidence for exemplary medical care. J Clin Epid 1995;48:45–57.

25. Cappelleri JC, Ioannidis JPA, Schmidt CH, de Ferranti SD, Aubert M, Chalmers TC, et al. Large trials versus meta-analysis of smaller trials. JAMA 1996;276: 1332–1338.

26. Moher D, Cook DJ, Eastwood S, Olkin I, Rennie D, Stroup DF for the QUOROM Group. Improving the quality of reports of meta-analyses of randomized

controlled trials: The QUOROM statement. Lancet 1999;354:1896–1900.

27. Irwig L, Tosteson ANA, Gatsonis C, Lau J, Colditz G, Chalmers TC, et al. Guidelines for meta-analyses evaluating diagnostic tests. Ann Intern Med 1994; 120:667–676.

28. Stroup DF, Berlin JA, Morton SC, Olkin I, Williamson GD, Rennie D, et al. For the Meta-Analysis of Observational Studies in Epidemiology (MOOSE) Group. Meta-analysis of observational studies in epidemiology: A proposal for reporting. JAMA 2000;283:2008–2012.

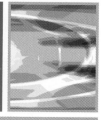

Knowledge Management

It is astonishing with how little reading a doctor can practice medicine, but it is not astonishing how badly he may do it.

— William Osler

Finding the best available answer to a specific clinical question is like finding a needle in a haystack. Essential information is mixed with a vast amount of less credible data, and it is a daunting task to sort the wheat from the chaff. Yet that is what clinicians need to do. Critical reading is only as good as the information found.

Knowledge management is the effective and efficient organization of knowledge (valid, useful information, as opposed to information in general). This was a difficult task in the days of print media only. Fortunately, knowledge management is a great deal easier now than it was just a few years ago. There are more and better studies on a broad range of clinical questions, widely available access to this information, and ways to rapidly sort information by topic and scientific strength. These opportunities followed the widespread availability of computers, the World Wide Web, and electronic databases for clinical purposes.

Finding information may seem to be a low priority for clinicians still in training. They are surrounded by information, far more than they can handle comfortably, and they have countless experts who help them to pick and choose the information they should take most seriously and that which they can disregard. However, developing one's own plan for managing knowledge becomes crucial later on, whether in practice or academe.

Even with recent developments, effective and efficient knowledge management is a challenging task. In this chapter, we review modern approaches to clinical knowledge management.

A BASIC CHOICE—DO IT YOURSELF OR DELEGATE?

Clinicians must first ask themselves, "Will I find and judge clinical research results for myself or delegate this task to someone else?" The answer should be both. Clinicians should be able to find and critique information on their own; it is a basic skill in clinical medicine. But as a practical matter, it is not possible to go it alone for all of one's information needs. There are just too many questions in a day and too little time apart from patient care. The question really is, "Which knowledge management tasks should I delegate and to whom?" When clinicians delegate, it should be to a trusted source, preferably the best available to them.

EXAMPLE

A patient sees you because he will be traveling to Ghana and wants advice on malaria prophylaxis. You are aware that the malaria parasite's susceptibility to antimalarial drugs varies across the globe and that it is continually changing. The textbooks in your office, though relatively recent editions, are out of date for this purpose, and it is unlikely that you will be able to track down an infectious disease consultant while the patient is waiting. Fortunately, you remember that the Centers for Disease Control and Prevention has a Web site (http://www.cdc.gov) with current information for travelers to all parts of the world. With it, you quickly find out which prophylactic drug this patient should take and for how long—before and after the trip. You are also reminded that he should be vaccinated for hepatitis A and B, yellow fever, and meningitis. The information you are relying on is the best available because it is a synthesis of the world's best evidence, is continually updated, and is available to you within seconds.

WHICH MEDIUM SHOULD I USE?

A rich array of media now exists by which one can obtain information. They range from printed books and journals to digital information on computers via the Web, CD-ROMs, and DVDs. There are audiotapes, videotapes, and more (Figure 13.1). The information is neither more nor less sound because of the medium by which it happens to come to you. Validity depends on authors and editors, not the medium. However, the availability of various media, with complementary advantages and disadvantages, makes it easier to find ones that match every user's preferences.

LOOKING UP ANSWERS TO CLINICAL QUESTIONS

One of the clinicians' information needs is to be able to look up answers to questions. They certainly

need this for things they do not know. Beyond that, sometimes they should look up answers to questions they think they know but might not, because the information base for patient care is always changing.

Criteria for Useful Clinical Information Sources

If an information source is to be useful, it must meet a very demanding set of criteria (Table 13.1).

Rapid Access

Clinicians must be able to obtain the information they need rapidly, usually within minutes. Even just a few extra minutes per patient adds a great deal of time to their workday and may not be feasible. Fast access to information allows clinicians to use what they have found to make decisions about the individual patient they are seeing at the time. Also, information acquired at the time it is most needed, called **just-in-time learning**, is more likely to be retained than information imparted out of context in, for example, a classroom or lecture hall, or in books or journals. Putting off answering the question to a later time is an unreliable substitute. Also, it is usually less helpful to the patient.

Up-to-Date

If a clinician is to make high-stakes decisions based on evidence, the evidence must reflect the state of knowledge at the time. True, older information is sometimes adequate. In many ways, recognition of an acute abdomen or an attack of gout has not changed much over the years. But other aspects of medicine such as choosing antiviral agents for patients with HIV infection, recognizing the clinical presentation of Hanta virus infection or SARS, state-of-the-art management of macular degeneration, or prescribing disease-modifying drugs for rheumatoid arthritis are changing rapidly.

Unfortunately, printed books contain relatively old information. Their contents are somewhat out of date by the time they are printed (having been written several months earlier) and only become more dated with time. Perhaps for this reason, books and journal reviews tend to be conservative in recommending changes in usual practice.

EXAMPLE

How do expert recommendations in books and journal reviews compare with the most rigorous available evi-

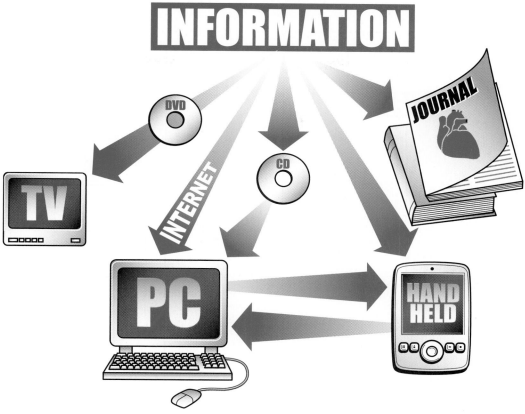

FIGURE 13.1 ■ The dissemination of the evidence base for medicine. Content matters while the media used for dissemination are a matter of convenience.

dence on a question? Figure 13.2 compares the results of a cumulative meta-analysis (see Chapter 12) of thrombolytic therapy for acute myocardial infarction with the recommendations of clinical experts who have written review articles and textbook chapters. (1) Although it was clear by the early 1970s that thrombolytic therapy was effective, it was not until 1985 that the majority of textbooks and journal reviews recommended it as usual care. Was this just for thrombolytic therapy? No, the same phenomenon was found for other treatments aimed at reducing the risk of death from acute myocardial infarction—drugs now widely accepted such as aspirin and oral beta-blockers. On the other hand, many experts still recommended lidocaine to prevent ventricular fibrillation after acute myocardial infarction at a time when 9 of 9 clinical trials had shown that the drug caused net harm (although none of the studies was statistically significant). Is lag between evidence and expert recommendations still a problem? Probably, but perhaps less so than in the past because of wider appreciation of evidence-based medicine, dissemination of systematic reviews, and availability of continually updated textbooks.

Tailored to the Specific Question

Clinicians want to find information that corresponds as closely as possible to the specific clinical situation they are in. If the patient is elderly and has several diseases, the research information should be about elderly patients with comorbidities. Medicine is such a personal experience that clinicians and

TABLE 13.1 ■ Criteria for Useful Sources of Clinical Information
Rapid access
Up to date
Can be tailored to specific questions
Can be sorted by scientific strength
Portable

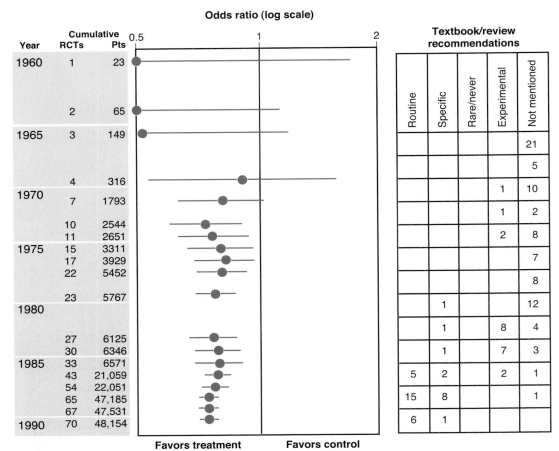

FIGURE 13.2 ■ Expert recommendations tend to be out of date. Comparison of the results of a cumulative meta-analysis of the effectiveness of thrombolytic therapy for acute myocardial infarction to recommendations by clinical experts in textbooks and review articles. RCTs = randomized controlled trials. PTs = patients. (From Antman EM, Lau J, Kupelnick B, Mosteller F, Chalmers TC. A comparison of results of meta-analyses of randomized control trials and recommendations of clinical experts: Treatment of myocardial infarction. JAMA 1992;268:240–248.)

patients want the evidence to match their specific circumstances as much as possible. Modern search engines make it possible to make precise matches between the clinical situation and research information, limited only by the level of detail in the information base.

Sorted by Scientific Strength

Clinical information needs to be sorted by its scientific strength. What the clinician needs is not *an* answer but the best available answer, given the state of knowledge at the time.

The clinician also needs to know just how credible that information is. The extent to which research information should drive practice decisions depends on its scientific strength. Clinicians need to locate the information on a spectrum of certainty, from just an idea based on reasoning, intuition, or custom to strong research evidence (Figure 13.3). If evidence for a practice is sparse, expert recommendations based on a plausible rationale or usual practice may be a useful guide, but the clinician has the latitude to try other approaches. On the other hand, if the effectiveness of a practice has been well established by strong research evidence, it would be irresponsible to ignore it except for very good reasons related to the individual patient's clinical situation and preferences.

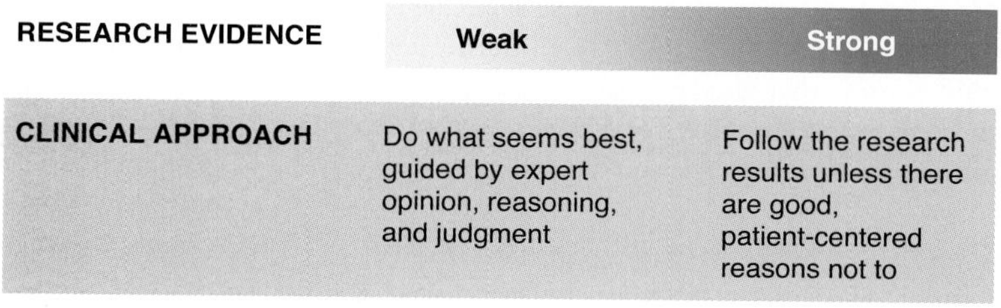

RESEARCH EVIDENCE	Weak	Strong
CLINICAL APPROACH	Do what seems best, guided by expert opinion, reasoning, and judgment	Follow the research results unless there are good, patient-centered reasons not to

FIGURE 13.3 ■ The certainty spectrum. Relationship between the strength of the research evidence on a clinical question and the latitude for clinical decision making.

Portable

Clinicians move around in their work. They travel from their office to home (where they take night and weekend call) and to hospitals and nursing homes. They need information sources that move with them. Print media, except those that fit in a pocket or brief case, are limited in this way. So are desktop computers, unless clinicians are always near terminals where the Internet can be accessed. Hand-held computers are less limited by memory than in the past but have small screens and keyboards, limiting displays of text, tables, and figures.

Modern Solutions

We will mention a few kinds of information sources that were available when this chapter was prepared. We have made no effort to be a comprehensive listing are shown below. Indeed, the options will change rapidly over time.

Electronic Textbooks

Information technology is rapidly making electronic textbooks a reality. For example, UpToDate, the electronic library of medicine (we are among dozens of its editors) is continually updated, contains the equivalent of more than 70,000 printed pages, and can be rapidly searched. Abstracts for citations are part of the database, as are graphics of all sorts, including video, illustrations, and audio. *ACP Medicine,* Harrison's *Textbook of Medicine,* and many other "textbooks" are now updated continually and available online. Search engines allow users to target very specific questions in seconds.

Clinical Practice Guidelines

Clinical practice guidelines are recommendations to clinicians for the care of patients with specific conditions. Besides giving recommendations, good guidelines also make explicit the evidence base and rationale for the recommendations. Like evidence-based medicine,

guidelines are meant to be a starting place for decision making about individual patients, to be modified by clinical judgment; that is, they are guidelines, not rules. High-quality guidelines represent wise application of research evidence to the realities of clinical care. But guidelines vary in quality. Table 13.2 summarizes some criteria for credible guidelines. A relatively comprehensive listing of guidelines can be found at the

---

TABLE 13.2 ■ **Criteria for Guidelines You Can Trust**

Attribute	Rationale
Diverse expertise of authors	Including different types of expertise enriches the possibilities and provides checks and balances on special interests.
Evidence based	Honesty and clarity are fostered when all recommendations are backed by an explicit statement of rationale, either the base in research evidence or reasoning from existing information.
Considers all of the consequences of recommendations	Clinical decisions take into account not just effectiveness but also risks, availability and costs.
Current	Guidelines tend to go out of date. Each version should be dated.
Sponsor	Guidelines tend to be more carefully prepared when the reputations of a sponsoring society or government organizations stand behind them.
External review	Review by other interested organizations provides checks and balances against omissions and narrow or self-serving agendas.

National Guideline Clearinghouse available online at http://www.guidelines.gov. A limitation of most guidelines is that they go out of date. In one study, more than three quarters of guidelines from one major government organization needed updating. (2)

The Cochrane Database of Systematic Reviews

Clinical scientists throughout the world have volunteered to review the world's literature on specific treatment questions, to synthesize this information in the Cochrane Database of Systematic Reviews, and to keep it up to date. The collection of all such reviews is available at http://www.cochrane.org. While the Cochrane Database is far from complete, given the vast number of questions it might address, it is an excellent source of rigorously selected information on the effects of interventions.

Clinical Evidence

"Clinical Evidence," a publication of the British Medical Journal, summarizes the best available evidence for the effects of common clinical interventions. Reviews are guided by the principles of evidence-based medicine. New editions of "Best Evidence" are published twice a year and available in print and on CD-ROM.

MEDLINE

MEDLINE is a database of more than 4,500 worldwide journals in 30 languages; half of these journals are published in the United States, and 89% of the articles are in English. It is easy to access MEDLINE (part of The National Library of Medicine) from any computer, and the Web site contents are available at no cost. MEDLINE can be searched by topic, journal, author, year, and research design at http://www.nlm.nih.gov. In addition to citations, abstracts are available.

MEDLINE is a valuable element of any comprehensive search of the literature. However, MEDLINE searches have two major misclassification problems. First, searches produce many false-positive results; that is, they find more citations than are actually wanted on the basis of scientific strength and clinical relevance. Second, they produce false-negative results; that is, they miss articles, such as randomized trials of the effect of an intervention, which really are wanted. Both problems can be reduced by better searching techniques. (3)

MEDLINE searches are a mainstay for investigators and educators who have the time to construct careful searches and sort through the resulting articles. But MEDLINE searches are too inefficient to be of much practical value in helping clinicians, especially when they need to answer day-to-day questions quickly. As one of many clinicians' resources, however, MEDLINE is essential, particularly for looking up whether rare events have been reported.

E X A M P L E

You are seeing a patient whom you thought had cat scratch disease and who now has abdominal pain. After ruling out other causes, you wonder whether the abdominal pain might be from abdominal lymphadenopathy. Has this unusual occurrence ever been reported? You do a MEDLINE search and find that in fact there has been such a case report. (4) Armed with this information, even though about just one case, you are more confident in your diagnosis and management.

SURVEILLANCE ON NEW DEVELOPMENTS

Keeping up with new developments in any clinical field is a daunting task. It is not that the pace of practice-changing discoveries is unmanageable. Rather, the relevant information is widely dispersed across many journals and mixed with a vast number of less important articles.

E X A M P L E

How widely are the best articles in a field dispersed among journals? The Editors of *ACP Journal Club* regularly review more than 80 journals and select scientifically strong (by explicit criteria), clinically relevant articles in internal medicine. The results are published in a bimonthly journal. This process provides an opportunity to estimate, at least for internal medicine, the degree to which key articles are dispersed among journals. Figure 13.4 shows the proportion of key articles a reader would encounter according to the number of journals read, starting with the highest yield journal and adding journals in order of descending yield. One would need to review regularly 9 journals to find half of these articles and 30 journals to find 90% of them.

Therefore, it is not possible for individual readers, even with great effort, to find all of the essential articles in a field on their own. They need to delegate the task to a trusted intermediary, one who will

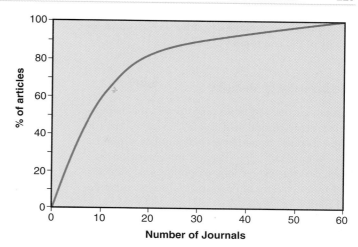

FIGURE 13.4 ▦ How many journals would you have to read to keep up with the literature in your field? The proportion of scientifically strong, clinically relevant articles in internal medicine according to the number of journals, in descending order of yield (Data from ACP Journal Club, January–June, 2004).

review many journals and select articles according to criteria they agree with.

Fortunately, help is available. Most clinical specialties have publications that summarize relevant articles in their field. These publications vary in how explicit and rigorous their selection process is. At one extreme, *ACP Journal Club* publishes its criteria for each kind of article (studies of prevention, treatment, diagnosis, prognosis, to name a few) with each issue and provides a critique of each article it selects. At the other extreme, many newsletters include summaries of articles without making explicit either how they were selected or what their strengths and limitations are.

JOURNALS

Journals have a special role in the health professions, at both the emotional and the practical level. Every clinician should subscribe to a few journals and look at them regularly, whatever else they do to manage information.

First, let us acknowledge what journals are not good for. Individual journals are not a reliable way of keeping up with new scientific developments in a field. The important articles are just too widely dispersed, as discussed above, so clinicians must rely on collections of articles across many journals. Access to a few journals is also not an efficient resource for looking up the answers to clinical questions; journals' contents are just not organized for that purpose.

What at least the best journals *are* good for is assuring that reports of original research, the foun-

dation of all clinical information, are sound. They also expose readers to all the dimensions of the medical profession, beyond the research information that clinicians believe they need for patient care.

Guardians of Science

Research reports are selected and improved before publication by a rigorous process involving critical review by editors who are guided by advice from scholars outside the journal offices (**peer review**). Often biostatisticians participate in reviews. Peer review is intended to select for publication articles that are about important, unanswered questions and are based on scientifically sound methods. Editors and peer reviewers provide suggestions for improvement to authors of submitted papers. Another agenda is to maintain ethical standards for such issues as duplicate publication, plagiarism, conflict of interest, and fraud. All articles undergo careful technical editing before publication to ensure that they are clearly expressed. Acceptance rates are as low as 6% of submitted manuscripts for some of the major journals, mainly because submitted manuscripts compete for a fixed number of published pages.

Peer review and editing practices, along with the research basis and rationale for them, are summarized on the official Web site of the World Association of Medical Editors, which can be accessed at http://www.wame.org. These practices have been shown to improve articles. (5) Nevertheless, published articles are far from perfect, so readers should be grateful for the journals' efforts to make articles better but also maintain a healthy skepticism of the quality of the end result.

The Diversity of Medicine

Journals are one way of keeping up with the many dimensions of a clinical field. Table 13.3 summarizes the kinds of issues covered in general journals. Opinions, stories, untested hypotheses, commentary on published articles, expressions of professional values as well as descriptions of the historical, social, and political context of current-day medicine and much more, reflect the full nature of the profession. One would not otherwise encounter this kind of information with even the best plan for looking up information and maintaining surveillance on new scientific developments. The richness of this information completes the clinical picture for many readers. For example, when we were editors of *Annals of Internal Medicine*, we began publishing stories about being a doctor. (6) Many readers remarked that while reports of research and reviews were essential, the experience of being a doctor was what they cared about the most.

"Reading" Journals

The ability to critique research on one's own is a core skill for clinicians. But this skill is used selectively and to different degrees, just as the completeness of the history and physical examination, which is part of a clinician's repertoire, is used to a varying extent from one patient encounter to another. A compressed version of critical reading, based on an in-depth understanding of the more complete approach, is more feasible. In this form, it can be practiced throughout a clinician's workday.

How can critical reading be simplified responsibly? It is not necessary to read journals from cover to cover, any more than one would read a newspaper from front to back. Rather, one can read in layers, according to the time available and the strength and relevance of each individual article.

Approaches to streamlined reading vary. It is a good idea to at least survey the titles (analogous to newspaper headlines) of all articles in an issue to decide which articles matter most to you. For those articles, one would dig more deeply, but only as deeply as is justified by their importance (Figure 13.5). The abstract is the best place to start, and many responsible readers stop there. If the conclusions are interesting, the methods section might come next; there, one finds basic information bearing on whether the conclusions are credible. One might want to look at the results section to see a more detailed description of what was found. Key figures (such as a survival curve for the main results of a randomized trial) may communicate the "bottom line" powerfully. A few articles are so important, in relation to one's particular needs, that they are worth reading word-for-word, perhaps in preparation for a journal club.

Structured abstracts are organized according to the various kinds of information that critical readers depend on when deciding whether or not to believe the results. Table 13.4 summarizes the headings of a structured abstract. The headings make it easier for readers to find the information they need. Thus, one might look at "Setting" and "Patients" to see how generalizable the results are, "Intervention" to see what was tested, and "Design" to see if the study appears to be scientifically strong. The headings also force authors to include this information, some of which might otherwise have been left out if the abstract were less structured.

One approach to reading journals, and it is unfortunately common, is to set goals that are higher than can be achieved because one feels that one must spend a lot of time with each issue and look at each article in detail. Too often, this results in postponing reading and perhaps never getting to it at all. It also generates a lot of anxiety and self-reproach. If such negative feelings are associated with reading medical journals, something is wrong.

TABLE 13.3 ■ The Diverse Contents of a General Medical Journal	
Science	**The Profession**
Original research	Medical education
Preliminary studies	History
Review articles	Public policy
Editorials (for synthesis and opinion)	Book reviews
Letters to the editor	News
Hypotheses	Stories and poems

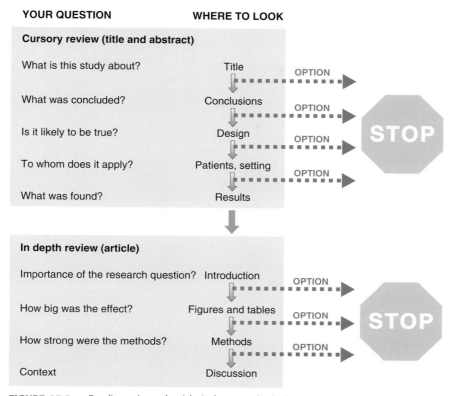

FIGURE 13.5 ■ Reading a journal article in layers. Individual readers can progress deeper into an article or stop and go on to another, according to its scientific strength and clinical importance to them.

TABLE 13.4 ■ **The Organization of a Structured Abstract**

Heading	Information
Context	Burden of suffering from the disease/illness? Why is the research question important? What is already known?
Objective	What the investigators wished to learn
Setting	The setting to which results can be generalized, such as community, primary-care practices, referral centers, and the like
Participants	What kinds of patients (regarding generalizability)? How many (regarding statistical power/precision)?
Design	How strong is the study? How well is it matched to the research question?
Intervention (if any)	Is the intervention state-of-the-art? Feasible in your setting?
Main outcome measures	Are the outcomes clinically important?
Results	What was found?
Conclusion	Do the authors believe that the results answer their question? How convincingly?

PUTTING KNOWLEDGE MANAGEMENT INTO PRACTICE

We recommend a break with the past. The mainstays of keeping up have been looking up information in print textbooks, subscribing to a few journals, and (for physicians in practice) continuing medical education, and advice from colleagues. These sources remain valuable but are no longer good enough on their own. Much better options have become available. Also, the pace of change in medical knowledge has accelerated, and expectations for being up to date have increased.

Clinical epidemiology, as described in this book, is intended to make clinicians' professional lives easier and more satisfying. Armed with a sound grounding in the principles by which the validity and generalizability of clinical information are judged, clinicians can more quickly and accurately detect whether the scientific basis for assertions is sound. For example, they can see when confidence intervals are consistent with clinically important benefit or harm or that a study of the effects of an intervention includes neither randomization nor other efforts to compare like with like. They are better prepared to participate in discussions with colleagues about patient care decisions. They have a better basis for deciding how to delegate some aspects of their knowledge management plan. They can gain more confidence and experience greater satisfaction with the intellectual aspects of their work.

A workable approach to knowledge management must be active. Clinicians must invest time to create a plan that meets all of their information needs. They need to set aside time periodically to revisit the plan, to learn about new opportunities as they arise, and to acquire new skills as they are needed. There has never been a time when the evidence base for clinical medicine was so strong and accessible. Why not make the most of it?

REVIEW QUESTIONS

Read the following and circle the best response.

13.1. You are finishing residency and will begin practice in a small town. You want to keep up with new developments in your field even though there are few professional colleagues in your community. All of the following might be useful but which will be *most* useful to you?

A. Subscribe to a few good journals
B. Buy new editions of printed textbooks
C. Subscribe to a service that reviews the literature in your field
D. Search Medline at regular intervals
E. Keep up contacts with colleagues in your training program by e-mail and telephone.

13.2. You can rely on the best general medical journals in your field to:

A. Provide answers to clinical questions
B. Assure that you have kept up with the medical literature
C. Guarantee that the information they contain is beyond reproach
D. Expose you to the many dimensions of your profession
E. Accept all submitted articles that meet a certain level of quality

13.3. Many children in your practice have attacks of otitis media. You want to base your management on the best available evidence. Which of the following is the *least* credible source of information on this question?

A. A clinical practice guideline by a major medical society
B. A systematic review published in a major journal
C. The Cochrane Database of Systematic Reviews
D. The most recent research article on this question
E. Clinical Evidence

13.4. Medline is especially useful for which of the following:

A. Finding all of the best articles bearing on a clinical question
B. An efficient strategy for finding the good articles
C. Looking up reports of rare events
D. Keeping up with the medical literature
E. Being familiar with the medical profession as a whole

Read the following statements and mark each one as True or False.

Peer review and editing assure readers that:

_____ **13.5.** Articles meet all criteria for scientific strength.

_____ **13.6.** Articles are better than when they were first submitted.

_____ **13.7.** All important new developments in the journal's field are covered.

Answers are in Appendix A.

REFERENCES

1. Antman EM, Lau J, Kupelnick B, Mosteller F, Chalmers TC. A comparison of results of meta-analyses of randomized control trials and recommendations of clinical experts: Treatment of myocardial infarction. JAMA 1992;268:240–248.
2. Shekelle PG, Oritz E, Rhodes S, Morton SC, Eccles MP, Grimshaw J, et al. Validity of the Agency for Healthcare Research and Quality clinical practice guidelines: How quickly do guidelines become outdated? JAMA 2001;286:1461–1467.
3. Haynes RB, Wilczynski N, McKibbon KA, Walker CJ, Sinclair JC. Developing optimal search strategies for detecting clinically sound studies in Medline. J Am Informatics Assoc 994;1:447–458.
4. Losanoff JE, Sauter ER, Rider KD. Cat scratch disease presenting with abdominal pain and retroperitoneal lymphadenopathy. J Clin Gastroentrol 2004;38:300–301
5. Goodman SN, Berlin J, Fletcher SW, Fletcher RH. Manuscript quality before and after peer review and editing at Annals of Internal Medicine. Ann Intern Med 1994;121(1):11–21.
6. Lacombe, MA, ed. On Being a Doctor. Philadelphia: American College of Physicians, 1995.

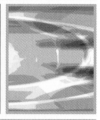

Answers to Review Questions

CHAPTER 1

1.1 D. Samples can give a misleading impression of the situation in the parent population, especially if the sample is small.

1.2 E. Generalizing the results of a study of men to the care of a woman assumes that the effectiveness of surgery for low back pain is the same for men and women.

1.3 A. The difference in recovery between patients who received surgery versus medical care may be the result of some other factor, such as age, that is different between the two treated groups and not the result of surgery itself.

1.4 B. The two treatment groups did not have an equal chance of having pain measured.

1.5 B. These are biases related to measurement of the outcome (recovery from pain).

1.6 C. The other medical conditions confound the relationship between treatment and outcome; that is, they are related to both treatment and recovery and might be the reason for the observed differences.

1.7 C. The observation that histamines mediate inflammation in hay fever leads to a promising hypothesis that blocking histamines will relieve symptoms, but the hypothesis needs to be tested in people with hay fever. The other answers all assume more about the causes of symptoms than is actually stated. For example, histamine is only one of many mediators of inflammation in hay fever.

1.8 True. Samples may misrepresent populations by chance, especially when the samples are small.

1.9 True. In nearly all situations, populations are too large to study without sampling.

1.10 True. When they are possible, random samples are best because they remove bias, although chance differences between samples and population may remain.

1.11 True. Generalizing from younger to older patients is a matter of personal judgment based on whatever facts there are that bear on how the two might respond to treatment, until a study of older patients becomes available.

1.12 False. Internal validity is about whether the results are correct for the patients in the study, not about whether they are correct for other kinds of patients.

1.13 False. Both bias and chance affect internal validity, which in turn affect whether the results are true for anyone, young or old.

CHAPTER 2

2.1 D. Ordinal

2.2 B. Dichotomous

2.3 A. Interval—continuous

2.4 E. Interval—discrete

2.5 C. Nominal

2.6 C. This approach, called construct validity, is one of the ways of establishing the validity of a measurement.

2.7 D. All except D are reasons for variation in measurements on a single patient, whereas D is about variation among patients.

2.8 D. Because clinical distributions do not necessarily follow a Normal distribution, abnormality should be defined by whether or not they do.

2.9 False. Naturally-occurring distributions may or may not resemble the Normal curve.

2.10 True. This is a property of the Normal distribution.

2.11 True. Normal distributions do have a single hump (mode) and are symmetrical around that mode.

2.12 False. Being associated with disease or response to treatment are sounder definitions of abnormality than statistical unusualness.

2.13 True. This is a reason for regression to the mean.

2.14 True. This can happen because of moment-to-moment variation.

2.15 False. Simply being unusually high on one measurement is not a sound reason for calling a patient abnormal and considering treatment.

CHAPTER 3

First, determine the numbers for each of the four cells in Figure 3.2: a = 27; b = 35; c = 37 − 27 (or 10); d = 112 − 35 (or 77).

3.1 Sensitivity = 27/37 = 73%

3.2 Specificity = 77/112 = 69%

3.3 Positive predictive value = 27/62 = 44%

3.4 Negative predictive value = 77/87 = .89

3.5 Prevalence of strep throat in this emergency room = 37/149 = 25%

3.6 $LR+ = \dfrac{27/(27+10)}{35/(35+77)} = 2.3$

Pretest odds = prevalence/(1-prevalence)
= .25/(1 − .25) = 1/3

Posttest odds = LR+ × pretest odds
= 2.3 × 1/3 = .77

Posttest probability = posttest odds/(1 + posttest odds)
= .77/(1 + .77)
= .44 or 44%

(Another, simpler, approach is that posttest probability = positive predictive value +PV = 27/62 = 44%)

3.7 False. Accuracy of physician impressions is (27 + 77)/149 = .70 or 70%, which is better than a coin toss.

3.8 True. Knowing the results of the "gold standard" would likely influence the physicians' clinical impression of whether or not the patient's sore throat is due to strep infection.

3.9 True. If only certain patients with sore throats are selected for throat cultures, the spectrum of patients would be altered and may affect calculations of the test characteristics.

3.10 True or False, depending on the medical environment. In a medical setting in which throat culture is not available, such as in many areas of developing countries, clinical impression is better than nothing. However, in most clinical settings in the United States, this is an example of a test that is not accurate enough to stop testing. Either a throat culture, the gold standard, or a rapid antigen detection test with culture of negative results is used in these settings.

CHAPTER 4

4.1 C. Duration of disease = prevalence/incidence = 1/100 divided by 30/100,000 = 33 years.

4.2 A. Cumulative incidence

4.3   E. This number is not a rate because there is no information on the number of people in the population at risk (denominator).

4.4   D. Period prevalence

4.5   C. Point prevalence

4.6   B. Incidence density (because the U.S. workforce is continually changing)

4.7   A. Cumulative incidence

4.8   D. Prevalence studies do not have a time dimension.

4.9   A. A cohort is a collection of people having something in common at the beginning and who will be followed up for outcomes.

4.10   True. Chronic diseases have a long duration and so are likely to be prevalent.

4.11   True. Pretest probability is a prevalence.

4.12   False. Studies of cause and effect imply a time dimension and prevalence studies are cross-sectional in time.

4.13   False. Diseases that resolve rapidly will neither remain in the population nor be detected in a prevalence study.

CHAPTER 5

5.1   E. A good way to organize your thinking for this question is to create a 2×2 table of the incidence of DVT according to OC use (present/absent) and Factor V Leiden (present/absent). 0.8/10,000 women/year (Absolute risk of DVT in women who neither are heterozygous for the mutation nor are taking OC)

5.2   G. 3.0/10,000 women/year (Absolute risk of DVT in women who do not have the mutation but take OC)

5.3   B. 5.7/10,000 women/year (Absolute risk of DVT in women who are heterozygous for the mutation but do not take OC)

5.4   H. 28.5/3.0 = 9.5 (Relative risk of DVT in women who are heterozygous for the mutation and take OC, compared to DVT in women without the mutation who take OC)

5.5   F. 3.0/0.8 = 3.7 (Relative risk of DVT in women who take OC but do not have the mutation, compared to those without the mutation who do not take OC)

5.6   A. 5.7/0.8 = 7.1 (Relative risk of DVT in women who are heterozygous for the mutation but do not take OC, compared to those without the mutation who do not take OC)

5.7 In a population of 100,000 white women, all of whom take OC, the risk difference (attributable risk) for carriers of Factor V Leiden = absolute risk for women on OC who are heterozygous for Factor V Leiden (28.5/10,000 women/year); minus the absolute risk for women on OC who are not carriers (3.0/10,000 women/year) = 25.5/10,000 women/year

5.8 Population attributable risk = attributable risk (25.5/10,000 women/year) × prevalence of Factor V Leiden (.05) = 1.27/10,000 women/year

5.9 Using OC in a woman heterozygous for Factor V Leiden is an example of a risk factor with a substantial relative risk (prescribing OC to such a woman increases her chance of developing DVT 500% for a relative risk of 5.0) but a relatively small absolute risk—28.5 women out of 10,000 who have the mutation and use OC would develop DVT in the next year. Even more relevant for this patient is that her risk would rise from about 6 to about 28 per 10,000 over the next year. It is important for a known carrier who wants to take OC to understand that her risk is increased and to know how much that increased risk is in absolute terms. A prudent clinician would also want to be sure that the patient does not have other indications of increased risk of thrombosis such as age, smoking, or a family history or previous history of clotting. This kind of decision requires careful judgment from both patient and clinician. However, using absolute or attributable risk will clarify the risk for the patient better than using relative risk when discussing clinical consequences.

5.10 C. Retrospective cohort studies do not allow investigators the luxury of deciding what data to collect. They can only choose from the available data collected at a time before the study originated. Also, these data, which are often collected for clinical purposes, may not have been collected systematically and in the same way. For example, studying family history retrospectively from medical records is fraught with difficulties. Sometimes, there is no information recorded nor is it even clear whether or not the question was asked (or whether the answer was negative, if it was asked). When information is recorded, it is often incomplete, with such notations as "positive for breast cancer" but giving no indication as to which relative, at what age, etc.

CHAPTER 6

6.1 A. Another name for cohort study is incidence study.

6.2 B. Case-control studies have the advantage of efficiency: Exposure can be measured just in cases and a sample of controls.

6.3 C. As with all studies, both cohort and case-control studies can be done on a sample of the population.

6.4 C. No study can identify risk factors if data are collected before enough time has passed for disease to have developed from exposure.

6.5 B. A disadvantage of case-control studies is that they measure only odds ratio and do not provide any direct information on rates of disease in exposed and unexposed people.

6.6 D. The statement is true, but neither cohort nor case-control studies measure prevalence.

6.7 B. Cohort studies provide incidence rates in exposed and non-exposed people, from which one can calculate relative risk, but case-control studies only provide an estimate of relative risk.

6.8 D. Case-control studies do not provide information on incidence.

6.9 B. Sampling cases and controls from a population ensures that, on average, the two groups are similar except for exposure.

CHAPTER 7

7.1 C. Multivariable analysis is the only way to identify the combined effects of several variables at the same time.

7.2 B. Rigorous entry criteria may improve internal validity but tend to reduce generalizability; patients in the trial are different from most patients in the community.

7.3 C. This is a typical case series in which patients are prevalent cases in a referral setting and the investigators look back at their earlier characteristics.

7.4 False. The 30 patients in the study were followed up for various periods of time, so 30 is an inappropriate denominator for a survival rate at 5 years.

7.5 True. Only three patients are under observation at the end of 5 years. If one of them happened to have a recurrence, the estimate would have changed substantially.

7.6 False. The time-to-event method was developed to overcome this practical limitation.

7.7 True. If patients who left the study were substantially different from those who remained, the results would be biased.

7.8 True. Time-to-event analysis is intended to make full use of whatever follow-up data are available. In contrast, follow-up of a full cohort, while conceptually simple, is often impractical.

CHAPTER 8

8.1 D. One strength of intention-to-treat analysis is that it reflects the consequences of a management decision, taking into account all the events (favorable and unfavorable) that follow the decision. Another strength is that the groups being compared are truly randomized.

8.2 **C.** Severity of disease is a characteristic that exists before randomization, so patients with it will be randomly allocated along with all other baseline characteristics.

8.3 **A.** Stratified randomizations help guard against "bad luck" in randomization, especially in small trials. If a variable that was known to be strongly related to prognosis happened to be unequally distributed in the treatment groups, it might bias the comparison.

8.4 **C.** The distinctive feature of randomized controlled trials is that randomization produces, on average, treatment groups of similar prognosis before the treatments are given. Observational studies, on the other hand, must apply a variety of methods to control for differences between groups, and even so are vulnerable to unmeasured differences.

8.5 **E.** Strict entry criteria improve the chances of finding effects for patients in the study, but improvement comes at a price: Those patients will be systematically different from most patients in ordinary settings.

8.6 **True.** The investigators would have assigned patients to treatment groups before the drugs are taken and their effects noticed.

8.7 **False.** The patients may be able to tell that they are on a beta-blocker because of its side effects and physiologic effects.

8.8 **False.** If the physicians are asking patients how they feel or are monitoring pulse and blood pressure, they may discover changes that may be attributable to the drug and can discern which of their patients are on the beta-blocker.

8.9 **True.** Investigators can assess stage fright without asking about other symptoms.

CHAPTER 9

9.1 The relative risk reduction of colorectal cancer mortality is the absolute risk reduction divided by the cancer mortality rate in the control group. (Chapter 8, page 136)

The colorectal cancer mortality rate in the screened group = 82/15,570 = 0.0052665

The colorectal cancer mortality rate in the control group = 121/15,394 = 0.0078602

Absolute risk reduction = 0.0078602 − 0.0052665 = 0.0025937

Relative risk reduction of colorectal cancer mortality due to screening = 0.0025937/ 0.0078602 = .33 or 33% reduction

The number needed to screen is the reciprocal of absolute risk reduction. The absolute risk reduction was 0.0025937. The reciprocal (1/0.0025937) = 386. Therefore, 386 people must be screened for 13 years to prevent one cancer death.

9.2 (1) *Lead-time bias* might be the reason why survival, but not lung cancer mortality, improved. (2) *Overdiagnosis*, detection of lesions that would not have caused clinical symptoms or morbidity, is another possibility because more lesions were detected in the screened group than in the control group, but the mortality rate was not different. The large difference in median survival times between the screened and control groups, without improvement in mortality rates, also suggests that screening was picking up very early lesions in some patients, perhaps some of which would not have gone on to cause morbidity or death.

9.3 Several important questions are to be considered when assessing a new vaccine, at least two of which are: (1) Has the vaccine been shown to be effective (preferably in a well-done randomized trial with important end points)? If you prefer, you could ask, (2) has the vaccine been shown to be *efficacious* (did it work under ideal circumstances when everyone in the intervention group received the vaccine and no one in a comparable control group did) and was it *effective* (under every day circumstances, in which some people in the intervention group did not receive the vaccine). Other questions include (3) Is the vaccine safe? (4) Is it cost-effective? (5) Is the burden of suffering of the condition the vaccine protects against important enough to consider a preventive measure?

9.4 A good screening test should be highly sensitive, highly specific, simple, safe, inexpensive, acceptable to patients and clinicians, and able to produce positive or no labeling effects.

9.5 **False.** Both diagnostic and screening tests require a gold standard to determine sensitivity and specificity.

9.6 **False.** Disease prevalence is lower in presumably well people (screening) than in symptomatic patients (diagnosis).

9.7 **True.** The incidence method and the detection method can be used for calculating sensitivity in cancer screening tests.

9.8 **False.** Positive predictive value and related false-positive results are important for diagnostic and screening tests. Because prevalence is low in screening situations, PPV tends to be lower for screening tests.

9.9 **True.** In a screening program, the first round of screening will detect *prevalent* disease— disease that may have begun recently or may have been present for a long time. On the second and subsequent rounds, screening detects mostly disease that has occurred since the last round of screening (*incident* disease). Therefore, the total number of cases is higher on the first than on subsequent screening rounds.

CHAPTER 10

10.1 **D.** Examination of findings in subgroups is a responsible thing to do as long as it is made clear how it is being done.

10.2 **C.** This is how the *P* value is interpreted.

10.3 **E.** Without knowing the statistical power of this study, one cannot know how likely the conclusion of "no difference" is to be misleading by chance alone.

10.4 **D.** This is how the confidence interval is interpreted.

10.5 **B.** One begins with a choice of how small an effect is clinically unimportant, then sees whether the confidence interval is consistent with (or rules out) this effect.

CHAPTER 11

11.1 **C.** Randomized controlled trials evaluating interventions that are believed to be harmful are unethical. If there were reason to believe that cell phones might be protective against brain cancer, an RCT would be ethical. E is incorrect. Theoretically, an RCT is the strongest research design to answer the question. A, B, and D are common problems in RCTs, but are not the most important reason to reject the idea of an RCT to determine a causal relationship. An RCT looking for a rare outcome (incidence of brain cancer is low) would be large and expensive, and it might take a long time to determine an effect. Also, people may be hesitant to participate if it meant not using a cell phone for several years.

11.2 **A, B, C, and D.** All are consistent with the results given. Although a relative risk of 1.0 was found, which suggests no effect, the confidence intervals were wide enough to include the possibility of a 50% increase or 40% decrease in risk (95% CI, 0.60 to 1.5). Also, because the results were for all types of tumors combined, the authors looked for an association with each type of tumor, and none was found.

11.3 **A, B, and C.** Evaluating a possible causal association can be strengthened by examining whether larger exposures lead to higher rates of disease (dose-response), searching for biologic plausibility (which in this case means determining whether the side of the brain most exposed to the cell phone might have higher tumor rates), and strength of association, which might be different according to different ways of measuring cell phone use. Therefore, all these approaches increase the methodologic strength of the study. The authors included all of these methods.

11.4 If you believe a 50% increase or a 40% decrease in risk is important, the study did not have enough power to exclude these possibilities (that is, the study was underpowered). Negative studies should exclude possibilities that you believe are clinically important. Studies rarely are able to exclude very small differences or associations, but if the results cannot exclude a 5% increase in risk, most clinicians (and patients) would believe that such a small difference is clinically unimportant.

11.5 Measurement of exposure is often a source of bias in case-control studies. In this study, patients and controls were asked about past use of cell phones. It is possible that the two groups systematically differed in the way they answered. For example, it is at least theoretically possible that patients with malignant brain tumors did not remember their cell phone use as well as control patients. To deal with the possibility that people with brain problems would have memory problems, the control patients had benign brain tumors. But even so, there could have been a systematic difference in answering the question.

11.6 According to Table 11.2, this case-control study is a II-2. As pointed out, several features were well done. Because the study was under-powered to exclude clinically important results, probably it would not be given the top grade of "good" but rather a "fair" grade. Therefore, the final grade would be II-2-fair. Note the somewhat subjective nature of assigning "good," "fair," or "poor."

11.7 If RCTs are not ethical because of intentionally assigning people to a perceived danger, nonrandomized trials in which the investigator assigns the intervention would also be unethical. All other types of studies listed in Figure 11.11 are possible. Some are more feasible than others. Note that the highest grade these individual studies could achieve is II-2. However, if several different types of studies, such as case-control, cohort and multiple time series, find no association and are large enough to exclude important clinical effects, the total evidence against cell phones causing brain cancer would be strong.

CHAPTER 12

12.1 E. When justified, pooling study results does provide a more precise estimate of effect size than any of the individual studies alone.

12.2 E. Because alcohol cannot be randomized, observational studies are the only feasible way of studying whether alcohol is a risk factor for breast cancer. All the other responses describe true limitations of a search strategy that includes only a MEDLINE search.

12.3 B. The main advantage of patient-level meta-analyses is that it is possible to place each patient into clinically important subgroups and to have enough patients within those subgroups to provide a relatively precise estimate of effects.

12.4 True. The cumulative meta-analysis shows how evidence is accumulated and the summary effect changes over time.

12.5 True. If the underlying assumptions are met, the summary effect size is the best estimate of effect from all of the trials as a whole.

12.6 False. One would need to look elsewhere in the report to decide how confident he or she is that the studies were all of the same question.

12.7 True. In the typical forest plot, one can easily form a visual impression or count the number of trials that met inclusion criteria.

12.8 False. These graphics summarize studies without regard to whether or not they are scientifically sound. For that, the reader would need to look at the authors' criteria for including studies.

12.9 True. These graphics typically show the confidence intervals for all available studies at the time each new study is added to the rest.

CHAPTER 13

13.1 C. When it comes to keeping up with new developments, important articles are so widely dispersed among journals that there is no substitute for getting some help with surveillance of the literature as a whole in your field.

13.2 D. General journals typically have a rich array of articles, exposing you to the many aspects of your profession as a whole. Although they publish their share of research articles and reviews, they are not in themselves a particularly good solution for keeping up.

13.3 D. The most recent articles are part of the information base on a clinical question, but they may or may not make the most important contribution. Currency alone is not an especially strong credential.

13.4 C. MEDLINE contributes to all of the listed tasks, especially for researchers and teachers; but for clinicians, it is uniquely valuable for finding out whether unusual events have been reported.

13.5 False. Peer review and editing improves articles, on average, but do not make them perfect.

13.6 True. Peer review and editing do improve articles.

13.7 False. Journal editors review what is submitted to them, and the journals themselves do not necessarily cover all important new developments in a field.

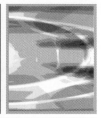

Additional Readings

1. INTRODUCTION

Clinical Epidemiology

Feinstein AR. Clinical Epidemiology. The Architecture of Clinical Research. Philadelphia: WB Saunders, 1985.

Feinstein AR. Clinimetrics. New Haven, CT: Yale University Press, 1987.

Gehlbach SH. Interpreting the Medical Literature. 4th Ed. New York: McGraw-Hill, Appleton, 2002.

Hulley SB, Cummings SR. Designing Clinical Research. An Epidemiologic Approach. 2nd Ed. Baltimore: Lippincott Williams and Wilkins, 2000.

Jenicek M, Cleroux R. Epidemiologie Clinique: Clinimetrie. St-Hyacinthe, Que., Canada: Edisem, 1985.

Riegelman RK. Studying and Study and Testing a Test. 5th Ed. Philadelphia: Lippincott Williams and Wilkens, 2004.

Sackett DL. Clinical Epidemiology. Am J Epid 1969;89:125–128.

Sackett DL, Haynes RB, Guyatt GH, Tugwell P. Clinical Epidemiology: A Basic Science for Clinical Medicine. 2nd Ed. Boston: Little, Brown and Company, 1991.

Spitzer WO. Clinical epidemiology. J Chron Dis 1986;39:411–415.

Weiss NS. Clinical Epidemiology: The Study of the Outcomes of Illness. New York: Oxford University Press, 1986.

Evidence-Based Medicine

Evidence-Based Medicine Working Group. User's Guide to the Medical Literature: A Manual for Evidence-Based Practice. Guyatt G, Rennie D, eds. Chicago: American Medical Association, 2002.

Sackett DL, Straus SE, Richardson WS, Rosenberg W, Haynes RB. Evidence-Based Medicine: How to Practice and Teach EBM. 2nd Ed. London: Churchill Livingstone, 2000.

Epidemiology

Friedman GD. Primer of Epidemiology. 5th Ed. New York: Appleton and Lange, 2003.

Hennekins CH, Buring JE. Epidemiology in Medicine. Boston: Little, Brown and Company, 1987.

Gordis L. Epidemiology. 4th Ed. Philadelphia: WB Saunders, 2004.

Greenberg RS, Daniels SR, Flanders WD, Eley JW, Boring JR III. Medical Epidemiology. 4th Ed. New York: Lange Medical Books, 2004.

Jekel JF, Elmore JG, Katz DL. Epidemiology, Biostatistics and Preventive Medicine. Philadelphia, W. B. Saunders, 1996.

Last JM. A Dictionary of Epidemiology. 3rd Ed. New York: Oxford University Press, 1995.

Rothman KJ. Epidemiology: An Introduction. New York: Oxford University Press, 2002.

Related Fields

Kassirer JP, Kopelman RI. Learning Clinical Reasoning. Baltimore: Williams and Wilkins, 1991.

Sox HC. Blatt MA, Higgins MC, Marton KI. Medical Decision Making. Boston, MA: Butterworth, 1988.

White KL. Healing the Schism: Epidemiology, Medicine, and the Public's Health. New York: Springer-Verlag, 1991.

2. ABNORMALITY

Feinstein AR. Clinical Judgment. Baltimore: Williams & Wilkins, 1967.

Feinstein AR. Clinimetrics. New Haven, CT: Yale University Press, 1987.

Streiner DL, Norman GR. Health Measurement Scales—A Practical Guide to Their Development and Use. 3rd Ed. New York: Oxford University Press, 2003.

3. DIAGNOSIS

Elasy TA, Gaddy G. Measuring subjective outcomes: Rethinking reliability and validity. J Gen Intern Med 1998;13:757–761.

Heckerling PS. Confidence in diagnostic testing. J Gen Intern Med 1988;3:604–606.

Ransohoff DF, Feinstein AR. Problems of spectrum and bias in evaluating the efficacy of diagnostic tests. N Engl J Med 1978;299:926–930.

Reid MC, Lachs MS, Feinstein AR. Use of methodological standards in diagnostic test research. JAMA 1995;274:645–651.

Whiting P, Rutjes AWS, Reitsma JB, Glas AS, Bossuyt, PMM, Kleijnen, J. Sources of variation and bias in studies of diagnostic accuracy: A systematic review. Ann Intern Med 2004;140:189–202.

4. FREQUENCY

Morgenstern H, Kleinbaum DG, Kupper LL. Measures of disease incidence used in epidemiologic research. Int J Epidemiol 1980;9:97–104.

5. RISK: LOOKING FORWARD

Feinstein AR. Scientific standards in epidemiologic studies of the menace of daily life. Science 1988;242:1257–1263. Response by Savitz DA, Greenland S, Stolley PD, Kelsey JL. Scientific standards of criticism: a reaction to "Scientific standards in epidemiologic studies of the menaces of daily life" by Feinstein. Epidemiology 1990;1:78–83.

Goodman SN. Probability at the bedside: the knowing of chances or the chances of knowing. Ann Intern Med 1999;130:604–606.

Samet JM, Munoz A. Evolution of the cohort study. Epidemiol Rev 1998;20:1–14.

6. RISK: LOOKING BACKWARD

Bogardus ST Jr, Holmboe E, Jekel JF. Perils, pitfalls, and the possibilities in talking about medical risk. JAMA 1999;281:1037–1041.

Gigerenzer G. Calculated Risks. New York: Simon and Schuster, 2002.

7. PROGNOSIS

Justice AC, Covinsky KE, Berlin JA. Assessing the generalizability of prognostic information. Ann Intern Med 1999;130:515–524.

Laupacis A, Sekar N, Stiell IG. Clinical prediction rules: a review and suggested modifications of methodologic standards. JAMA 1997;277:488–494.

8. TREATMENT

Friedman LM, Furberg CD, DeMets DL. Fundamentals of Clinical Trials. 3rd Ed. New York: Springer-Verlag, 1998.

Jones B, Jarvis P, Lewis JA, Ebbutt AF. Trials to assess equivalence: the importance of rigorous methods. BMJ 1996;313:36–39.

Sackett DL, Gent M. Controversy in counting and attributing events in clinical trials. N Engl J Med 1979;301:1410–1412.

Vandenbroucke JP. In defense of case reports. Ann Intern Med 2001;134:330–334.

Yusuf S, Wittes J, Probstfield J, Tyroler HA. Analysis and interpretation of treatment effects in subgroups of patients in randomized clinical trials. JAMA 1991;266:93–98.

9. PREVENTION

Harris RP, Helfand M, Woolf SH, Lohr KN, Mulrow CD, Teutsch SM, et al, Methods Work Group, Third U.S. Preventive Services Task Force. Current methods of the U.S. Preventive Services Task Force: a review of the process. Am J Prev Med 2001;20 (April Supp 1) 21–35.

Rose G. Sick individuals and sick populations. In J Epid 30:427–432.

U.S. Preventive Services Task Force. Available at: http:// www.ahrq.gov/clinic/uspstfix.htm. Accessed Dec 28, 2004.

Wald NJ, Hackshaw AK, Frost CD. When can a risk factor be used as a worthwhile screening test? BMJ 1999;319:1562–1565.

10. CHANCE

Concato J, Feinstein AR, Holford TR. The risk of determining risk with multivariable models. Ann Intern Med 1993;118:201–210.

Gardner MJ, Altman DG, Bryant T, Gardner M, Gardner MJ, Machin D. Statistics with confidence. 2nd Ed. London: BMJ Books, 2000.

Goodman SN. Toward evidence-based statistics. 1: The *P* value fallacy. Ann Intern Med 1999;130:995–1004.

Goodman SN. Toward evidence-based statistics. 2: The Bayes Factor. Ann Intern Med 1999;130:1005–1013.

Greene WL, Concato J, Feinstein AR. Claims of equivalence in medical research: are they supported by evidence? Ann Intern Med 2000;132:715–722.

Jones B, Jarvis P, Ebbutt AF. Trials to assess equivalence: the importance of rigorous methods. BMJ 1996;13:36–39.

Katz MH. Multivariable analysis: a primer for readers of medical research. Ann Intern Med 2003;138:644–650.

Rothman KJ. A show of confidence. N Engl J Med 1978;299:1362–1363.

Ware JH, Antman EM. Equivalence trials. N Engl J Med 1997;337:1159–1161.

11. CAUSE

Buck C. Popper's philosophy for epidemiologists. Int J Epidemiol 1975;4:159–168.

Chalmers AF. What Is This Thing Called Science? 2nd Ed. New York: University of Queensland Press, 1982.

12. SYSTEMATIC REVIEWS

Irwig L, Tosteson ANA, Gatsonis C, Lau J, Colditz G, Chalmers TC, et al. Guidelines for meta-analyses evaluating diagnostic tests. Ann Intern Med 1994;120:667–676.

Lau J, Ioannidis JPA, Schmid CH. Summing up the evidence: one answer is not always enough. Lancet 1998;351:123–127.

McAlister FA, Clark HD, van Walraven C, Straus SE, Lawson FM, Moher D, et al. The medical review article revisited: has the science improved? Ann Intern Med 1999;131:947–951.

Pogue J, Yusuf S. Overcoming the limitations of current meta-analysis of randomized controlled trials. Lancet 1998;351:47–52.

13. KNOWLEDGE MANAGEMENT

Cook DA, Dupras DM. A practical guide to developing effective Web-based learning. J Gen Intern Med 2004;19:698–707.

Ebell MH, Barry HC, Slawson DC, Shaughnessy AF. Finding POEMs in the medical literature. J Fam Pract 1999;48:350–355.

Godlee F, Pakenham-Walsh N, Ncayiyana D, Cohen B, Packer A. Can we achieve health information for all by 2015? Lancet 2004;364:295–300.

Shiffman RN, Shekelle P, Overhage JM, Slutsky J, Grimshaw J, Deshpande AM. Standardized reporting of clinical practice guidelines: A proposal from the conference on guideline standardization. Ann Intern Med 2003;139:493–498.

Winker MA, Flanagin A, Chi-Lum B, White J, Andrews K, Kennett, RL, et al. Guidelines for medical and health information on the Internet. Principles governing AMA Web sites. JAMA 2000;283:1600–1606.

INDEX

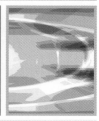

*Page numbers in *italics* denote figures; those followed by a *t* denote tables.